BLEEDING
Fabulous

BIOGRAPHY

MARK WARD is fifty-five years young and lives near Brighton. He was born with severe haemophilia and grew up in Hertfordshire—where he was the first severe haemophiliac to attend a 'normal' school, enabling special needs education to be established. At school and in hospital, they tried to dissuade him from his chosen career in aviation. But this never stopped him from dreaming, and then proving them all wrong: he joined the British Airways Youth Training Scheme at sixteen. He worked within the airline across a variety of departments on the ground and in the air, before his health declined and he medically retired.

Mark then became the 'Door Whore' for G-A-Y at the London Astoria, working with some huge stars and even performing as a drag queen. He's been an HIV and LGBTQ+ activist for over thirty years and has volunteered for charities including Terence Higgins Trust, the West Midlands Lesbian & Gay Switchboard, and Open Door in Brighton. In 2004, he addressed the World Federation of Haemophilia Congress in Bangkok with his ground-breaking booklet, 'You Don't Have to be Straight to Take Factor 8'; he was then asked to join the newly-established Tainted Blood ccommittee in 2006, and has since become an experienced campaigner, media representative, and core participant in the Infected Blood Inquiry.

In 2013, in order to provide sexual health education and help tackle stigma, he created the support network Haemosexual for those with a bleeding disorder who identify as LGBTQ+.He's been an active member of The Haemophilia Society for more than twenty-five years, and in 2019, he became the world's first ever LGBTQ+ Ambassador for Haemophilia.

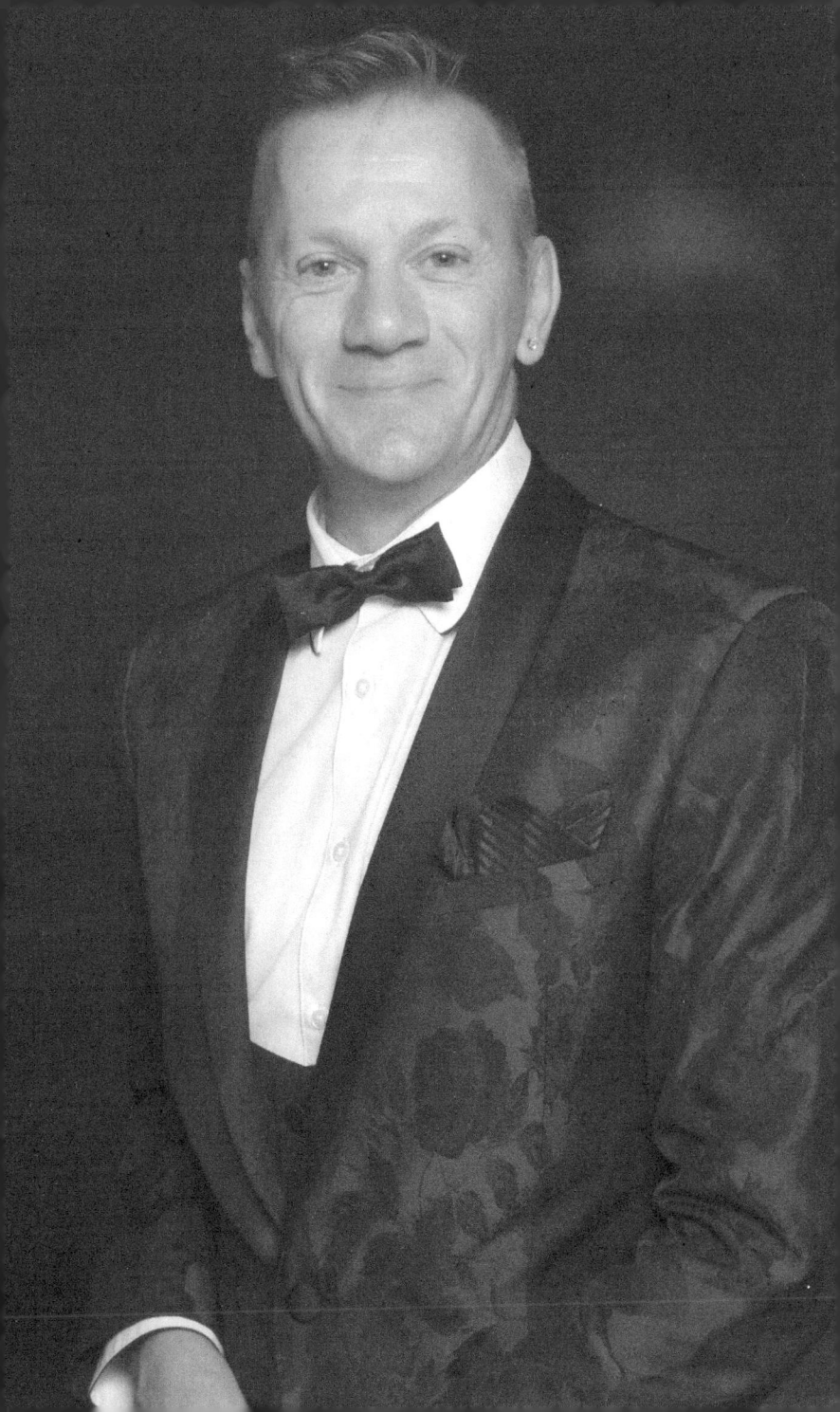

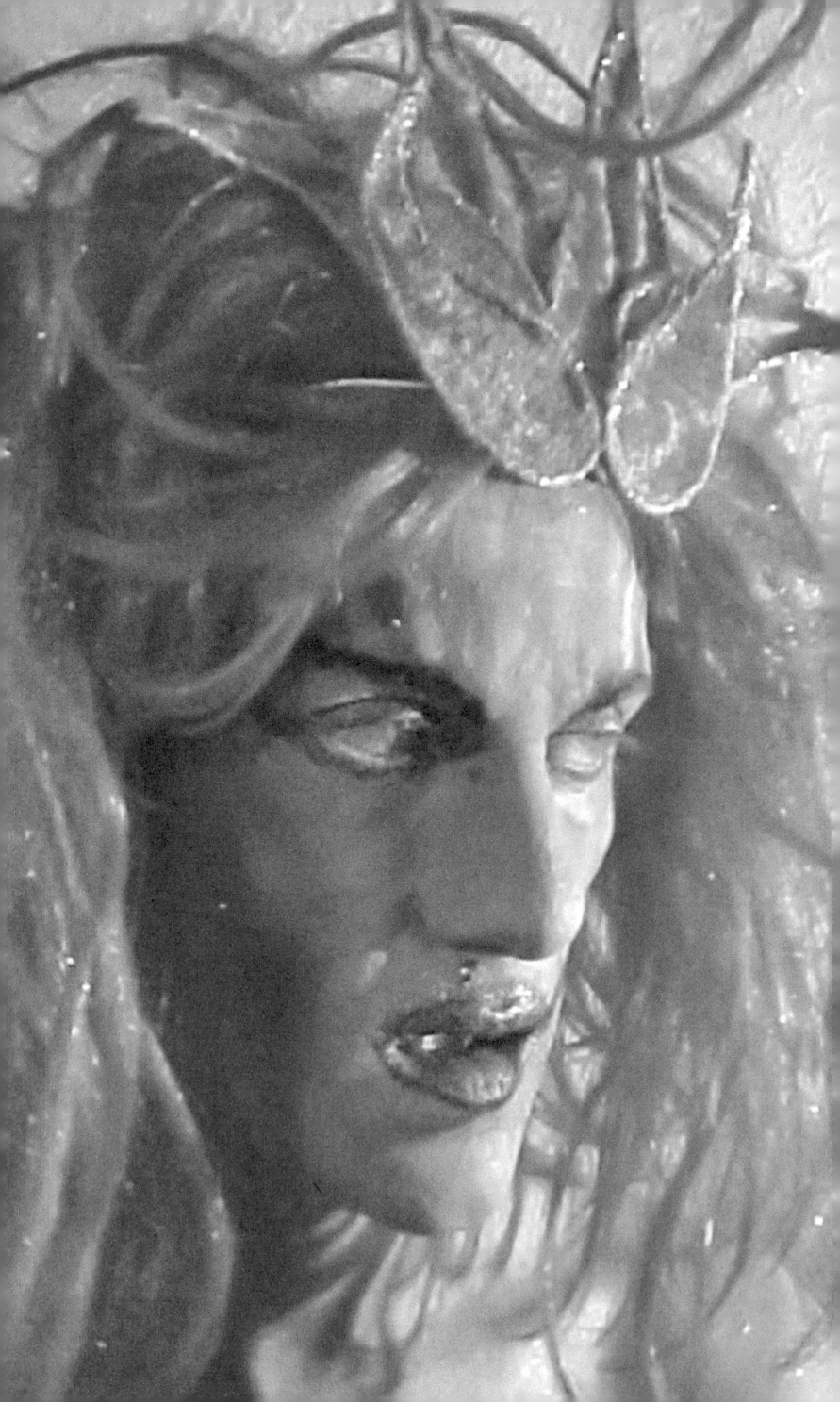

Praise for Mark Ward and *Bleeding Fabulous*

'This is a remarkable book—brave, funny and honest. Ward is a gifted writer with a profound story to tell and he does it beautifully.'
PETER MOFFAT

'This is a story of one of the worst cover ups of our time, and the author's part in the fight to expose it, but it is also the story of a human being who managed to live a life filled with joy despite the mistreatment he endured. An inspirational tale.'
ELKAN ABRAHAMSON
Director of Covid Enquiry Department
Jackson Lees Law Group

'This is a profound and important book from a courageous individual who has lived through the darkest episode of medical history, and contributed to the resolution for the thousands impacted in the UK'
BRIAN O'MAHONY
CEO of Irish Haemophilia Society

Inkandescent
First published by Inkandescent, 2024
Text Copyright © 2024 Mark Ward
Cover Design Copyright © 2024 Justin David

Mark Ward has asserted his right under the Copyright,
Designs and Patents Act 1988 to be identified as the author of this work.

This book is memoir: it reflects the author's present recollections of experiences over time. Some names and characteristics have been changed, some events have been compressed, and some dialogue has been recreated.

Every effort has been made to represent events accurately but if anything has been inadvertently overlooked or misrepresented, the publishers would be glad to be informed about it.

While every precaution has been taken in the preparation of this book, the publisher assumes no responsibilities for errors or omissions, or for damages resulting from the information contained herein.

A CIP catalogue record for this book
is available from the British Library

Printed in the UK by TJ Books, Cornwall

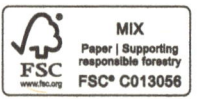

ISBN 978-1-912620-33-3 (paperback)
ISBN 978-1-912620-34-0 (ebook)
ISBN 978-1-912620-37-1 (audiobook)

1 3 5 7 9 10 8 6 4 2

www.inkandescent.co.uk

for Mum and Richard

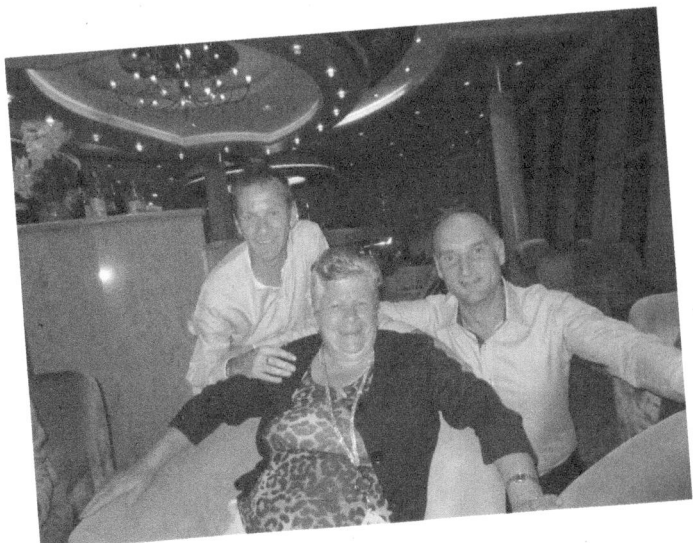

BLEEDING
Fabulous

~~MARK WARD~~
Mark 💋

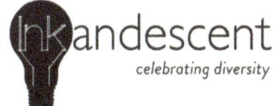
Inkandescent
celebrating diversity

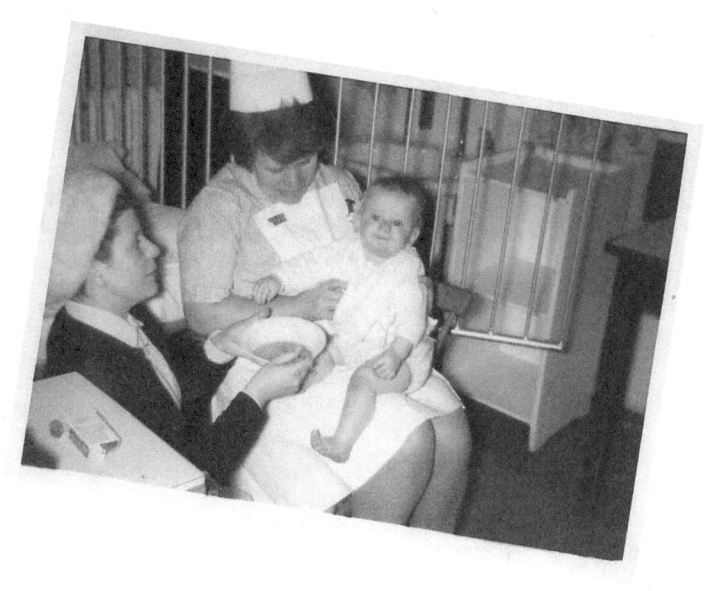

From the day I was born, hospital has been my second home

CONTENTS

	Foreword	13
	Prologue	19
1.	A Special Little Boy	23
2.	A Wonder Drug?	35
3.	And Lift Off	45
4.	Watch Out World, Here I Come!	55
5.	Finding Myself	65
6.	Busy Being Happy	75
7.	To Hell and Back	85
8.	Life and Death	95
9.	Queen of Hearts	105
10.	Dark Days	119
11.	High on a Hill was a Lonely Goatherd	129
12.	On the Campaign Trail	137
13.	Fighting On	145
14.	Pirates and Popping the Question	157
15.	Digging Deep	165
16.	The Truth, at Last	173
17.	The 'C' Word	181
18.	A First-Class Future	191
	Epilogue	201
	Acknowledgements	211

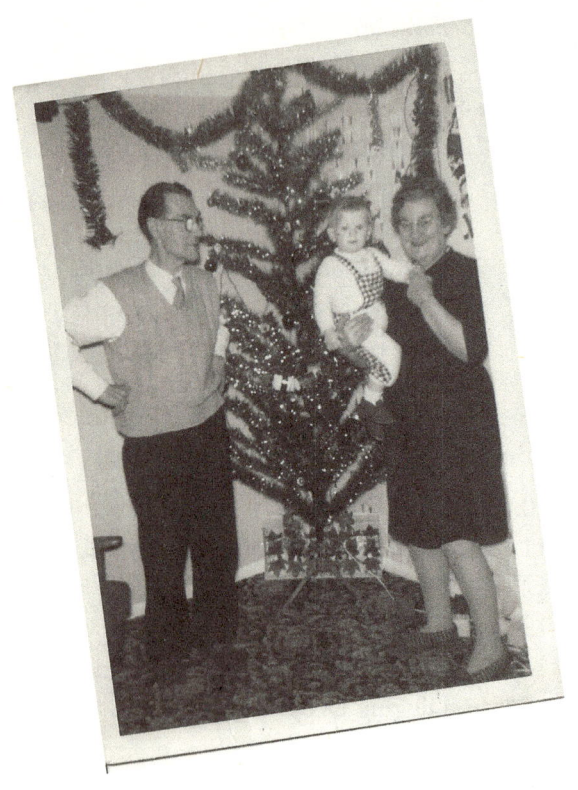

A very seventies Christmas—with Nana & Grandad Ward

FOREWORD

It is hard not to hero-worship Mark Ward; he's a survivor, literally, of the HIV pandemic visited upon him through contaminated blood, and rather than just revelling in the simple FACT of LIFE, he has dedicated himself to making sure that life remains possible for others. Mark's the guy you want around when the s**t has really hit the air-circulating mechanism, the flight attendant you'd want to be there in any disaster.

As a self-styled haemosexual and founder of the online support and information resource haemosexual.com—which supports everyone with a bleeding disorder, no matter what their sexual orientation—Mark has taken on the task of educating the world, and especially the less economically wealthy world, of the dangers of blood-borne viruses and about the need for gay haemophiliacs to understand the risks and thereby protect themselves. Mark's attention to detail and his determination to ensure that gay men who are haemophiliacs can enjoy a safe and varied sex life means that he does not avoid discussion of *any* possible variation of sexual congress. The aim of Mark's work and website cannot be better explained than by the man himself:

> 'Sexuality and disability is a subject still not often spoken about and many people are, unfortunately, not provided with the support they need from the haemophilia professional community. Sometimes, this is due to a lack of awareness, or information, or a person to confide in who really understands.
>
> Haemosexual has been designed to offer practical advice and information to patients, medical professionals and other organisations. Our aim is for those who are vulnerable to become properly protected—which means communicating with them as people, and not as a condition.'

Mark has lived through the horrors of multi-viral infection—with HCV and HIV—and the threat of bovine vCJD infection, as well as the many consequential dreadful effects on his body. But I wonder whether the most wounding of the many medical barbs thrown at him has been the conflation of his infection via contaminated blood products with his sexuality; unless, like Mark, you have lived through this, it is nearly impossible to understand. HIV was known as the 'Gay Plague' and was originally called 'GRID', an acronym for Gay Related Immunodeficiency Disorder; when Mark asked, as a teenager, whether there 'were many gay haemophiliacs', he was told that there weren't any, and instead he was led to believe that he had been 'infected with his homosexuality, just like his other viruses.'

Mark's work began when exposing the scandal that led to the contamination of so many haemophiliacs, including himself, in the 1970s and 80s; this occurred even though the risk of blood and blood products carrying infection was well known to the medical community for decades before the mass infection of the haemophiliac community.

It was the invention of specific blood products which could supply the missing clotting factor required for haemophiliacs which was the game changer; the Infected Blood Inquiry is expected to describe the fact that the medical profession managed to ignore the obvious dangers of using potentially virus-laden blood products and see only immediate treatment effects. The hows and whys of what happened are not for this foreword, and it is sufficient to say that the use of contaminated blood came close to eliminating the problematic and expensive treatment of haemophiliacs once and for all. A cynic, and all haemophiliacs I know are such, would say that *could* look like the intention was to wipe out the entire haemophiliac community.

Mark is one of the early HIV infected haemophiliacs (1982); with effective HIV treatments only having started in 1990, it is astonishing that he is around at all. Mark's evidence* before the Infected Blood Inquiry is a testament to his personal strength and mental resilience; the number of times he has been told that he is likely to die 'pretty soon' would by itself have killed off a lesser man: he is correctly described as a medical miracle. It is my belief that he celebrates the fact of his unlikely survival by living an outwardly vivacious life—seeking to help others around the world understand what has happened to haemophiliacs in the UK, and taking the positives learned from the British scandal to turn them into lessons for other countries. In doing this, he is supported and loved by Richard, his partner (who he loves right back); together Mark and Richard are a dynamic duo.

In November 2019, Mark's work was recognised: he officially became the world's first LGBT Ambassador for Haemophilia (for the UK Haemophilia Society). Mark's standing within the community has grown over many years, and he is now regularly invited to speak to parliamentary committees, and around the world.

I work with, and for, Mark as his representative KC before the Infected Blood Inquiry, having been briefed by the formidable Ben Harrison from Milners Solicitors. I would like to sign off by saying that Ben and I are proud to represent Mark, and very proud to be able to claim friendship with both Mark and Richard. All I can hope is that some of Mark's sparkle and strength might one day rub off on me!

Sam Stein KC
January 2022

*https://www.infectedbloodinquiry.org.uk/sites/default/files/documents/WITN1591001%20Written%20Statement%20of%20Mark%20Ward%20.pdf

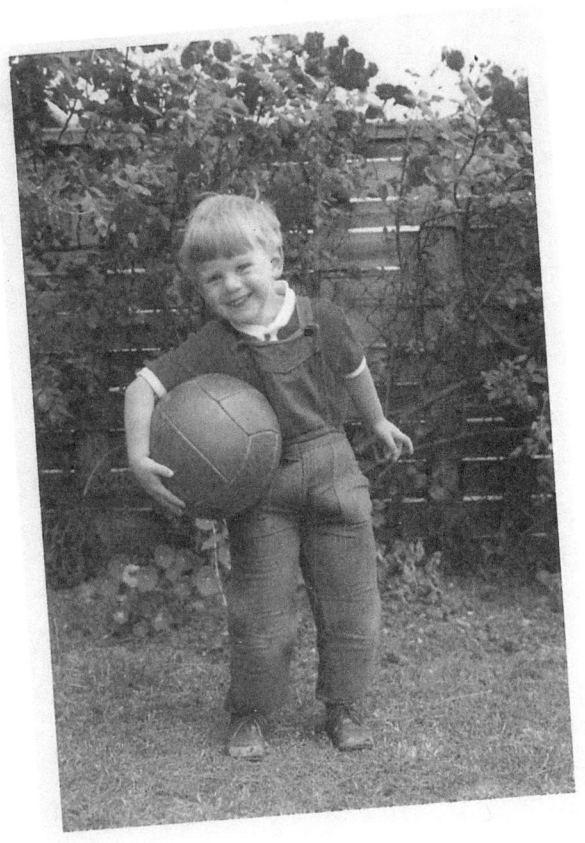

Wrapped in cotton wool

PROLOGUE

This little boy loved to play with his train set. He visited the zoo, fed the ducks and caught sticklebacks in the river. He loved going on the Tube and bus rides with his Nan, who always answered his question, 'Where are we going?' with 'There and back again to see how far it is.' She knew it always made him giggle. Everywhere they went was an adventure. On warm summer evenings, he sat in the garden with his grandparents, staring up at the skies in wonder as planes flew over, starting their descent into Heathrow—or London Airport, as Nan called it.

His dreams of working with aeroplanes started in that garden and became the driving force behind everything he did after Nan and Grandad took him on a visit to Heathrow airport. He had so many hopes and dreams, as all little boys do. But he also knew he was different to the 'normal' boys he'd met in school.

That difference wasn't the fact that he was born with a severe and rare genetic blood disorder called haemophilia, oh no.

You see, this little boy was used as a guinea pig to experiment on—because the specialists who were meant to care for him had decided to carry out their research on him. So they knowingly injected him with highly-infectious products made from the blood of donors—including drug addicts, prostitutes and prisoners—known to have health conditions and bodily contaminants.

They harvested the blood, with its hidden pathogens, sexually-transmitted diseases, and traces of drugs. And as if that wasn't enough, they then drained the blood from dead bodies and sold it for profit to infuse into little children—little children like the one in the picture before this introduction.

All he needed was to be cared for.

All he wanted was to live without fear.

All he deserved was protection and dignity.

He was failed, and nobody wanted to know why.

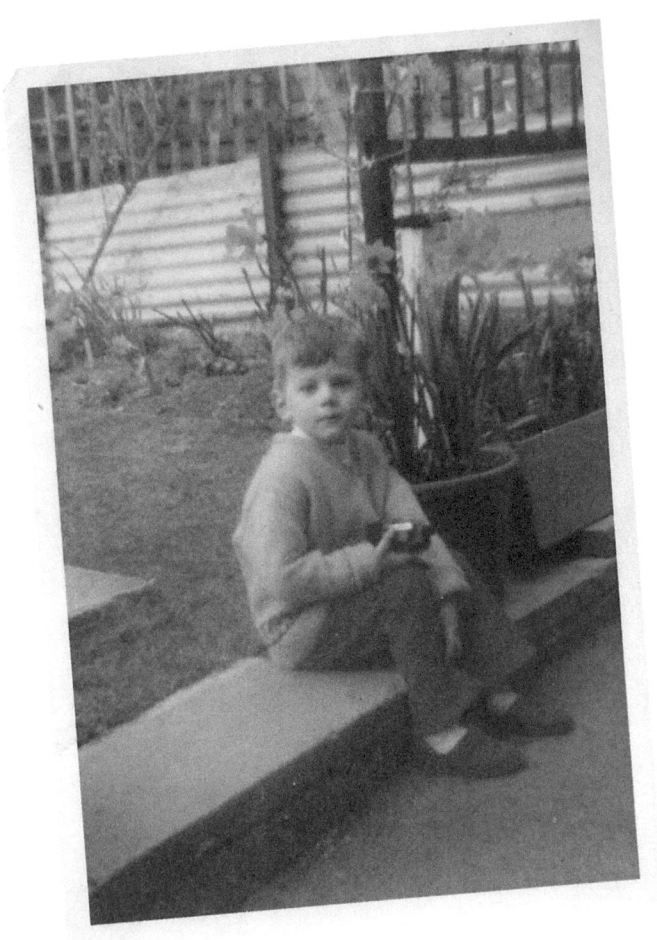

Gay as a daffodil

A SPECIAL LITTLE BOY

Looking back now, the word I would use to describe my childhood is 'exciting'. This may not seem the most fitting description for a childhood that began with a death sentence, but then there's nothing like the nearness of death to make you want to live. And to live your very best life. As you'll see, that's what I've always tried to do. Faced daily with my own mortality, I chose to live fabulously—each of my fifty-five years has been full of love, laughter, adventure, friendship, and feather boas. As a child, I was helped in this by a wonderful mum, who is at the heart of my story, and by fantastic grandparents, who were determined that their grandson would not miss out on anything. If I couldn't do ordinary things, like climb trees, then I would be given the chance to do extraordinary things, like be the first boy in our school to fly on a plane.

I was born in a terraced house in Letchworth (the first garden city!) on 24th April 1969. My dad was from a big family, who I grew up surrounded by. I was always close to Dad's Sister, Rose and her four, daughters Beverly, Deborah, Tracey, and Claire, but I think it's fair to say my dad and I have not had the easiest relationship. He was a very good provider, who worked hard for the gas board, so that we wanted for nothing. He is of the generation where the woman stays at home and cooks dinner while the man goes out and digs holes, comes home for food, and then goes out again to the pub. My mum, Doris, or Dot, more than made up for any emotional connection that I lacked with my dad. Mum and I were always extremely close—she was my support, my champion and my best friend through thick and thin.

Mum wasn't actually a stay-at-home housewife—she used to work on the switchboard at Marmet Prams (favoured by royalty, don't you know!). After taking time out to have me, she went back to work, leaving me in the good care of her friend, Rosie. One afternoon after work, Mum found Rosie in a right old state.

'I don't know what's the matter with Mark,' wailed Rosie. 'Look at his side!' Mum was horrified to see a huge dark-purple bruise, which seemed to have appeared without any explanation. I was about eight months old at the time. Retrospectively, my parents think I probably just leaned on the side of the pram, which caused an internal bleed. At the hospital, they diagnosed me with Christmas disease, said there was no treatment for it, and sent me home.

My second misdiagnosis occurred when another internal bleed caused my whole arm to turn black. This time, they said it was a disorder called Von Willebrand's disease and that they weren't going to treat it because there was a chance I may have become immune to the treatment. So once again, nothing was done.

The signs were all there if you knew what you were looking for. But of course, my parents didn't know. As a baby starts crawling, haemophilia really starts to show itself—because the baby gets bleeds in the knees. When Mum went to the clinic to check on my weight and health, she couldn't understand why she was being asked so many questions. Later, she realised they obviously thought there might be abuse because of all the bruises.

People often assume that, as a haemophiliac, blood spurts everywhere. However, it's more that you bleed normally, but the bleeding doesn't stop. On one occasion as a baby, my mouth started bleeding—in the area between my lip and gum. When it wouldn't stop, we went to the hospital; they packed the bleeding with gauze and sent us home. I wouldn't stop screaming. Mum knew I was hungry, but every time she tried to feed me, I would be sick. So there I was—starving, bleeding, and screaming.

I've often thought about the impact this would have had on my parents—how terrifying it must have been, especially for my mum. I guess this was just one of the many times she felt helpless because she couldn't ease my pain. Back at the hospital, a doctor examined me; Dad saw him take something out of my throat and put it in the bin. When the doctor left the room, Dad told Mum what he'd seen, and Mum looked in the bin. The gauze was there—it had obviously become dislodged and gone down my throat. No wonder I couldn't eat. When the doctor came back in, Dad asked him about it. 'It's nothing for you to worry about,' said the doc. That was it for my dad: it was like a red rag to a bull for him. He pinned the doctor up against the wall and snarled, 'It *is* something for us to worry about. Now, what's just happened?'

'It looks like some gauze went down his throat,' admitted the doctor. 'But he should be okay now. We'll do some tests.'

'You're not mucking about with him anymore. He's coming home.' And that was Dad's final word: there was no messing with my father once he saw red. He had a terrible temper; he believed in tough love and ruled the roost with an iron fist.

We spent all our time walking on eggshells hoping he wouldn't start.

Dad was also of the generation who didn't do feelings. I would disappear off to hospital not knowing if I would ever be home. But Dad just carried on like nothing had happened. It was only when *he* came home from the pub late at night that he would get Mum to wake me up and try to do fatherly things—like teach me how to tell time.

I was finally diagnosed with haemophilia, thanks to my nan's trip to the hairdresser. Mum's mum, Nanny Banham, was having her hair done when she got chatting to a lady about me and my inexplicable bruising. The lady said she'd heard on LBC radio that Great Ormond Street Children's Hospital was the best in the world, that Harley Street doctors worked there, and that people flew in for treatment from all across the globe.

So that's how, one day after my third birthday, on 25th April 1972, I was taken to Great Ormond Street by Mum and Nanny and Grandad Banham.

I can picture myself holding my mum's hand in a dimly lit corridor, as we found our way to the right department, to meet a man who would change my fate forever. The world outside was becoming smaller as the new 747 jumbo jets heralded a new era of aviation. And my world was about to be catapulted into a whole new direction.

I had a diagnosis within three hours. It was severe haemophilia A, a rare bleeding disorder in which the blood does not clot properly. At the time, life expectancy for haemophiliacs was not good; if you lived beyond twenty-one, you were lucky.

What a bombshell that must have been for my parents. Our family's lives were changed forever, as we were plunged into a completely abnormal way of living. But at least we now had

BLEEDING *Fabulous*

a diagnosis, and I was being cared for at a world-renowned hospital. As a haemophiliac, the slightest bump could give me an internal bleed that would require urgent hospital treatment. My mum was given a direct number for ambulance control, which she was to call any time, day or night. We soon got to know every ambulance driver in Hertfordshire; they were very kind to us, and they became my aunties and uncles.

One standout memory is from Christmas 1977, when 'Auntie Pam' told me she had a treat for me as she drove me home from the hospital. She took me all around Oxford Street and Regent Street in the ambulance so I could see the Christmas lights, which were a spectacular laser-beam display that year. Little things like that made a huge difference.

For haemophiliacs, pain becomes a familiar part of life. You want to try and avoid internal bleeds, but that's impossible if you also want to have any semblance of a normal existence. If I banged my arm or leg at nursery or at school, the bleeding wouldn't show itself immediately but I would get the feeling of something brewing. It's difficult to describe—a tightening and a sort of fuzzy sensation, followed by the area heating up, then the pain. The bleed would start to show itself by the evening, and sometimes, if there was a build-up of blood in a joint, it was such agony that I would tell Mum to shoot me.

My days were taken up with long ambulance journeys to the hospital in London. My poor mother spent half her time in the back of an ambulance—sometimes I might spend five out of seven days in hospital. In addition to the internal bleeding, I also suffered from nosebleeds, which added another level of danger to my condition. I would come downstairs with blood running from my nostrils and Mum would try to keep me calm as we waited to see if it would stop. Sometimes they did and on other occasions Mum would have to call the pub to let Dad know, then call the ambulance to rush me off to hospital before I literally, bled to death.

I remember lying in the back of an ambulance, blood running everywhere, hovering in and out of consciousness, and looking into my mum's eyes. She too, was covered in my blood, and even as she tried to keep me calm, I could see her fear of watching me bleed to death in front of her.

There was one occasion when the situation became even more critical because the ambulance broke down—smack-bang in the middle of Staples Corner. We couldn't have caused any more chaos. The ambulance man told Mum to flag down a black cab because their two-way radios would allow them to call the police for us. Then all of a sudden, a motorbike policeman with a white leather helmet pulled up, found out what was going on and said to me, 'Don't worry, son, I'll sort it.' Sure enough, a big white London ambulance arrived, and I was wrapped in a red blanket and swept inside. A police convoy also turned up and escorted us to Great Ormond Street, all sirens blazing. There was a team waiting at the door as we arrived, and then it was straight onto a trolley. It was so dramatic and scary. By the time I got to hospital, I had lost about a quarter of my life-blood, and if help hadn't arrived when it did, it could have been a very different story.

I'm still haunted by how frightening and lonely it felt, as a small boy, to be taken to hospital and then left there on my own. Especially at night. In those days, parents weren't allowed to stay with their children. I can't imagine my mum's anguish as she handed me over to the doctors and walked away from her son, knowing I would wake up at some point and call out for her. It was just like in the movies: I lay there, cold and almost lifeless, watching the hospital staff, rushing in slow motion to stick needles in me, to give blood transfusions and the haemophilia treatment needed to stop the bleeding.

Today, some of their practices could almost be described as torture. Picture a toddler, frightened and in agony, arms splinted and literally tied to the side of the cot to ensure he didn't move or attempt to pull the needles out. One of the worst forms of torture was the cauterisation process that followed a nosebleed. This involved gauze that had been soaked in snake venom, which was pushed up my nose to numb it. Then while the nurse held my head, the doctor would take a huge matchstick and cauterise my vein by burning it. Even today, it makes me shudder to think about it. By any standards, it was barbaric. It could never happen now.

Neither could a doctor nowadays tell parents to give their toddler Guinness to drink! During my nosebleeds I would lose a lot of blood—which gave me anaemia on top of everything else. So along with the iron tablets and the vegetables, I had a daily Mackeson Stout, as I couldn't stand the texture of Guinness.

Great Ormond Street wanted to send me to Lord Mayor Treloar School in Hampshire, where many other haemophiliacs went. But my parents said *no*, I didn't need a special school because there was nothing wrong with my brain. They wanted to keep me at home and send me to our local school. There were infant and junior schools right at the end of our road, so my mum argued that if anything happened, she would be right there on the doorstep..

My parents stuck to their guns, so the council had to make provisions for me, and I was the first haemophiliac to attend a non-specialist school. A welfare assistant was employed to be with me at all times—never more than six feet away from me in classroom or playground, where I had to walk around the edge holding my assistant's hand. Before I started infants, the kids were given a talk explaining that a 'special' little boy was joining and that they couldn't touch him because he would bleed if they did. Apparently, one girl went home and told her mum that they were getting a boy who burst if you slapped him!

I have fond memories of infant school, and I made some nice friends there. Kids of that age are more accepting. But I became more of a freak at junior school, where no one likes being different. I think there was another reason that I felt different to other boys, but I couldn't put it into words and I didn't really understand it. I just knew that, aged seven or eight, I enjoyed looking at all the men getting changed when we went to the disabled swimming club on a Sunday.

I could swim, but I couldn't play football or cricket—I had to play rounders with the girls instead. There were so many things I couldn't do in case I bled. It was instilled in me from a young age that there were dangers lurking everywhere. We were told that the two biggest danger areas were my head and stomach: if I banged my head, then I could DIE DIE DIE, or if anything happened to my stomach, I could have an internal bleed. So from the age of three, I was told not to do certain things—like climb trees, roller-skate or ride a pushbike: all the things kids want to do. Mum would tell me to read a book instead; I did as I was told because I didn't want to end up in hospital again. Dad wanted me to be able to play but was so paranoid about me banging my head that he bought me a little crash helmet to wear whenever I did. He even got Mum to sew padding into my dungarees so there would be cushioning if I fell over. That was his version of wrapping me up in cotton wool; every parent of a child with a bleeding disorder will find his protective instinct totally understandable.

To me, it was quite normal to be constantly reminded that I must be careful not to hurt myself. Even the simple joy of licking a yoghurt pot lid was not allowed in case I cut my mouth. Instead, Nanny Banham would hand me the pot with the lid already off; my whole family was one step ahead of me, always looking out for me.

I spent a lot of time with my grandparents: Nanny and Grandad Banham, who lived in Surrey, and Nanny and Grandad Ward, who lived in Letchworth. Both my nans were my biggest fans; the sun shone out of my backside as far as they were concerned. I could have shot someone right in front of my Nanny Ward and she would have sworn I didn't do it. And I was especially close to my Nanny Banham, who would always come and see me after work if I had a long stretch in hospital. They all wrapped me up in their love.

But despite everyone's best efforts, I did end up with a lot of bleeds and so missed quite a bit of school. I didn't mind, really. By juniors, I didn't like school that much anyway, and teachers treated me as though I was stupid because I was so often absent. But I was far from stupid; I was getting a different kind of education.

In hospital, I read all the books my grandparents brought in. And I used to ask the lab technicians if I could borrow their biology books too. I devoured them: as a six-year-old, I could tell you all the different parts of the heart. Then I would go back to school, and they would be talking about stupid stuff like Jesus walking on the Sea of Galilee. I remember our teacher, a former nun, asking me how Jesus was able to walk on water. My reply, 'It was frozen over,' got me sent out of the classroom.

I was always firm in my beliefs and never afraid to express them!

In many ways, being in hospital was an education in itself because you were thrust into a world where you had to talk to eminent people. When I first injured my knee I was examined by a Harley Street doctor, who treated me with great respect and asked me to describe my pain in great detail. I was really listened to. I think these sorts of experiences set me up well for adulthood and gave me the confidence to talk to anyone from any walk of life.

My grandparents' attitude was, 'Okay, you can't roller-skate, but you can use your brain.' They frequently took me to museums, and they instilled a sense of curiosity in me—a thirst for the kind of knowledge you can't get in the classroom. I remember my grandad telling me there was a lot more out there than we know; he was a big influence because he spoke to me like an adult.

Grandad Banham used to work on the trains at Nine Elms. One time, he took the day off work and took me to the National Railway Museum. There they had the Mallard, a steam locomotive that holds the world speed record. Grandad lifted me over the barrier, stuck me on the footplate and let me pull the whistle. I was standing on the footplate of the world's fastest steam locomotive! No wonder I said my childhood was exciting.

Once, we went to the Natural History Museum to see an exhibition about volcanoes. Dad was trying to film Nanny Banham on his cine camera, but she kept hiding and he kept teasing her. It was good to see him being so light-hearted, and when I saw those exhibits on volcanoes and other natural wonders, it made me want to go and see them for real.

It was at my Nanny and Grandad Banham's house in Surrey

that my love of aeroplanes began. Their house was on a hill, which was on the flight path for planes coming into Heathrow, so you could stand in the back garden and watch the aircraft come over and then stand at the front door and watch them as they began their descent. We would watch them every night, and twice a night when Concorde came over! I wondered where they had come from, those amazing flying machines. All those incredible places—I wanted to see them.

I wanted to see the whole beautiful world.

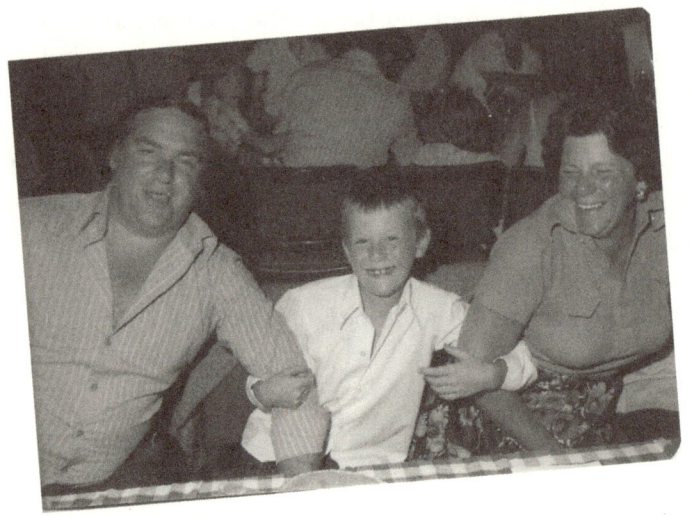

Oompah, Oompah—with Mum & Dad at the Pomme D'or

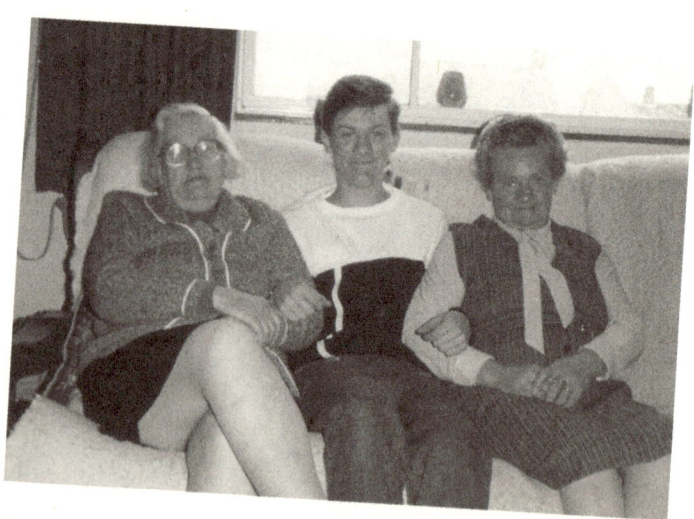

The love for two Nans—Ward on my right & Banham on my left

A WONDER DRUG?

When I was seven, I slipped on an icy playground. When the welfare assistant tried to help me up, I smashed my knee on the concrete. This triggered a really bad bleed that put me in hospital for a couple of weeks. They pumped me full of treatment to stop the bleeding and put my leg in a plaster cast. When Mum came to take me home, there wasn't an ambulance available, so we had to travel on the train. I was mortified because I was in a giant-sized buggy—like a giant-sized baby. When we arrived at Letchworth station, there was no one to help, so my poor mum had to get me and the hateful buggy up all the stairs. We got outside to discover there had been a power cut, so there were no lights, no buses—nothing. Mum had to push me all the way home in that sodding buggy. But though I did feel sorry for Mum, I must confess I was also a little bit excited about the pair of us having an adventure alone in the darkness.

That first incident with my knee was the beginning of many years of treatment and pain as my knee weakened. I had to spend more and more time in hospital, so I was living a kind of double life between there and home.

It wasn't long after I hurt my knee that the hospital started mentioning that they were going to change my treatment. From the age of three, whenever I had a bleed, they gave me a treatment called cryoprecipitate ('cryo' for short), which replaced the clotting protein in my blood. In 1976, Sister Kay told Mum that the cryo was being phased out, and we were going to have to swap over to Factor 8 treatment, from America. This new, all-singing, all-dancing wonder drug was going to change our lives forever because we could keep the treatment at home in the fridge and administer it ourselves. Mum would be taught how to inject me, and I could be treated straight away, rather than spending hours being rushed to hospital, so this would reduce the risk of trauma and damage. On paper it all sounded great.

But my dad was having none of it. He told the hospital in no uncertain terms that he did not want me 'put on that American muck until we know it's safe'. My dad had a general mistrust of Americans anyway, but he and Mum both agreed—rightly, as it turned out—that not enough was known about this new treatment. My parents wanted me to stay on British cryo for as long as possible, and they made their feelings clear.

The year 1977 is imprinted on my brain. In April, I had a humdinger of a nosebleed and so went to Great Ormond Street at night. Mum couldn't stay overnight, of course; a doctor gave me my treatment, and the following day Mum came to take me home again. As far as anyone knew, it was all the same old routine. But three days later I had another bleed, so when we went into hospital again, the nurse went to get my treatment from a little side room and as she was making it up, my mum could see that it was different from normal. Instead of the big bag of frozen cryo, she could see little bottles.

'What's that?' Mum asked the nurse.

'Factor 8,' came the reply.

Mum was horrified. 'No, we said he was to stay on the cryo.'

'But he had it the other night,' said the nurse. 'He's now on Factor 8.'

So that was it—a fait accompli, a sly switch that went completely against my parents' wishes.

How much more horrified would my parents have been if they had known the full truth about Factor 8? But *that* horror would only be revealed later. For now, they just had to go along with what the hospital had decided for them. What else were they going to do? The medics took advantage of parents' fear by saying, 'We can care for your children and help them survive with our treatment.' No parent wants to see their child in agony, or bleeding to death—so they handed us over, little knowing we were lambs to the slaughter.

I was now on Factor 8. My mum was totally amazing: she was forced to overcome her fear of needles so she could inject me at home. She had such a phobia of needles that she used to faint if she saw one. But because she loved me so much, she learnt to use one. The hospital gave her syringes so she could practice on oranges, and she actually became very good at it. I used to call her 'Jab-Happy Mammy,' because it seemed as if she couldn't wait to inject me. If I came home from school limping because my feet ached a bit, it would be, 'Do you need a jab?' I don't blame her at all, when I look back. The hospital always said, 'If in doubt, do a treatment.' And obviously, my mum was just anxious about her boy—because she cared so much about me.

To be honest, having the Factor 8 did change our lives. It gave us more of a sense of normality because we didn't have all those hospital visits. And it wasn't just better on a day-to-day basis. For the first time ever, we could travel, which meant going on planes—an absolute thrill for me. So while being a haemophiliac had always made me different, there was now also a sense of being genuinely special.

We flew to Jersey, which became a regular thing for several years. Before we went, Dad took me to Burton's, where he had a three-piece suit made, complete with a tie, for me to wear on the flight over. Everyone remarked on it. I remember sitting there, this smartly dressed seven-year-old, looking out of the big plane window at the propellers. I thought I'd died and gone to heaven, especially when Dad gave me a sip of his Bacardi and Coke. This was where I wanted to be. Poor Mum meanwhile, was terrified of flying and given a choice, would rather have gone by boat.

We had brought my treatment in an old-fashioned cool box with ice packed on top, and when we got to customs, we had to declare the blood products. As the officer spoke to Mum, she just stood looking at him blankly. We couldn't understand what was the matter with her. Then the customs officer asked her if she was drunk, and the penny finally dropped—she still had cotton wool in her ears from the flight over! It was so funny.

There was one night in Jersey when we went to the Pomme d'Or Hotel on the harbour front. It was a very posh hotel, and during the German occupation of Jersey in World War II, it became the Nazi headquarters. When we were there in the 70s, the hotel used to have a German Oompah night every week (get your head around that!), and my dad asked the manager if I was allowed to go. Dad explained that, as a haemophiliac, I couldn't be left with anyone else. The manager wasn't keen, as children weren't normally allowed, but my dad assured him I was very well behaved. Which I was. So I was allowed in, with a warning that if I misbehaved, we would have to leave. It was brilliant fun, and in the end, it wasn't me who got us into trouble. At the end of the night, Dad had probably had one beer too many, and he got so carried away that he stood on a chair and dropped his trousers. We were kicked out! We've never let him forget it.

Something else I'll never forget is going to Malta and having breakfast on a jet, which—loving planes as I did—I thought was fabulous. Because of my haemophilia, we often got special treatment while travelling. We were always boarded first, and I would be shown around the aircraft. Oh, the thrill of being on the flight deck! And Dad brought me a model aircraft on the plane which started a life-long collection; I now have over six hundred.

When we arrived at customs, Mum gave the Maltese officer the hospital letter which explained we had medication with us. He nodded to the cool box; Mum opened it. He looked inside and then tipped *everything* out on the table; Mum looked close to tears. Only when he'd opened every box and examined every bottle, did he wave his hand for us to go.

Not everyone was so contemptuous: one year when we were in Jersey, we had to come home following a bad bleed in my knee and the steward on the flight couldn't have been kinder to me. As we were boarding, he came to the terminal door, carried me out to the plane and gently placed me in my seat. He treated me with such care and respect. I knew at that moment I wanted to work on planes—not just to fly to wonderful places, but so I could make a difference to someone in the way that this steward had made a difference for me.

Someone else who made a difference was my beloved Grandad Banham: he had always been such a wonderful, positive influence. But not long after that trip to Jersey, we lost him. I went to visit him in hospital, not knowing it was the last time I would see him before he died of kidney failure.

Tragedy was never far away. As I was spending time in hospital with some very sick children, death was all around me. Although I wasn't really conscious of it; the little boy you were drawing with one day just wasn't there the next. But my first real encounter with death had a profound effect. I was ten years old and the oldest patient on the ward—which meant I got to watch the portable telly for a little bit longer than the younger children. As I was watching, I could hear a baby screaming, and there was something about this baby's cry that just didn't sound right to me. I didn't know if he was in pain or lonely, but the cry had this plaintive pitch that made my heart ache. When the nurse came into the ward, I asked if I could hold the baby. 'Please let me give him a cuddle; he sounds so lonely,' I pleaded. After a lot of persuasion, the nurse finally agreed to let me hold him for five minutes. So she plumped up my pillows and brought him over to me. Gradually the crying stopped, and the baby was gurgling happily in my arms as I watched the TV. Time went by; it started getting dark, and I was still holding the baby, who was completely quiet and settled. Then the nurse came back, realised I still had the baby and took him off me. Not long after, all hell broke loose. The curtains were closed around the baby's cot, and everyone was running around. I didn't know what was happening, but I managed to get to sleep.

The next morning, the nurse came and sat next to me on the bed and told me that the baby had gone to heaven. 'But I want you to know that the last thing he knew was that he was in the arms of someone who cared about him,' she said. I have never forgotten that. I've always wondered what that baby would have grown up to be. I never knew his name, but I had this strong connection to him. I'm so glad I was able to give him comfort. I carry him in my heart always.

Not every hospital experience was quite so sad. There was one magical day when I met the most beautiful princess. Mum and I were at Great Ormond Street, trying to get to our appointment, but we could hardly move for crowds in the corridors. We had never seen so many people milling around. When Mum stood on a policeman's foot by mistake, we decided it would be best to wait until the crush had passed, so we stood in a doorway. Five minutes later, Princes Diana appeared, along with her entourage. She spoke to everyone as she walked along the corridor, and when she crouched down and said 'Hello' to me, I thought I was going to explode. She asked what was wrong with me, and when I told her, she asked if I spent a lot of time at Great Ormond Street. When I nodded, she said, 'Take care of yourself' and kissed me on the cheek. I was thrilled. She was so beautiful. And the way she smiled at you and spoke to you made you feel as if you were the most important person in the world. I fell in love with her.

I hated it when I moved up to secondary school. For a start, I was completely abandoned and had no welfare helper. I had to find my way on my own with the big boys and girls. We know how cruel teenagers can be when they see vulnerability or difference. And boy, was I different. When the other boys did metal or woodwork, I was doing cookery and needlework with the girls—which made life hell. (But who was the winner here? I can sew on a button, and I can cook dinner!) When the boys played football and rugby, I just had to walk around the edge of the pitch, often in the freezing cold. Until I was eventually allowed to go and have a swim at the local leisure centre instead.

My arm didn't help. When I was 11, my right arm fused

because of all the bleeds that it had suffered. Whenever I had a bleed, I had to rest my arm, so I spent a lot of time with it in a sling. And that's the shape the arm fused into. The doctors said it was better not to operate and that we should just leave well alone because if they tried to straighten it, I might not be able to move it at all. My arm may have been bent, but at least I could move it. I couldn't hide it from fellow pupils, though. It looked like the spout of a teapot or one of John Inman's camp gestures in *Are You Being Served?* So there were lots of jokes about me being gay; I was called a 'poof' and various other derogatory terms. Secondary school was often a very lonely place.

In October 1982, I went into hospital to have four teeth removed. Once haemophiliacs were on Factor 8, there was a huge spike in dentistry because now we could have procedures that had previously been deemed too dangerous due to the potential for severe bleeding. There was a sneaking suspicion that they were taking out the teeth simply because they could, rather than because they should. A lot of haemophiliacs at that time seemed to need four teeth out, and they told us they were taking out four of *my* teeth. But when I woke up—with a face so swollen I looked like a gorilla—they had taken out thirteen of them. Only four remained. My mum was so shocked. She asked why on earth they had done it, once again without any consent. And they said it was to make room for my wisdom teeth. So I went back to school looking like Bugs Bunny.

As if I needed another reason to be bullied.

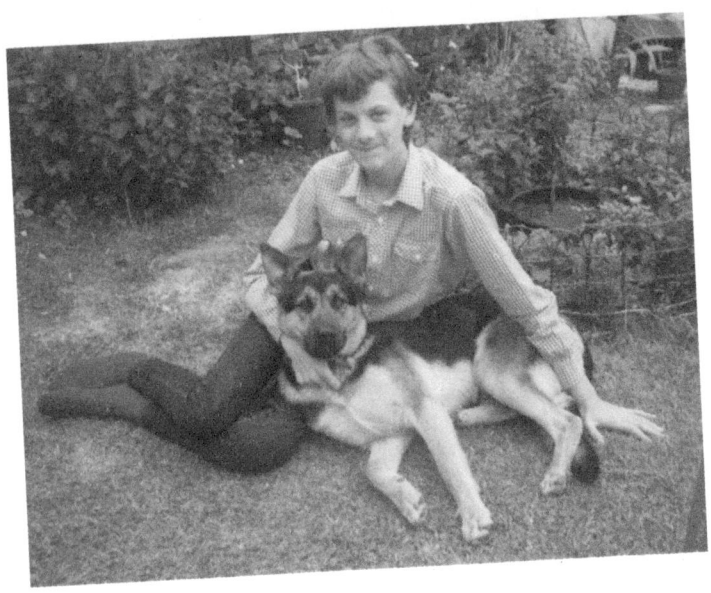

Sabre—in my eyes he could never be 'runt of the litter'

AND LIFT OFF

My misery at school deepened as the condition of my knee worsened. I was in constant pain and it eventually got so bad that you could see it bulging like a small football in the middle of my leg. On the rare days I wasn't in hospital, I had to travel to school in the giant baby buggy—imagine the fun everyone had with that. And when I was in school, the other kids used to slam doors as I was going through them and kick my crutches out from under me.

Life was just shit.

So when the hospital told me I needed to have an operation or I would end up in a wheelchair, I knew I had no choice: I had seen severely disabled older people and I was terrified by the prospect of ending up in the same predicament. As with everything else to do with my medical care, I was controlled by fear. I had already set my sights on a career with aeroplanes and there was no way I was going to miss out on that: I needed to sort my knee out.

In order to have the operation, my care had to be transferred from Great Ormond Street to the Royal Free in Hampstead. So in June 1983, the transfer went ahead and I saw a pleasant Harley Street surgeon called Mr Madgwick, who arrived with his entourage and spoke over me, as lofty consultants tend to do. Many years later, I read the notes he'd written, and he was complimentary about me, saying that I was a very bright young man with, 'I believe, homosexual tendencies'. This was quite astonishing to me as I wasn't even sure at that point that I was gay (despite being as camp as a row of pink tents), and what did my being gay have to do with my knee? What business was it of anybody else's? Which is to say, I experienced a culture shock after spending so long at Great Ormond Street. At the Royal Free, you were treated like an adult, which I wasn't: I was a frightened fourteen-year-old boy about to have a huge operation.

A couple of months before the op, I was out in the car with Dad, and he said we were going to see some puppies. 'I'm telling you now, we're just going for a look. We are not having one,' he said firmly. We arrived at a house, and a woman let us in. She pointed us towards a cupboard that was so dark you couldn't see anything inside. I put my hand in, felt around, and scooped up a little bag of bones—a pup so tiny and so skinny it was barely alive. I just looked at Dad. 'No,' he said. The woman tried to knock the pup out of my hand and said that it was the runt and that if it didn't die soon, they were going to kill it. That was it for me. I pleaded to be allowed to take him home, just for a bit, so I could see if I could keep him alive. 'Oh, let him have it if he wants it,' said the woman. 'It won't last the night.' I snuggled him inside my padded jacket and off we went. But before we got home, Dad pulled in at the vet's. 'We've got a dog now; the vet needs to check him,' he said. Despite his gruff we're-not-keeping-him bluff, Dad was a dog lover. He had been a dog handler when he was out in Malaya doing his national service, and he'd had a German Shepherd called Bruno. So he wasn't going to let a dog suffer. The vet checked the pup over and then put his hand on my shoulder and said, 'Son, take my advice, take him back because he isn't going to live.'

But I was not going to let him die.

When we got home, Mum took one glance at him and said, 'Is he supposed to look like that?' We explained that the vet thought he wouldn't last the night. 'We'll see about that,' she said, then went out for a bit and came back with some Heinz baby food. We fed him and made him a bed in our outhouse. There was a thunderstorm that night, and I spent all of it sitting on the outhouse floor with the dog in my lap. I had decided to call him Sabre after the dog in *The Secret Diary of Adrian Mole*, which I was reading at the time.

That dog lived for thirteen and a half years! Sabre was the love of my life; I totally adored him. He gave me a reason to get through my knee operation and to be up and walking again as soon as possible. This was probably why Dad agreed to keep him.

My parents took me in to the Royal Free on a Sunday evening; I was going to spend six weeks there. The operation went well, and I wasn't in too much pain, unlike the man in the bed next to me, who'd had the same operation. He was in so much agony that I ended up rubbing his foot for him. We became great friends and would go down to the hydrotherapy pool together—in fact, we were the first to use the pool before it was officially opened. My friend smoked in his hospital bed—you could in those days—and the fag ash would drop onto his chest. I was constantly watching him to make sure he didn't set his bed on fire. I didn't sleep very well, so when I could get out of bed, I would sit with the nurses and watch this poor old love called Alice, who had dementia, wander around naked with her Zimmer frame.

It was quite an eye opener for a fourteen-year-old.

Then came the day—and a throwaway remark—that would once again throw my life into a completely new direction. I had been discharged from hospital, and my parents were wheeling me out to the car, which was parked just outside the haemophilia unit. As we passed through reception, a haemophilia sister popped her head out and called to my parents, 'Do you want to know Mark's HIV results?' We were stunned because we didn't know what that meant. We had no idea I'd been tested for anything, let alone HIV. 'He's positive. See you next time,' she said casually. That simple sentence, so cruel in its carelessness, dropped a bomb on our lives. It seems almost inhuman that this is how the news was broken to us. I'd spent six weeks in the hospital and had obviously been secretly tested, yet not a word had been spoken to Mum or Dad until that moment.

I can't remember the car drive home, but I remember going to see the consultant a couple of days later. He told us that 'if I was lucky', I probably had two or three years to live, but probably I wouldn't live long enough to leave school. This was a particularly cruel blow because the Factor 8 had given us a sense that I finally had some sort of future, that I could live beyond the predicted age of twenty-one. But now that hope had been snatched away again. Mum asked the consultant how it could have happened. He said it was because the Factor 8 manufacturers had sourced blood from homosexuals and that it had accidentally got into the treatment. So that was the narrative we were given: the gay community was being blamed, which immediately turned haemophiliacs against homosexuals. What he didn't tell us was that while my earlier treatment, cryoprecipitate, was made from the blood of up to ten British donors, Factor 8 concentrate could contain blood from up to a hundred thousand American donors. And because they were often paid for their blood, American donors were frequently from dubious sources. These so-called 'skid row donors' were desperate people, including prisoners, drug addicts and prostitutes. So their blood was full of pathogens and contaminants, and that blood went right around the world and was put straight into the veins of little boys like me.

But nobody would admit that at the time.

The consultant also told us not to tell anyone about my HIV status, as they couldn't guarantee our safety. He told us that in America, kids with haemophilia were being shot at and their homes set on fire. After we were told all this, I had a feeling that I might now describe as grief—a profound sense of loss. I suppose I had lost my future. But at the time, I didn't quite understand it—I just had all these emotions going mental inside me.

At home, we didn't talk about it; we just buried it as best we could. It was a case of, 'Yes, you are going to die; now, peas or beans for tea?' But this was the peak of the AIDS crisis, and it was everywhere. We were watching horrible TV footage of row upon row of gaunt gay men dying of AIDS. But it wasn't just the gay community being blamed; the news kept telling us it was caused by the three Hs: homosexuals, haemophiliacs and heroin addicts…

At school, I remember people saying that I must be really scared of AIDS because I was a haemophiliac. The teasing became even worse; I did my best to ignore it but it felt like I had a huge target on my back. Everyone knew about my haemophilia, so I couldn't hide like others with HIV did. Mum had to go and tell the headmaster about my status. He was a decent man and said I could carry on attending, but he also said that things might change if someone complained.

Sometimes, it felt as if I was in the eye of a hurricane. I was still only fourteen. But in the midst of all the horror, there was a beautiful bright spot. When I woke up from my knee surgery, my dad was waving a Concorde timetable at me. Mum had seen in the paper that BA did charter flights over the Bay of Biscay, and Dad had worked night and day. He said, 'You are going on Concorde, but you have to make me one promise. You have to walk up the steps yourself; you can't be carried or in a wheelchair.' So along with Sabre, this was my incentive to work hard in physio. There was no way I was missing a trip where I'd be travelling twice as fast as the speed of sound. I did indeed climb up those Concorde steps—alone—and enjoyed the most amazing flight. I was given caviar and a sip of champagne; I stood on the flight deck while the plane was going at Mach Two.

This was the stuff of my dreams.

I think I always knew, somewhere deep down, that I was gay. But it was not something I was really conscious of, or understood. And because I was teased about being gay, I suppose I resisted the idea of being gay, to some extent. I'd been born different to everybody else, so I wasn't sure if my feelings towards boys were just because I was a haemophiliac. But those feelings must have been becoming more pressing because when I was fifteen, I asked a nurse if there were any gay haemophiliacs, and she said no, there weren't. I then asked one of my doctors, who told me that, if there were any, she was sure they lived a solitary life and perhaps turned to faith. I told her I thought I might be gay, and she looked at me and said, 'Well, you do have HIV.' In other words, being HIV positive was causing my homosexual feelings. Apparently, I had been infected with homosexuality, just like I'd caught all the other infections. Even at fifteen that didn't sit quite right with me.

But I had the 'gay plague', so I hated myself anyway.

Time and again, I was treated with a lack of compassion by so-called carers who were supposed to have my best interests at heart. One time, when I was fifteen or sixteen, I had to go to the hospital for a review, and I needed treatment. The haemophilia nurse just plopped the syringe tray down in front of me and said, 'You know what you're doing; get on with it.' But I had never gone through the training process of giving myself injections.

I didn't have a clue how to do it. I just freaked out and said to Mum, who was in the waiting room, 'Come on, we're going.' When I told her what had happened, she wondered why they hadn't asked her to do it, seeing as she had been giving me my treatment from the age of eight.

At my next appointment, I was given a severe bollocking and told I was selfish for wasting money. It was always about the money. 'Do you know how much the treatment cost? Don't you know how lucky you are?' It was brutal. There was no attempt to try and understand what I was going through emotionally, how frightened and vulnerable I felt. It's no coincidence that I have always tried to treat people with kindness, dignity and respect—I know all too well how it feels when those qualities are missing, and I don't want anyone else to feel as valueless as I so often felt during those medical meetings.

As I approached the school-leaving age of sixteen, I had a chat with a careers officer and told him I wanted to work with aeroplanes. 'They wouldn't look at someone like you,' he said dismissively. 'You need to get your head out of the clouds. What about working in a shop?' When I said, 'I don't want to work in a shop; I want to work with aeroplanes,' he just rolled his eyes. I could see he was thinking, 'What's the point? This kid is going to die.' So much for a motivational chat.

Fortunately I had the most amazing form tutor, Mr Christodoulou, who was aware of my circumstances *and* supported my ambition to work in aviation. He advised me which subjects I should be taking to have the best chance of leaving school with qualifications. I didn't let him down: I left in May 1985 with better results than some of the kids who never missed a day of schooling.

I immediately applied to all the airlines for one of Margaret Thatcher's youth training schemes. I was offered an interview with Britannia at Luton, sat the exam and was offered a place on the spot. I think I floated out of there. I had only been home for a few minutes when the phone rang. It was a lady from Britannia, who said she wanted to confirm a few details. She asked about my haemophilia, including what it was. I told her it was a bleeding disorder, but that I had treatment for it. Then she said she was sorry but there had been a mistake; they had given out more places than were available, and they couldn't offer me one after all.

To say I was heartbroken didn't really cover it.

But I wasn't giving up—that door had closed for a reason. I firmly believe I was destined to work for British Airways because it kept popping into my life. As an eleven-year-old, I was interviewed on Great Ormond Street Hospital's radio station, and they asked me what I wanted to do when I grew up. I said I wanted to work with aeroplanes, so they gave me a postcard of a Concorde and a BA keyring. Then after our first trip to Jersey, I came home to a big box—it was a gift from my parents, a radio in the shape of a BA jumbo jet. I've still got it.

And of course it all began with those joyous moments in my grandparents' garden, watching Concorde make its majestic descents. So I was full of hope when I got an interview with BA at Heathrow.

I aced the test, passed with flying colours, and the lovely lady who interviewed me said the only thing she was worried about was the long journey from Letchworth to Heathrow. Thinking quickly, I asked if they had a YTS at Gatwick because my nan and auntie lived near there. (They actually lived in Surrey and Worthing, but hey, it was southern England!). She said they did and sent my file over to Gatwick—where I was interviewed by an amazing human being called Tricia Hercoe. Once again I found the test a piece of cake, and in my interview, Tricia asked what I would bring to the role. 'All I can offer you is me,' I said. 'If I had to, I would happily sweep the runway with a toothbrush—that's how much this means to me.' Tricia quickly made a phone call. She had already allocated her twelve places but liked me so much that she wanted to create a thirteenth. So that's what she did. I joined BA in September 1985.

Thirteen's always been my lucky number.

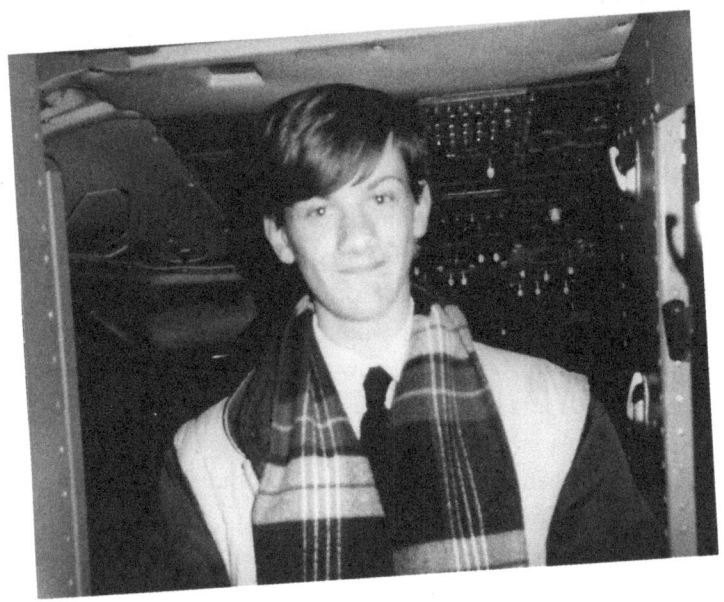

It may have only been a 737, but I'm in heaven.

WATCH OUT WORLD, HERE I COME!

My first placement on the YTS was in a department called the aircraft library, and I couldn't have got a better introduction to the world of BA. The job involved going on every aircraft to pick up and drop off the pilots' airport manuals, which had to be updated constantly. On my first day, my colleague Len said, 'Right, I'm going to show you everything,' and it just so happened that most of England was fogbound that day—except for Gatwick, which suddenly had all these extra planes on diversion. Talk about a kid in a sweet shop! I was going onto jumbo after jumbo. I will never forget Len stopping at the steps of a BA Tristar whose registration was Bravo Papa; I remembered watching Tristars at Heathrow with my Grandpa, and how he'd said they looked bow-legged. BA did the ground handling for a number of airlines, and when I stepped on board a Pan Am jumbo jet, I thought I was going to explode; it was like stepping into one of my childhood Airfix models. Len walked me up and down the aisles and showed me the flight deck. And of course, I got to meet all the crew and the captain. I was beside myself with excitement. Here I was, actually onboard a plane I had only ever seen in the air!

Len knew I wanted to be cabin crew eventually, so he kindly arranged a familiarisation flight to Lanzarote on Boxing

Day. I worked the flight there and back, serving people their refreshments; it was such a thrill.

I was so dedicated to the job that I didn't mind the long journeys I was having to make to get to work. I was living with Nan in Surrey and travelling back and forth by train. Fortunately, I went through a phase of very few bleeds, but if I needed treatment, I went to hospital or home for Mum to inject me. And I would always go home on Fridays, getting the coach from Gatwick to Luton airport, where my parents would meet me and take me back to Letchworth. Then at 4 a.m. every Monday, I would be driven back to Luton to get the coach to Gatwick to start my day's work. I was earning the princely sum of £12 a week on the YTS, plus some travel expenses, but that didn't include the coach, which my parents paid for. This was my routine, week in and week out, and I took it all in my stride. I was just so happy to be working for BA.

Once I'd completed my first block, I went to college for three months. Then I was sent to different departments, including lost and found, cabin services, and human resources. When I was in cabin services, Len had taken a real shine to me and had arranged another familiarisation flight. It was to Lanzarote again, but this time on the first plane in BA's new livery, so there was lots of pomp and ceremony about it arriving at Gatwick. The interior of the plane was so brand-spanking new it smelled like a new car, and here was this panel falling off! We were rather embarrassed and just propped it by the door so everyone could disembark, and then put it in the hold for the return journey because the Spanish engineers couldn't fix it. On the way back, we had an extra busy flight because an Air Europe 757 had broken down, and we had to take all their passengers, too. We were awash with babies; I think there were about sixty on board, and I had to step over various little people as I was walking down the aisle with food. As we were arriving at Gatwick, it was announced that I was a YTS trainee, and everyone clapped while I took a bow! I thought my heart would burst with pride. But I was brought back down to earth as we disembarked: I had to search the toilets for the false teeth that a lady had left there.

'All part of the service, madam!'

The YTS was only supposed to last a year, but luckily, Margaret Thatcher extended the scheme to two years. Wonderful Tricia pushed for us trainees to have a second year because she thought we were really good. So three of us were kept on. In September 1986, Tricia arranged for us to go on a familiarisation flight to Toronto. I was going to be working as cabin crew there and back. It was such an exciting prospect for me and my family were so proud that they all came to the airport to wave me off. I worked the flight across to Toronto, and I could scarcely believe it was actually happening. Here I was, walking up and down a jumbo in my smart uniform as part of the cabin crew. Never before had the words, 'Chicken or beef?' meant so much. To me, it meant that I'd made it. I was practically floating down those aisles.

Then, we had five fantastic days in Toronto. One of the trainees had family there, so Steven, Lewis and I stayed with them. The family had two daughters; one of their friends joined us, and together we went to drive-in movies and on rollercoasters—six teenagers having an absolute ball. We'd worked the British Airtours charter flight on the way out; Tricia arranged for us to work a scheduled flight coming back so that we could see the difference. I was so excited to go upstairs into the pilot's bubble and take it all in. On my break, I sat in club class, listening to music on my headphones. A Steve Winwood song, 'Higher Love', came on, and in that moment, I knew I was living my best life. There I was, at seventeen, working on a jumbo jet as it traversed the Atlantic.

I couldn't have been happier.

My aim was to be the first haemophiliac to work as cabin crew. And, while I was never contracted in that role, I did have many unofficial opportunities to do the job during my years at BA, particularly when they were shorthanded, such as during the Gulf War. As a trainee, I would take my uniform with me on a flight, explain to the CSD that I was a trainee on the ground but wanted to be cabin crew and ask if I could give them a hand. They were always only too happy to have extra help. When my two-year training ended in 1987, I got a six-month contract with flight enquiries thanks to Tricia, who interviewed me (no favouritism there!).

But I think I repaid Tricia's faith in me. One day, I took a call from a man who wanted to report an accident: he said a plane had crashed on the Balcombe Road. I asked for details and thought I recognised the voice on the other end of the phone. I thanked him for the call and went straight to my supervisor to relay what I'd been told. I also told him that I recognised the voice as one of the managers from upstairs. My supervisor couldn't stop laughing. He said, 'I never expected that! Well done, Mark.' Apparently, it had been a drill, and we went through all of the protocols that should happen in such a situation. A few days later, I was called into a meeting with the airport duty manager, the BA station manager and Tricia. I had no idea what to expect. They told me that because of my reaction to the phone call and how I had dealt with the situation, a letter of commendation had gone onto my file. They also sent me to Heathrow for EPIC (Emergency Procedure Information Centre) training to handle a real plane crash, which was an amazing experience and meant that I would be one of the people taking calls from the public in such an emergency.

I happened to be on shift on the night of October 15th when a hurricane-like storm hit Britain. On my way home to Nan's, our train was hit by a tree, which scared the life out of me. I woke up the next day to devastation. I was due into work, and I knew I had to get there: I'd a feeling I would be needed on flight enquires like never before.

So I packed a bag, told my nan I didn't know when I would be back and managed to get a very slow train into Gatwick. I was the only one who made it in. I started work at 2.30pm and went right through to 6.30 the following morning. I wasn't allowed to work any more hours on that shift, so my boss arranged for me to go to the nearby Hilton hotel to freshen up and get a few hours' sleep. Then, I went back in again until 10pm. These were the days before smartphones and internet, so a lot of anxious people were trying to find out what was going on post 'the great storm'. It was absolute bedlam in flight enquiries—and I absolutely loved it.

After six months, an opportunity came up in cargo as senior cargo assistant. I had already worked in cargo during my YTS training; I really enjoyed it because it was like a little family, and I had such a good rapport with everyone. So I was delighted to go back there, but this time as a fully employed member of staff. In cargo, you are dealing with the public—passengers with excess baggage—and freight brought in by lorries from all over the place. We were trained to do everything involving imports and exports. Cargo was a very male-dominated department, and there were some huge characters; it is where BA would send you if you weren't pretty or blonde enough to sit on the check-in desk. So while we all worked really hard as a team, we also had a lot of fun. The men in the warehouse used to tease me mercilessly, especially one great character called George Dance, whom I would frequently find with his trousers round his ankles—shouting *will you have my babies?* or *I love you*—when I went to look for a piece of freight. One time, they tied me to a chair and pushed me around the warehouse. It sounds like homophobic bullying, but it wasn't. Those men accepted me for who I was, and they cared about me. If a lorry driver or anyone gave me any shit, they would always step in to protect me. I loved my boys, and they loved me.

It was all change in 1988 when BA and British Caledonian merged. At Gatwick, there was a massive love-hate relationship between staff from the two airlines. It's not exaggerating to say that if a BA staff member was in a lift and saw a British Caledonian employee approaching, the BA person would push the button to close the doors on them. And vice versa. That's how fierce the rivalry could be. When the merger happened, many BA staff left Gatwick to work at Heathrow rather than be forced to work with their rival. I was very happy to stay within cargo, where I was now a permanent member of staff—wearing the brand-new uniform by Roland Klein, designed to fit the *putting people first* ethos rolled out across the airline by Lord King.

The merger meant that I was thrown together with a lot of British Caledonian folk, and so I had to learn to do things the British Caledonian way. It was sink or swim; I swam with the tide. And suddenly I was surrounded by all these women. I loved it. They used to call our section of the office the 'rabbit corner' because we would all sit and have a good old natter—once we had done our work, of course. Working such long hours, colleagues became friends. I became particularly friendly with two women, Debbie and Mandy. I was especially close to Debbie, who would become like a sister to me. We were a work family.

After a year as an employee, I became eligible for staff travel, which meant I could get flights very, very cheaply. You could fly to Europe for eight pounds, and a long-haul trip was just fifty pounds. My boyhood longing to see the world had never diminished, and I intended to make the most of every opportunity for adventure. On my first staff trip, I flew out to Malaga and stayed in an apartment owned by some lovely family friends, Janet and Keith. Janet was absolutely terrified of flying, so I said I would sit with her on the plane, and she could hold my hand. She nearly broke it! Having managed to arrive there in one piece, we had a lovely week—spending the whole time laughing and drinking. It was great to have a break after I had been so work focused. I literally lived and breathed BA and picked up as many extra shifts as I could.

In October 1988, Debbie and I made the first of our many visits together to Dubai. It only cost fifty pounds to get there with our ninety per cent staff discount. We had such a wonderful time that we made a pact that we would try and go away together every month if we could.

So friendships were being built; my career was blossoming; I was jetting off for fabulous cheap holidays, and all was going well. I was so happy to be a fully-fledged member of cargo. I got all the licences I needed; for example, you need a licence to send hazardous or radioactive materials, or animals by freight. It was a very responsible job. If you put your signature on a piece of paper but hadn't done your job properly, you could bring down an aircraft.

I loved my job. But hovering at the edges of my happy life was the darkness of my regular hospital visits, when I was constantly told that I was going to die of AIDS. I could be lying on a beautiful beach, but the experience would be tinged with sadness because I didn't know if I would ever see such beauty again. Every day was precious because I was so aware that I may not have many more ahead of me.

And of course, I was carrying around a secret that no one at work could know.

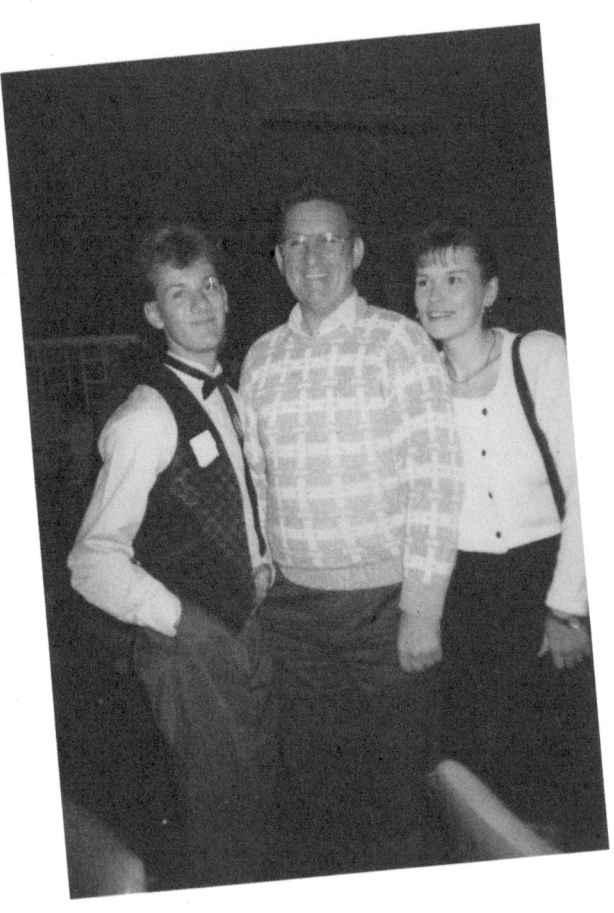

Coming of age—with Drew & Denise at my 21st birthday party.

FINDING MYSELF

Following the merger between BA and British Caledonian, when a lot of BA staff left, there was a big recruitment drive, which brought some new faces to Gatwick. One of these was Luke, who was to play a very important part in the discovery of my sexuality. Although everyone around me assumed I was gay, I still wasn't sure. Bearing in mind that I was also HIV+, I was just happy to bury myself in work and friendships and to try to live each day as fully as possible. I don't know how long I would have carried on in blissful denial if Luke hadn't come along. He asked me if I had ever been to a gay club, and when I said I hadn't, he said he would arrange for us to go to one with some of his friends.

So we went to London and met his friend Kevin in The Royal Oak—a well-known gay venue at that time. You had to knock on a hatch door to get in, and once through the door, it was just WOW. I felt like Bob Hoskins in *Who Framed Roger Rabbit?* when the curtains first open up and he goes into the glorious technicolour of Toon Town. We went from the grey London pavements into this amazing pub full of glitz, glamour and gay men.

'Good evening, girls.'

We were greeted by a marvellous old queen called Dolly,

who was wearing a top hat, tails and shorts covered in sequins. I was gobsmacked. It's hard to put into words just how good it made me feel and how important this moment was to me. It was as if I had gone into another world, another dimension, where I wasn't judged and I was the same as everyone else. I felt so comfortable, and when they played the unofficial gay anthem, 'I Am What I Am', I knew I had come home.

We had a brilliant night and went back to Kevin's flat, where we were staying. He put on the film *Torch Song Trilogy*, and it was like receiving a gay education. I was so naïve, and there was so much I didn't know. But I did, at last, know for sure I was gay. I was eighteen. It wasn't a coming out, exactly—more a confirmation of what I already knew deep down.

Going to London with Luke became a regular thing; we would go clubbing, and then stay with Kevin. I was so naïve it never occurred to me that Luke was gay. He was married with children—how could he be gay? So naïve was I that, even though Luke shared a bed with Kevin while I slept on a blow-up mattress in the living room, I didn't twig. Then one day, I asked Luke if we were going to London that weekend, and he said, 'Okay, but we can't stay with Kevin.' When I asked why not, he said, 'Because I've dumped him.'

My face must have been a picture.

Luke became my best friend, and my only gay friend. There was never anything romantic between us. I was still so unworldly and really not ready for any kind of relationship, physical or otherwise. He was such a tart, but everything just went on around me: I was happy simply being in the gay world, and having a scream. It was at this time I discovered my love of drag: I could put on a mask and hide behind it. I was changing, and my musical tastes were developing in response to all the amazing music I was hearing.

I could feel myself becoming more comfortable with being gay; I could never forget my HIV status, however. Every trip to the hospital was a reminder. When I was on the YTS at Gatwick, I'd fitted in getting my bloods done around work because I was determined that nothing was going to interfere with my career. From the age of sixteen, my appointments had become increasingly intrusive when an all-female medical panel started asking me about sex. Was I sexually active? Did I use condoms? Did I masturbate? Because AIDS was so new, I went from being a person to a research object.

Over the years, my sexuality—or speculation about it—is repeatedly mentioned in my medical records, which I found unnecessary and offensive. I began to feel as if my sexuality was having a negative effect on how medical staff at the Royal Free were treating me. I wasn't spoken to as a person; that's not how they did things. They had a strict style of nursing—sometimes verging on hostility. And you couldn't question the doctors. If you did, you were made to feel small. Or stupid.

But if the hospital was an inhospitable place for me, work was most definitely my happy place. I loved it when I stood on the platform at Clapham Junction in my BA uniform and Concorde flew over us. People would look at the plane and then at me, and I felt so proud. We were part of the same thing.

I almost got to fly Concorde to Florida; my cousin Beverly now lived there and I would get out to see her as often as possible. If I was having a particularly rough time at home or just needed to escape for a little while, I felt safe there with Bev and her husband, Kenny who was like a big brother to me; he had a gay cousin so I could be completely open with him.

I had arranged my next visit with Beverly. And travelled to

Heathrow to try to get on the British Airways flight to Miami. But I was told that flight was oversold; this is one of the perils of staff travel. So a lovely lady at the ticket desk did some checks; BA had a reciprocal agreement with other airlines, and she suggested I go to Gatwick and fly Air Inter across to Paris Charles de Gaulle. 'Air France have flights to Miami with seats and you're more than likely to get one of those,' she said. So that's what I did.

Air France had two check-in desks; one of them had the Concorde sign above it. As I approached, I was shaking with excitement at the prospect of flying to Miami at twice the speed of sound, and the twenty minutes I had to wait felt like hours; when she handed me my boarding card my heart sank a little, but I was to get other staff perks aboard the jumbo jet.

The noise aboard the plane was deafening—people draped over seats, laughing, moving around. The girl in the seat next to me said we were travelling with a French orchestra, who were going to the United States to perform. I couldn't help noticing a handsome steward; he looked at me and carried on walking, and then he came back again. 'Are you airline staff?' he asked in broken English. When I responded in the affirmative, he asked which airline, and he smiled when I told him British Airways. 'Oh, in that case...' When he came back and asked me to follow him with my bags, I thought I was going to be offloaded because the flight was now full, but instead he walked me into first class and said, 'There's your seat.' Before I was able to sit down, he had a glass of Champagne waiting.

He served me lobster for dinner, and after—while passengers watched movies and crew went on their breaks—I went to the galley to thank the handsome steward who had made my flight so perfect. He smiled at me again, and maybe it was the champagne, but I thought it was only right to give him something in return for his hospitality.

I joined the Mile High Club that day, and when Beverly collected me in Miami, neither the jet lag nor the hangover could take the smile off of *my* face.

My twenty-first birthday in 1990 was also very special, thanks to a lovely man called Drew Ronaldson and his family. Drew was one of the duty managers, and he took me under his wing when I was on the YTS. I also became friends with his daughter Denise, who worked in check-in. I loved and respected Drew so much, and he obviously saw something in me.

Our friendship grew and deepened. Then one day, he said to me out of the blue, 'You have your twenty-first coming up, and we wondered if you would like to celebrate it by coming to Australia with us?' Did I! Even the question gave me goose bumps. It had always been my dream to go to Australia.

Drew, his wife, Bet, and Denise were travelling to Sydney to stay with friends and then going on to Perth, where their eldest son David lived. I had a party for my birthday, and the next day, I flew to Australia. I managed to get a staff standby flight to Sydney, not knowing if Drew and his family were even on it. As a manager, Drew was entitled to travel in club class, but there was never any guarantee with staff travel; it all depended on how busy the flight was on the day. We were well on our way to Singapore when I went to the loo and spotted Drew—not in club as he'd hoped, but way back in economy.

Following a stop to refuel in Singapore, we all managed to sit together for the rest of the journey to Sydney. When I got off the plane, it seemed like such a personal moment of triumph—a response to all those people who had put me down, said I couldn't do so many things and thought I would never make it to twenty. I had just walked off a jumbo jet in Australia, using staff travel that I'd earned—working hard for the world's favourite airline. So my arrival in Oz felt like a 'Fuck yer!' to all those doubters.

We were met by Drew's friend Rob, who we were staying with. Rob drove us two hours into the outback. It was incredible to wake up the next morning to the sound of kookaburras and to see Sydney as a tiny black speck on the horizon. I had to pinch myself.

We went into Sydney, where I couldn't wait to go and see the opera house. Drew said he always touched the opera house walls, and I touched its walls on that first visit. This became a ritual that I repeated on every subsequent trip to Australia: whenever I arrived in Sydney, one of the first things I would do was go and touch the opera house, as if to say, 'Hello, I'm here again.' I would also try to do the same before leaving—not a *goodbye*, but a *see you next time*. After spending time in Sydney, we then flew to Perth, where we had a great time. All in all, it was the most brilliant trip.

Not long after returning from Australia, Debbie and I went on one of regular jaunts to Dubai. But there was nothing regular about our return journey.

Out in Dubai, we had stayed at the Sheraton Hotel, where we had spent a lot of time hanging out with the BA crew. We'd just boarded the flight home when the steward warned me and Debbie that we might be diverted on the way home. But we had an uneventful flight; the crew gave us champagne and really looked after us. We weren't diverted, after all; we went straight to Gatwick.

Debbie and I waited for everyone else to disembark so we could say goodbye to the crew. We couldn't believe our ears when the captain emerged from the flight deck and said to us, 'You're never going to believe what fucking happened!' The captain swearing!? Then, we learned why, as he told us the full story. Apparently, we had been due to divert to Kuwait City, where a BA jumbo jet had broken down. We were meant to arrive on the stand next to it and take its passengers to London with us. But after take-off, the captain was told to go straight through to London because Saddam Hussein had invaded Kuwait. So we'd been happily sipping our bubbly, completely oblivious to the fact that we were flying over a war zone. What's more, the broken-down jumbo jet in Kuwait that we were supposed to have helped had been blown up—our plane was meant to have been standing in the bay next to it.

Debbie and I just looked at each other—and we also swore. 'Fuck!' It was horrific afterwards to see pictures of that destroyed plane. That could so easily have been our fate, too.

By that time, I'd started to do some treatments myself, but mainly I was still going to Mum, or to the hospital. In 1991, I attended a medical review at the Royal Free with my consultant. My notes were on the desk, and I remember seeing her filling in a form that had separate boxes with different titles. One said 'HCV' on it, and I asked her what that meant, assuming it was some kind of HIV. 'Oh no,' she said. 'That's your hepatitis C. But you don't need to worry about that.' She explained that when I was infected with HIV, the hepatitis C piggybacked. 'So if you have one, you also have the other. But because it affects your liver over such a long period, you won't have to worry about it because you will have died of AIDS.' This was the first I had heard about having hepatitis C, and no further information was provided for me. Once again, the news was broken to me with no compassion or regard for my feelings.

Having later obtained my medical records, I found it astonishing and impossible that there were absolutely no references to hepatitis in any notes from either Great Ormond Street or the Royal Free. This was a time when the risks of hepatitis viruses had been well-researched and documented. So it's impossible to believe I wasn't tested during this time. My notes had been purged, or destroyed. There *is* a note, dated 22nd May 1991, which states that I had not been tested for hepatitis C. The way it is written suggests we had a cosy little chat about hepatitis C, and then I agreed to be tested, which is completely untrue.

The truth of the matter is, I had received another death sentence—alone, and with no counselling. Is it any wonder I was always fighting my own exhaustion in order to simply go on living? And having been informed of my hepatitis C status, I now had something else that I was terrified people might discover. Hepatitis C was associated with drug addicts, so it was another guilty secret I had to keep, especially from people at work—my career was everything to me.

So I was forced to continue living a double life.

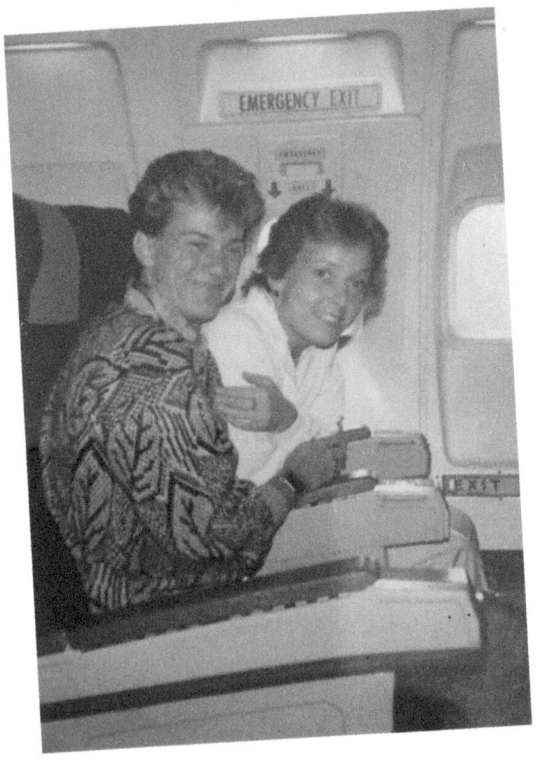

Chocks away Ginger—Debbie & me, off on tour

BUSY BEING HAPPY

I was always scared of people finding out about my HIV, but there was one work colleague I really wanted to tell. Debbie and I had become very close as we stuck to our pact to try to travel somewhere together every month. We would use our staff travel to fly off to Dubai, Mauritius, Sri Lanka and we would very often share a double bed in hotels. It really was like a brother–sister relationship, and so the fact that I hadn't told her my secret was tearing me apart. I loved Debbie, but how could I call it love if I wasn't telling her the whole truth? I found my opportunity one night while we were in Dubai. We were getting something to eat in Burger Queens, and Debbie sensed there was something up. When she asked me if I was okay, I just went for it and told her everything. I was terrified of what her reaction would be, but I just thought *if she runs away, I will have to deal with it*. I had a feeling, a deep hope, that she wouldn't run. And of course, she didn't.

'Why didn't you tell me before?' she asked.

'Because I was afraid you wouldn't want to know me,' I replied.

Debbie's eyes filled with tears. 'You daft sod, come here,' she said, giving me a cuddle. 'This doesn't change a thing, Mark.'

I was so glad I'd told Debbie; it made our friendship even

stronger. We used to come back from Dubai and go to her house in Crawley, where she lived with her parents. We would go up to their bedroom, and her brother Tony would make us all tea, and then we would just sit in her parents' bedroom together, drinking tea and telling them all about our trip. I even used to call Debbie's mother 'Mum'. I felt like a treasured member of her family, which was lovely.

Through BA, I was able to rent my own house in Crawley in 1992. So, I moved out of Nan's and was living on my own for the first time. It was something of a shock to the system—working shifts and running a home. I was used to having everything done for me by my mum or my nan. I wasn't used to being alone. Being alone reminded me of being in hospital. Fortunately, I was never on my own that much; people were always coming to stay with me, and I loved the company.

One night, there was a knock at the door, and it was Luke. His wife had chucked him out. I told him he had a room with me for as long as he wanted, so he moved in. We became as thick as thieves, going clubbing in London and flying off abroad whenever we could. We went to Sitges, and we were back and forth to Gran Canaria, where we had such fun in the clubs. In those days, there was a famous club on the island called Café La Belle, which had a fantastic drag show. Tourists would be bussed out to watch the show, and it was a real riot. The gay men would stand around the edge of the room, watching the (mainly) straight tourists enjoying the entertainment, while the drag queens played up to all the homos across the bar with lots of in-house jokes.

Pure-living me suddenly started smoking and drinking, but that's as far as my party lifestyle went. My fun was never sexual because I was terrified of 'infecting' anyone or hurting them, and I was scared of being labelled sleazy—such as going into the dark rooms that were in most gay bars. There you could hook up with strangers. That was not for me, though I didn't judge anyone else for doing it. We all had our own ways of enjoying ourselves. I was just happy to laugh and drink and dance.

Then things got a bit messy with Luke and his family. By then, I'd met his family a few times and one night, we were both working a late shift when, out of the blue, the bell rang and I found Luke's four kids sat in reception. 'What are you doing here?' I asked them. It seemed that their mum, Susan, had brought them and said they had to stay with their dad. It was no doubt meant as a punishment.

Luke went ballistic when I called him to reception and he saw the kids. I told him not to worry, that we would sort something out. I left work early, took the youngsters home and fed them. I had no idea how to look after children; they were all under eight and one was a two-year-old toddler, but I took some time off work, and we managed somehow. Then Luke went to London to speak to Susan, and after five days with us, they returned home to their mum.

It was maybe three or four weeks later that I was at home when suddenly a brick came flying through the window. I looked out in time to see Susan driving off. I thought to myself, *hang on, I've just looked after your kids, what exactly have I done wrong here?* It turned out that Susan knew someone at British Airways. Because Luke was staying with me, the assumption at BA was that I had turned him gay. The fact that he was gay long before he met me and had been shagging his hairdresser for ten years was neither here nor there. No doubt this person had passed on the rumour that I was responsible for splitting up her family.

Sadly, that wasn't our last run-in with Susan. We had gone to Gran Canaria and were in Café La Belle one night when Luke grabbed me and pulled me round the corner. 'Susan's here!' he hissed. 'Look!' Sure enough, there she was, sitting at a table with some friends. And there we were, dressed up like a couple of poofs. Not the best situation to meet a vengeful ex-wife. We went over to say hello; Susan fairly bristled with hostility. We stayed sitting there until the interval of the drag show, when we excused ourselves and headed for the bar upstairs so Luke could say hello to a guy with whom he'd had a liaison earlier.

Afterwards he raced downstairs, hoping to avoid Susan. There was a limit to how fast I could go in my Cuban heels, and I was still negotiating my way down the stairs when I heard the sound of something snapping. Luke was already at the bottom; Susan had swung around the corner and slapped him across the face with such force he went flying. Luckily, I slipped in my heels and went arse over tit before she could start on me. I could not afford to take a beating like the one she was giving Luke because it could have triggered a bleed. So those Cuban heels really did me a favour. Eventually, one of Susan's friends turned up and pulled her off Luke, whose face was quite a mess. Why was Susan in a gay club in Gran Canaria? It seemed to be pure spiteful troublemaking on her part, but we decided to avoid Café La Belle for the rest of our holiday. Having managed to stay out of Susan's way, we were walking down the aisle of our homeward-bound plane when who should be sitting there but our nemesis. We could feel Susan's eyes boring into us all the way to Gatwick.

If I was playing hard, I was probably working even harder. During the Gulf War, when people didn't want to fly, a lot of airlines went into the red. But BA avoided this by filling flights up with freight. So in cargo, we were very busy and also short-staffed; I did loads of overtime. Sometimes, Debbie and I were the only ones in, and we often worked sixteen-hour shifts. With such a tough schedule, going away to Dubai or Gran Canaria gave me the chance to recharge my batteries.

Then, one of our supervisors left BA to help set up a cargo operation in Dubai. Having seen Debbie and I at work, he said he was very impressed with our dedication and skills, and he offered us both positions—helping him set up the new Emirates operation. He told us to go away and think about it. It was a tempting offer, but there was no way I could contemplate it seriously. Dubai did not recognise haemophilia, so there would be no medical care, and to my horror, I found out years later, it is illegal to enter UAE if you are HIV+.

The next time Debbie and I visited him in Dubai, he took us to the Meridian Hotel—and there was Simon Le Bon strolling past in his Speedos with Yasmine! It turned out that Duran Duran were playing a concert there that night. Debbie and I were beside ourselves with excitement. I turned down the job offer, using the excuse that my grandad wasn't well. Debbie didn't go because she'd had some devastating news: her brother Tony had died suddenly. Tony was such a gorgeous man; it was heart-breaking for everyone

There was an occasion after this when I was able to bring a smile back to Debbie's face. She was seeing a chap who worked for BA's courier department, and she would do jobs for him, which sometimes meant going to New York on Concorde. She had one of these courier trips booked, and I said I would go with her, just for the supersonic ride. But when the day arrived, I was offloaded due to bad weather. (I couldn't help wondering if my seven and a half stone would really have made such a difference.) I was disappointed because we'd planned a special trip, including a helicopter ride over New York. I'd also planned something special for Debbie en route. Not to be thwarted, I asked one of the crew if they would do me a favour during the flight. 'Will you take this red rose and note?' The note asked Debbie to marry me. I wanted her to be able to say she'd been proposed to at twice the speed of sound! Later, she called me from New York. 'You daft bugger,' she said. I could hear the smile in her voice. And all was not lost for me: I cashed in my Concorde ticket and went back to Australia instead.

I was still living a double life. In between my fulfilling career and travel adventures, there was still the constant doom and gloom of my regular hospital trips. My holidays were certainly good for my emotional health, and they seemed to be boosting my physical wellbeing, too: tests showed that my CD4—which measures your immune system—always went up after a trip away, and my viral load would drop. So my health was stable, and I was having fun. It couldn't last, though. One night, trouble came a-knocking…

It was the end of 1992, and I was living alone again. I was always accommodating when Luke brought guys back. But he wanted a place of his own, and he didn't want me to get dragged into what had become a messy divorce. So Luke had moved out and gone to live in Horsham. On hearing a knock at the door, I opened it to find a woman standing there in floods of tears.

'My husband has just attacked me with a carving knife.' she sobbed. 'Can I come in?'

I said, 'Of course' and ushered her inside. 'Do you want to call the police?' I asked her. Perhaps the fact that she said no should have rung some alarm bells, but domestic violence is a very complicated thing, and I was a very naïve twenty-three-year-old.

It turned out that Patty, an American, lived at the end of our road. She had a very strange domestic set-up, because she lived with both her husband and ex-husband, as well as her son. It was Simon, the current husband, who had attacked her.

That's what Patty told me, anyway.

She also worked for BA, in reservations, though she was signed off sick; she was morbidly obese. She said she came to my house because she recognised my BA uniform. I said that she could stay in my spare room that night.

The next day, I went to her house and spoke to her ex-husband, Rob. I asked if he could guarantee her safety. He said he could, so he came to take her back home. A few days later, Rob stopped by with a gift from Patty as a thank you for helping her.

After that, Patty and I chatted on the phone fairly regularly. Then one afternoon, she came round and said that things had deteriorated with the husband. She wanted to leave him, but she was terrified that he would kill her. Feeling sorry for Patty, I told her she was welcome to my spare room until she found herself somewhere permanent.

Our friendship grew and developed. Patty seemed like a really nice person; she was funny and supportive while I was finding my feet as a gay man. At that time, I was becoming more distant from my parents, so Patty was filling the emotional gap.

Dad thought I looked down on him for working for the gas board—who he had been fighting for years, following his diagnosis of vibration white finger. He had recently taken early retirement, which I believe triggered depression, but he would never have admitted that. He was also struggling to cope with the AIDS stuff. It was always conflated with homosexuality. And 'people don't like it,' Dad told me. He was always bothered about what people thought of him. So I suppose I was trying to hide from him. I didn't want to feel like I was letting them down again.

Patty introduced me to her gay hairdresser and his partner, and we all went to a club night called Kinky Gerlinky. It was held at the Empire Ballroom in Leicester Square and was a fabulously glamorous event, filled with fashionistas and famous faces. You could only gain admittance if you were a celebrity or in drag/fancy dress. My mum made me a wonderful costume without my dad knowing. We had a great night, and we became great friends—frequently going out to clubs in London.

At home, we got into a pattern; I would return from work to find Patty's ex, Rob, cooking dinner for us. Patty treated him like a servant—she was incredibly lazy and incredibly controlling, and seemed to use her illness as a way of getting what she wanted. The warning signs were there, if only I'd noticed.

But I was too busy having fun: for my twenty-fourth birthday I dressed up as a fairy ('Surely not,' I hear you cry!) with wings and blond hair. It was such a good party that a neighbour complained about the noise. I seem to remember the track 'No Limit' was pumping when I opened the door to the environmental health officer. I recognised him because he sometimes came into cargo to check certain perishable goods; he seemed shocked by my appearance, but let me get away with simply turning down the volume.

The day after the party, I moved over the road to Patty's place. It had been her suggestion: the troublesome husband had left by then, so there was plenty of room for all of us, and Patty had said it would cut costs if we lived together. It seemed to make sense at the time, so I gave up my own house and I moved in.

And so began my descent into hell...

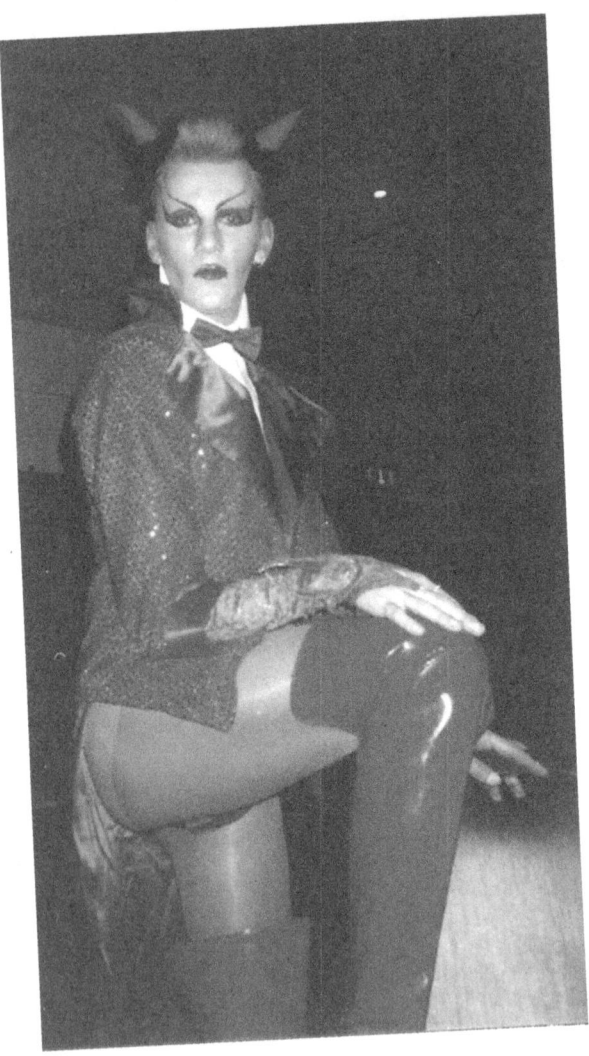

The devil gets the best legs.

TO HELL AND BACK

A week after my party, I came home from work to find Patty not there and Rob acting very strangely. When Patty finally came home, she was clearly wound up and I had no idea why. Out of the blue, she accused me of 'changing' and of 'going behind' her back. I was totally dumbfounded—I hadn't a clue what she was talking about. As far as I knew, I hadn't changed my behaviour around Patty, and I certainly hadn't gone behind her back. I asked her what she was accusing me of, and it turned into an argument, during which she grabbed her car keys and went flying out of the door. I ran after her and grabbed her keys off her as she was sat in the car. 'Please, stay and talk to me. I don't know what I've done. You need to explain,' I implored. Patty's response was to pull out her spare car keys and drive off. Devastated and confused, I cried my eyes out. What on earth had happened to make her behave like this? I barely slept that night, and Patty didn't come home.

The following day, I was at work—on secondment in passenger services, sitting at a check-in desk—when a supervisor called me upstairs. I was greeted by two police officers, who arrested me. It was like a nightmare.

It turned out that Patty had said I'd attacked her with a carving knife—the carving knife was her modus operandi—

and that I had tried to infect her with AIDS. I couldn't believe my ears when I heard her lies. Why would she do this to me when I had only ever been kind to her? I felt as if I'd been punched in the stomach. Not only had she falsely accused me of violence, but she'd also revealed my HIV status. Being the fool that I was, I had trusted Patty enough to tell her my full story; at that point, I still believed I was the lucky survivor of a medical accident and I still trusted people. What kind of person would hear my story and then betray that trust, pick up the phone and tell my employer?

And now that the HIV cat was out of the bag, I dreaded what the consequences would be.

I was taken to Crawley police station and had to take off my tie and belt before being put in a cell. It was all so unreal; I was in a state of utter shock. I still couldn't understand how it had come to this—me being treated like a common criminal when I'd done nothing at all. During my police interview, I explained why I couldn't have attacked her in the way Patty had alleged. She said I'd punched her and attacked her with a knife. I showed them my fused right arm and explained that it was impossible for me to straighten it, let alone punch someone. Also, if I had punched her, the buckle ring my dad gave me for my 21st, which I always wore, would surely have left a mark. Patty also claimed that I had climbed in through the open car door and tried to strangle her. I explained that with my weak knee, there was no way in the world I would have been able to do that. I was physically incapable of attacking Patty in the way she said. The policemen just looked at me contemptuously—to him, I was a snivelling man who hits women.

I was released without charge, but that was not the end of it, because Patty then tried to press more charges against me.

It was unbelievable. I went to stay with my parents, who were having their house rebuilt due to a defect and were, at that time, living on a boat. Only to find that Patty—who'd come with me when I went to visit on one occasion—had sent them pictures of me at Kinky Gerlinky. Given my dad's attitude to my HIV status, and given the dark secret of my sexuality bubbling beneath the surface, this was like taking the pin out of a hand grenade and chucking it in the middle of us. I will never forget the image of Dad bobbing up and down on the boat, waving the photos at me and shouting, 'Why are you doing all this shit and bringing it to my door?' I just couldn't understand Patty's motives in wanting to destroy me and my career. When the boys in the warehouse heard what Patty had done, they wanted to go around and beat the hell out of her, but I stopped them.

My parents and my friend Terry came with me to get my stuff from Patty's house. Half of it had disappeared, and the other half was strewn on the lawn. I couldn't get out of there quickly enough.

Now homeless, I moved in with my friend Trixie and his boyfriend, who had a spare room in their Bethnal Green flat. They lived on the Roman Road, and I remember watching out of the window as the funeral procession of Ronnie Kray passed by. It was extraordinary to see thousands of people lining the streets to say their farewells.

I knew Trixie from the gay scene in London. Trixie (whose real name was Mark) was six foot four and weighed 18 stone; he was a skinhead who couldn't have been less like his menacing image. It was because of him that I ended up with the two cats who became such an important part of my life.

His female cat, a short-haired, exotic variety like the one in the Sheba ads, had three kittens—two boys and a girl. Trixie kept the girl and the other two were supposed to be sold. But I fell in love—how could I not? I'd watched them being born behind the telly. I'd held my breath when the tiny white one, the runt of the litter, was born struggling for life, and it was touch-and-go whether he'd make it through the night. Thankfully, he did survive; I named him Ghost, while his big handsome brother was Trojan. Having watched them grow over twelve weeks and seen their personalities develop, I became deeply attached. There was no way I could let them go to anyone else. I ended up giving Trixie two hundred quid and keeping them both. My boys, Ghost and Trojan, were to bring me huge amounts of happiness for many years.

Meanwhile, with a court case hanging over me and having been betrayed so badly, I hit the self-destruct button. In the clubs, I would take cocaine, acid and ecstasy, though never the hard stuff—I wouldn't have anything to do with needles. But if it could go up my nose or down my throat, I was having it.

I also had the most amazing time. When I went clubbing, I could leave all my troubles at the door. When I put a pill on my tongue, I was no longer Mark the haemophiliac 'criminal', but Bijoux (my gay nickname), the party animal. I would dance on the bar and table tops, and I'd forget everything. I don't regret a single moment of it; I had a fabulous time. I loved being off my face, meeting so many people, and laughing like there was no tomorrow. For me, it was possible that there was no tomorrow. But there in the clubs, I was so happy that it reminded me of my fierce desire to live. I really didn't want to die.

There were so many amazing club nights during that time, but one moment really stands out. The DJ had arrived with a new track he'd brought over from Amsterdam. It was by Robert Miles, and it was called 'Children'. When I heard it at the end of the night, I knew straight away that it was extraordinary. I get goose bumps even now when I hear it because it takes me back to those heady, wild nights when I danced my cares away.

I got to know so many wonderful people on the London gay scene. Some of the friendships I made will stay with me forever, including two great friends called Bev and Ronnie (Beverly and Veronica). Luke and I used to have such amazing, laughter-filled times with this beautiful couple. We were all so close that we'd go back to Bev's after clubbing and the four of us would share a bed. Bev's mum would bring us tea and toast; she was so cool and really made me feel part of the family.

Going to London Pride also became something of a ritual for us. I've always loved a costume, and we always made a big effort to dress up—including top hats and tails one year. And after that, top hat and tails became my signature outfit—which was me *tipping my hat* to Dolly at the Royal Oak. Being present at Pride was incredibly important to me because Section 28 legislation meant Pride was a protest: we still had such a long way to go in terms of fighting for equality. For me, sharing this experience with Bev and Ronnie, as well as Luke, made it even more special.

We were often doing daft things like going to Chessington Zoo and having pictures taken in big Victorian crinoline frocks. I think I inherited my theatricality, as well as my fighting spirit, from my Nanny Banham's side of the family. Her mum was a suffragette and cousin of the acclaimed actress Dame Ellen Terry. No wonder I was drawn to the limelight and to fighting for justice—it was in my genes!

Another great friend from those times was Terry, Luke's ex. We remained great friends after their split because Terry and I shared a very special connection. Sometimes, I would go to G-A-Y, the huge club in the London Astoria where Terry worked the door. One night, I got talking to the club's promoter, Jeremy Joseph, who asked if I would be interested in covering for Terry if he couldn't do the door. Of course, I said yes.

Eventually, Terry gave up the job, and Jeremy asked if I'd like to take over. I said I could help him out on Saturdays, but my job at BA prevented me from doing more. My official title was 'door whore': I would stand there, sometimes in full drag, greeting everyone. And flirting with them. Nobody said 'no' to a drag queen. I'd see a good-looking guy walk through the door and tell him he couldn't come in. When he asked why, I'd say, 'Because I haven't got your phone number,' or 'because I haven't felt your arse,' or if I really wanted to push it, 'because you haven't brought me a drink yet'. I was almost always successful, and one of the security guards took such a shine to Bijoux that we even went out on a date or two.

One Saturday evening, the manager of the Royal Vauxhall Tavern came into the club. We got chatting and he told me about the AIDS fundraiser they were having for Halloween. I asked if I could do anything to help and he said, 'Yes, please—in fancy dress.' So I asked my friend Brian if he would be up for it.

Brian and I met at the club, and he was on my guest list whenever he wanted after that. All that attention I was getting on the door, I didn't always know who was genuine. Brian would meet a guy, then disappear for a while, but without fail, he would show up again. And our friendship just kept growing.

That night at the Royal Vauxhall Tavern, I dressed as the devil (in drag) and Brian came as Bette Midler's character from the film 'Hocus Pocus'. We had a scream. By the end of the evening we'd raised five hundred pounds, and we were each given a bouquet of flowers. Then a lovely trans woman came up to Brian to ask why he was carrying an A to Z. He'd been using it to direct his mum, Della, who had dropped us off, and he'd stuffed it in his handbag as we got out of the car. It must have been poking from within all evening, but nobody had said anything; the trans woman thought it must be some kind of kink.

The kinky guys went to FF—which stood for First Friday, though it was actually on a Sunday. It was the complete opposite of G-A-Y. The club was in Farringdon, and instead of camp pop music the DJs played techno and trance. This was where the 'blokes' went to party—muscle men, skinheads in leather, rubber, uniform, the firemen, the builders and even the odd copper. It was said that if you could survive FF you were a true clubber.

One night in 1994, I was at the bar at the back of FF—which was the darkest place in the whole venue. We always went there to get off our faces and have a laugh. I noticed a man looking at me, and all I could see were these bright blue eyes. I thought he might be smiling at me, but I couldn't be sure. Then all of sudden, he waved me over.

He asked me my name and said he'd been watching me. 'You're a really good dancer,' he said. 'And I've noticed that lots of people come and speak to you, so you must be a really nice person.' Right from the start he had a knack for making me feel special.

His name was David. He bought me a drink and ended up coming back to my place in Bethnal Green, though nothing happened sexually. Then about a fortnight later, it was his thirtieth birthday and I bought him a big bouquet of roses. After that, we started seeing one another.

I did tell David about my haemophilia and HIV status, but it didn't faze him at all. In fact, our relationship wasn't based around sex; it was more like an old-fashioned courtship. David always used to shower me with compliments and ask me how I was, which I really wasn't used to: he always made me feel so valued. I felt a bit like a schoolgirl being wooed by an ardent suitor. For six weeks, I enjoyed this gentle relationship; we would go out for romantic dinners and there was no pressure to have sex. I loved sitting opposite this tall, dark, handsome man; I was developing strong feelings that I had never really experienced before.

When David turned up at the Bethnal Green flat on Christmas Eve with a teddy bear and a big bunch of red roses, I thought he had come to wish me a happy Christmas before we went home to our respective families. So I was stunned when David told me he couldn't see me anymore. The reason? He was also developing feelings for me, but he didn't want to fall in love with someone who was going to die and leave him.

When I'd told David about my health, he'd acted so grown-up; it hadn't *seemed* to bother him. But it clearly had. This was the first time I'd experienced what had felt like a proper relationship, even if it was only for six weeks. My newly raised barriers slammed shut, and I vowed that I wasn't going to let anyone else into my heart. I didn't want to feel such pain ever again. I had my friends, and they were all I needed.

But I was still being tortured by someone who I once thought of as a friend…

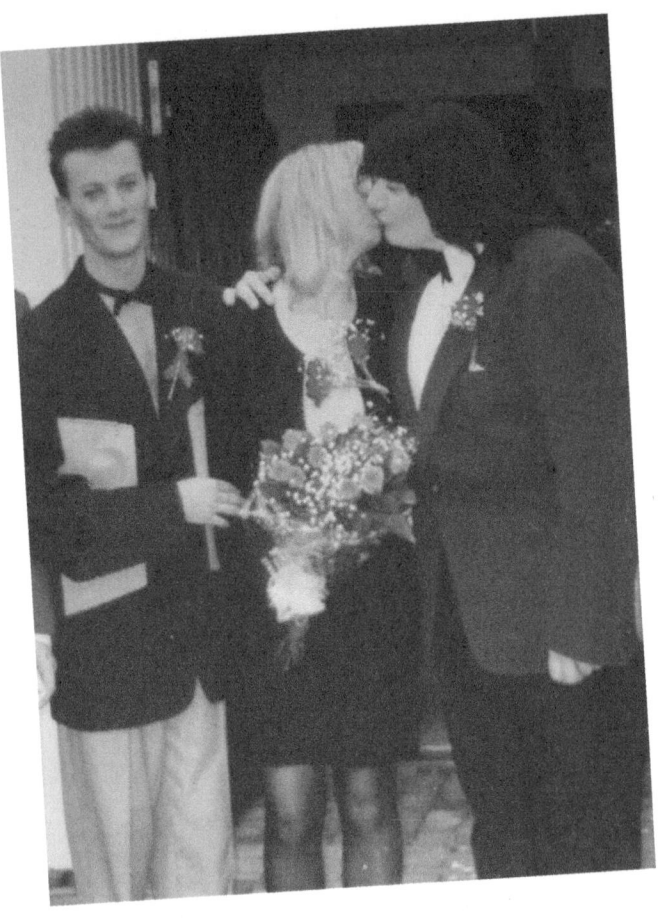

Making a bit of LGBT history—as bridesmaid to Bev & Ronnie

LIFE AND DEATH

I was on a late shift in cargo one night when the phone rang and a voice said, 'That's a lovely car you've got; it would be awful if something happened to it.' I recognised the voice as that of Patty's first husband, Simon, and I knew she must somehow be behind this barely veiled threat. I had been able to buy a really nice sports car because of some money I'd received, money that Patty knew all about because I'd opened up to her over every area of my life. And now she wanted to take some of that money from me.

In 1990, I'd received twenty thousand pounds from the Macfarlane Trust, a charitable organisation that had been established by the government to assist HIV-infected haemophiliacs and their families. We were seen by some as 'innocent' victims, who had been infected through NHS blood products, and the money was an ex-gratia payment. Then in 1991, an out-of-court settlement from litigation I knew nothing about meant that I was due to receive a further twenty-three thousand, five hundred if I signed a waiver saying that I wouldn't take any legal action if I became further infected with viruses or anything else. But this didn't sit quite right with me. Was it compensation or hush money?

I knew my life was worth much more than twenty 'k', and

at the time I was earning really good money but I knew there were people who needed it more than me. People were dying, and there were men with families who were desperate for the payout. No one would receive any money unless everyone signed the waiver. And in the end, that was why I signed. My dad urged me to take the deal, too. 'When are you ever going to get that much money again, boy? Take it,' he said. So I signed under duress, but I felt it was the right thing to do for everyone else's sakes.

Patty knew all about this. No doubt she hoped she would relieve me of some of my money by winning her trumped-up court case. And now, she had come up with another way to squeeze cash from me.

I was rattled by Simon's sinister phone call at work and immediately told my manager, Colin, that I was being targeted. I asked him to log the incident, which he did. Then I started receiving nasty little notes, such as 'I'm still here,' or just a series of question marks. Once, I found 'ha-ha-ha' written on my misted-up windscreen. It was meant to intimidate me.

But I was not going to let Patty defeat me.

One day, I found a note on my windscreen that said, 'I want your car' and a phone number. The duty manager called the number and spoke to someone who said that if I sold them my car for five hundred pounds, they would drop the charges. I told my solicitor, who advised me not to play their game. I had no intention of doing so. There was no way on earth I was going to give them nine thousand pounds worth of car for five hundred quid just to make their pack of lies disappear. The complete lack of evidence was surely going to do that, if and when we went to court.

While I held firm in my resolve not to be bullied, I did feel pretty shaken and scared knowing that they were watching me. So I went to stay with my cousin Beverly for a couple of weeks. When I returned, Mum handed me a letter saying that they were dropping the case due to lack of evidence. The sword that had been hanging over me for eighteen months had finally disappeared. It was such a relief; I could finally breathe again. It turned out that Patty had done a similar thing to her ex-husband Simon. She had accused him of attacking her, then moved on to Rob, and then to me. She was quite a piece of work. Thankfully, she disappeared after that, and I never had contact with her again.

The year 1995 was quite a mixed one. It was the year my nan was diagnosed with cancer and Bev's dad died, but in amongst the dark days, there were some wonderful times. In March, Bev and Ronnie got married in Amsterdam. It was still not legal for gay couples to marry over here, and the whole thing was filmed for German television. I was Ronnie's bridesmaid, so I was in my element—dressed in my finery, with a face full of slap, and a gorgeous bouquet. It was a fabulous day, filled with love and laughter.

For that year's London Pride celebrations, we did the march in the day, and then in the evening, we pulled out all the stops at G-A-Y. I changed into plumes and feathers—transformed into a Las Vegas showgirl to work on the door of the Astoria. I must admit, after a few sherries and glasses of fizz, I was feeling a little worse for wear as I welcomed in some five thousand people.

But I was also having the most glorious time. As well as taking people's tickets, part of my job was to go backstage to see if any of the stars performing that night needed anything.

I got to meet all sorts of well-known people; I was nearly always star-struck, but I couldn't show it because I had to appear professional.

On this Pride night, I was particularly star-struck because the headline act was none other than gay icon, Kylie Minogue. Kylie was co-hosting the show with G-A-Y's promoter Jeremy Joseph. One of them would introduce an act upstairs while the other was hosting downstairs, and then they would swap places. I was standing at the bottom of the stairs when something ran into me at breakneck speed. I turned and screamed, like an old fishwife: 'Stop fucking running!' Then I spotted the diminutive figure, receding. 'Kylie! I'm so sorry...' The next thing I knew, my stiletto slipped on the concrete floor and I went flying straight through the toilet door. Brian, who witnessed the whole thing, spat out his drink, laughing. He said all he could see was feathers flying, like a Tom and Jerry cartoon. Kylie just carried on running, oblivious to the carnage I was causing. All in all, it was a fantastic evening.

If the highs that year were life-affirming, the lows reminded me just how fragile my life was when I was suddenly taken ill and taken to hospital where they diagnosed Cytomegalovirus, which is a virus that attacks different parts of your body. It caused ulcers and affected my lungs, stomach and eyes, which meant I couldn't breathe, eat or see properly. My body was shutting down, and I went down to four and a half stone. My CD4 level was 0.002—so low they said I only had days to live. My consultant came to my bedside, and when I asked her how I had got the virus, she said that it was because of my lifestyle: I had contracted CMV because I was homosexual.

Years later, I found out that the hospital had been secretly testing for CMV, which is why they were so quick to diagnose it. At around the time I was ill, the Royal Free's Haemophilia Centre director had published a research paper highlighting the dangerous contaminants—including CMV—remaining in the Factor 8 product, which I was still using.

I was in a fight for my life. The hospital told my dad that they were going to admit me and make me as comfortable as possible for the little time I had left. But my dad said, 'No, if my boy's going to die, he's going to die at home.' He shut down the consultant's protests when she said I needed to be in hospital to properly receive the drugs. 'This ain't up for discussion; he's coming home,' said Dad. 'Dot's done his injections all these years; if she can't connect up a drip to a piece of pipe, then there's something wrong. I'm not arguing—just get the stuff we need. My boy's coming home.'

My parents were now back living in their house again. Mum hung my bag of treatment from a glass chandelier and connected me up to it. I was numb as life went on around me. My stomach felt as if someone was pouring boiling water down my throat, my mouth was full of thrush, and my teeth—the adult teeth that had regrown after my milk teeth were removed without consent—were breaking. As I lay in bed, I believed that this was how and where I was going to die.

Then after two days on the treatment and against all the odds, I started to eat again. And I mean EAT. I couldn't get enough food down me. I'd have a full English breakfast in the morning, a sandwich at lunch and then, after one of Mum's huge dinners, I still had room for a Chinese takeaway later in the evening. Plus, I'd eat whole trays of chocolate eclairs that Mum brought me. I put on half a stone in a week and when Dad took me to the hospital, they were shocked that I was still alive.

Once again, I had defied death.

I slowly got better, but I was signed off sick for months. This was the beginning of the end as far as British Airways were concerned. After Patty's accusations, BA had contacted the hospital, who'd confirmed that I had 'full-blown' AIDS—which put the first nail in the coffin of my career, a career that had once been full of such joy and promise.

HIV/AIDS caused me such deep emotional and irreversible damage; I felt I couldn't escape from it. Not only was it in newspapers, across billboards on television each time I turned it on, but every part of my life was impacted—friends I was clubbing with on Saturday night, who were dead by Monday morning, grounded cabin crew who never came back to work again. And every time I went to the hospital, another face had disappeared from the waiting room.

After the CMV, I became ill again with suspected MAI—which is basically bovine TB. I was told I needed immediate treatment or I would die before the results came through. It was another death sentence to battle through.

Which I did.

But after finding out about my diagnosis, Gatwick decided that they no longer wanted me working there, and they arranged for me to go to Heathrow, where I was put on twelve-hour shifts. Those long, draining workdays started having a detrimental impact on my health, and I was still burning the candle at both ends—going clubbing while working stupid hours. Not surprisingly, my health suffered.

My CD4 levels dropped, which confirmed to me that I did have full-blown AIDS. The hospital put me on AZT, an experimental AIDS drug that they had tried on cancer patients. It had been banned because it killed so many people. Perhaps the lives of those with AIDS were considered less valuable;

why else would they have used it on us, knowing how toxic AZT was?

Eventually I was summoned to a meeting at Heathrow and told that they no longer wanted me working there, due to my sickness record. They gave me a choice: I could either go back to Gatwick or think about resigning. They weren't going to get rid of me that easily. I had worked too hard and given too much of myself to BA to be brushed aside like a worthless piece of scrap. So I said I would go back to Gatwick.

I was put on light duties and four-hour shifts. I was working with a lovely man called Roger Moore (yes, really). It was just the two of us in the office, shuffling papers, and I ended up telling him everything that had gone on in my life. He was a real ally for me at a time when I didn't feel I had many friends at work; Debbie and I were still close of course, but she was off training, by this point.

I became a bit of a nomad, house-wise. I'd left Bethnal Green because of my failing health. Mum had taken the cats and I'd gone to live again with Nanny Banham, but since she'd been diagnosed with breast cancer, I felt I couldn't be there—she was so very poorly. So I went from place to place. Then Luke invited me to go and live in his house near Heathrow. 'You helped me out when I needed a home, so now it's my turn,' he told me. I was grateful to have a more settled place to stay.

I had just come back from Gran Canaria (again!) and was in our local pub when I noticed a bloke looking at me. He eventually came over and introduced himself as Hugh. He was tall, dark and very attractive. But after what happened with David, I was not letting anyone get close to me again. I did find myself drawn to him though, because he seemed so nice, and when he came back to mine, we spent the whole night talking.

I loved feeling that someone desired me, and I decided I would just enjoy the moment. It turned out that Hugh also worked for BA; he was an engineer in Birmingham. He just happened to be in that pub that night because he was down south visiting his family. Fate works in mysterious ways.

Next morning, Hugh left, saying he would call me. To save myself from any disappointment, I didn't hold out any hope. So I was pleasantly surprised when he did call. By this time, Luke had moved in with his boyfriend, who I didn't get on with: I think he was jealous of the closeness I shared with Luke. Sadly, this had driven a wedge between me and my good friend, so I was living in Luke's house alone. Hugh and I would talk on the phone. He would come and stay with me, and our relationship slowly developed. He became my first proper boyfriend.

By 1997, it was clear that the long, drawn-out ending of my career had reached its finale. BA called me in and gave me two choices: you can take early retirement and a lump sum, or the next time you go sick we will terminate your contract. I loved BA so much that I took the early retirement. The way I looked at it, I would still be on the payroll, which meant I was still part of this company whose uniform I had been so proud to wear, and I would keep my staff travel, so I could keep going on my adored jumbos.

My last flight as a fully-fledged employee was in January '97, when Debbie and I flew to Harare. We went on safari, saw Angel Falls and had a brilliant trip—though in the last couple of days I got sunburn. And because of the AZT medication, my hair was falling out again and my teeth shattering. I was a mess.

And I retired from BA shortly afterwards.

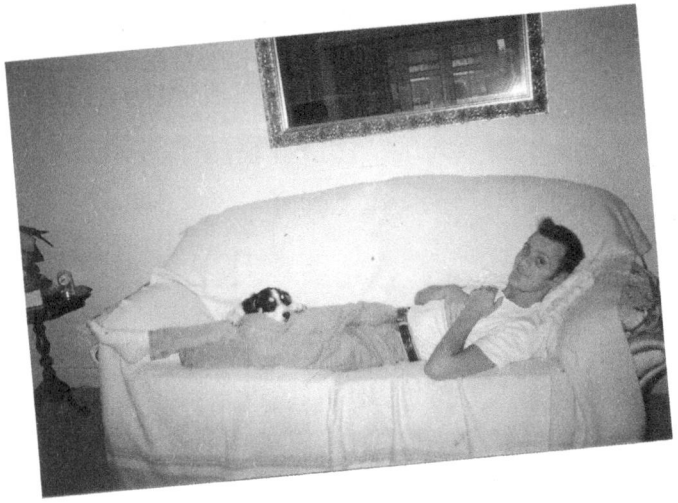

Simba—a bundle of fluff who gave me something to live for

QUEEN OF HEARTS

After I had retired medically from BA, there was no reason for me to stay in London, so when Hugh suggested I move to Birmingham, I agreed. I arrived in the spring of 1997. It was a big step, moving up north and into Hugh's flat, but I felt ready for it. Our relationship had been going very well, and I wanted to fill my life with positive things now that my career in BA was over. I kept my primary care at the Royal Free, though I also registered with the Queen Elizabeth Hospital (QEH) in Birmingham.

Hugh continued to be a supportive partner, especially when Grandad Ward died. I was determined not to be a kept man, living off Hugh's earnings, so I got a bar job in Subway City, a gay nightclub underneath the railway arches near Hugh's flat. I hated it. There was me on one side of the bar, stone-cold sober and run ragged, and then there was everyone on the other side of the bar, having a ball. I knew which side I wanted to be on!

I gave up that job and eventually got another temporary job in a call centre with Thomson Holidays. It was a far cry from BA, but it helped to pay the bills. And I was still doing my Saturday nights at G-A-Y, so I would drive down to London in the afternoon and stay overnight before driving back to Birmingham on the Sunday evening.

Saturday 31st August 1997 was a night I will never forget. I was standing at the bottom of the Astoria stairs, chatting to people, when Jeremy Joseph came up to me and said, 'She's dead; she's dead.'

'Who's dead?' I asked.

'The princess,' he replied.

'What princess?'

'Diana. Princess Diana has died.'

'Fuck off and don't be so nasty,' was my disbelieving response.

Jeremy went away and came back with a portable television. And there it was: the sad, extraordinary tragedy that had unfolded in Paris. I found it so hard to take in. After meeting her in the hospital all those years earlier, when she had been so kind to me, I felt a special connection with Diana. Then she had become the most famous person in the world. But she was always a genuine humanitarian and had done so much for so many charities. I have such a vivid image of her shaking the hands of AIDS patients at the time when they were being treated like lepers. She really was the Queen of Hearts.

The news went through the club like wildfire, and when it emptied out at 6am, there was none of the usual queenie silliness. Instead, we all left in a sombre mood. I walked down Old Compton Street with my friend Carlo, who also worked at G-A-Y, and there were loads of people sitting on the pavement, saying, 'Isn't it awful?' We shared a hushed, collective sadness. At Compton's café, which was normally closed for cleaning at this time, they let us in and gave us coffee and sandwiches. I think we were all in deep shock. Then I drove to my parents, woke them up and burst into tears.

Later, Hugh and I visited his mum in Ascot so we could go to Windsor and sign the memorial book. On the day of Diana's funeral, I was driving down the M1 to London, and the traffic came to a halt. We all got out of our cars and stood on the central reservation to pay our respects as the funeral cortege drove past. It was unspeakably sad. That night at G-A-Y, Carlo, Jeremy and myself stood on the stage, and with all the music stopped, we led a minute's silence for the Queen of Hearts. It was the least we could do for the compassionate woman who had been so supportive of the gay cause.

Hugh and I had been talking about a bigger place for both of us to live in, and in the spring of 1998, I bought a house in Birmingham using the lump sum I had received from BA and the money from the Macfarlane Trust. Hugh already owned his own flat, so the mortgage was in my name. I figured that it was something for my parents to have when I died, because it was all I could give them. I really wanted to leave my parents something, especially my mum, after everything she'd done for me. But because of my haemophilia, I couldn't get life insurance, so at least this way they could sell the house after I'd gone.

For my twenty-ninth birthday in April, Hugh surprised me with the most wonderful gift—a rescue puppy from Birmingham Dogs Home. I couldn't believe it when I saw this beautiful bundle of fluff on the living room floor. I was sat with him, trying to think of a suitable name, when an advert for 'The Lion King' came on the telly and each time the word 'Simba' was said, he yapped. So I tried it: I called out Simba; he turned and ran towards me. He chose his own name, and it was perfect for his character. I adored him, and he would be my faithful friend for fourteen years.

My monthly expeditions with Debbie had come to an end since I'd moved up to Birmingham, but we kept in contact via telephone. One night, Debbie suggested another trip; she checked a few flights to see what the passenger loads looked like and found available seats to Antigua. We had been there before and loved it; a week in the Caribbean would do us both good, and it would also give us a chance to properly catch up without certain people (Hugh) listening in on our conversation.

The first few days were beautiful—nice and warm, swimming in the sea, just like old times. We sat on the beach with a rum punch as we watched the sunset; the sky looked like it was on fire. But when we went back to our room to get ready for dinner, we noticed a letter had been pushed under the door. It was from the manager—requesting our mandatory attendance at a meeting the following day in order for him to advise us on the possibility of a hurricane hitting the island. Well, that really put us off our rum punch.

The following day, we did what was asked. And yes, we were told that Hurricane George was heading our way and the hotel staff would keep us updated on its progress. Then they told us to carry on enjoying ourselves, which wasn't the easiest of tasks.

Debbie and I both called home; I couldn't get through to Mum, but I was able to speak to Nanny Banham who, as always, assured me I'd be ok. I also couldn't get through to Hugh, and when I tried him at work, his supervisor told me he was on annual leave—he thought we were on holiday together. My partner had gone AWOL—just what I needed with a natural disaster around the corner. Fortunately, a British 'stiff upper lip' camaraderie was forming amongst hotel guests as we prepared for what could happen next.

When we got back to our room, there was another letter advising us to pack all of our belongings and put our suitcases up as high as possible. Then we were to meet in the hotel lobby where we would be escorted to their hurricane shelter.

The hotel staff were absolutely amazing: they had been preparing the shelter, which was actually the dining room; it was built into the side of a hill. The windows had been boarded up, and all the sun loungers had been taken from the pools and from the beach, and placed in rows in the shelter. We were asked to take a sunbed each and that's where we should stay. We could stand outside the door for a cigarette while the hurricane was still approaching. But once the manager had given the order, that was it. We wouldn't be allowed out after that, whether we smoked or not.

Another hotel guest had a small radio and we were listening to the local broadcast, which was advising us of developments, and as the hurricane came closer the sounds of devastation began. Crashing. Banging. Glass breaking. The noise was terrifying. Debbie and I said this is how it must have felt for the people who went through the Blitz in London during the Second World War. The wind was like a jumbo jet taking off right outside the window. Powered by Mother Nature. She ravaged the island for hours and all we could do was lie there, listening. We tried to sleep but found it impossible. Then the voice on the radio told us the eye of the hurricane was about to reach Antigua. And not long after, everything stopped. It all went silent. It was like somebody had flicked a switch and turned it off.

Just in case anyone felt tempted, the manager said that under no circumstances could we go outside because the worst was yet to come. As the eye of the hurricane passed over the island, the hotel staff frantically did everything they possibly could to reattach boards to windows and provide us with food until, all of a sudden, a door started gently banging. Debbie looked at me and said, 'It's coming.' And then again, just like a switch had been flicked, the roar returned.

In all, we spent thirty-six hours in that hurricane shelter. When we finally emerged, it was to pure carnage—a car in reception, palm trees ripped up, and where beach huts had been, only foundations remained. We were advised to go back to our rooms and check on our cases. Debbie was particularly concerned for my welfare because broken glass would be a hazard with my haemophilia. But thankfully, all we had was sand in our room. So we got brooms, and we swept out the sand. And then we helped the hotel staff clear other areas. Later that afternoon, we asked the manager if we could arrange a hurricane survivor's party with the British Airways crew we had befriended. We said we would man the bar so the staff who had looked after us could go and get some much-needed rest. He seemed shocked by our request. But then a look of gratitude crept across his face and he agreed. So that's what happened: with the stranded stewards and stewardesses of our flight back to London, Debbie and I ran around and did what we did best. We partied.

Then in September 1998, the CMV came back in my right eye; it made me almost blind. I ended up back in the Royal Free. One day, my consultant appeared at my bedside and told me that they were going to have to stop the HIV treatment they were giving me because it was causing crystallisation behind people's eyes, which in turn caused brain haemorrhages. I was sent home with a new treatment, which had an unfortunate side effect—it turned my pee bright red. This sent me into a panic when I first saw it. Incredible though it may seem, no one at the hospital had warned me that this might happen. It was only when I phoned the hospital that they said it was a standard side effect. I was more angry than shocked; it was yet another example of why the Royal Free's haemophilia centre was notorious for keeping patients in the dark.

During my two weeks in hospital, Hugh had not been to visit me once. He said it was because he had to look after the cats and dog, but it soon became clear to me that it was something more than that. He didn't even come to collect me when I was discharged, so I had to get myself home on the train.

After having been so supportive, Hugh became distant, and we started arguing a lot. He would come home from work and get angry that I hadn't hoovered or because he didn't like the food I'd cooked. There was no thought for my health. Then he became violent. You would have thought that would have been enough to make me walk away, but I hung on in there. He was my first love, and I suppose I just hoped that we could find what we'd once had. I had confided my relationship worries to some friends I'd made in Birmingham, and they suggested that we all go to Gran Canaria, where Hugh and I could perhaps rekindle our romance. I was persuaded, reluctantly, to go. But within three days, I wanted to come home. The deep cracks in our relationship were not going to be healed by some fun in the sun.

On the fifth night, we were out in a club and I really wasn't in the mood to party. For a start, I didn't exactly relish using public toilets when, because of my tablets, I was still pissing bright red. I just wanted to go home and lie down. Hugh had disappeared, so I asked our friends to tell him I'd left. As I made my way out of the club, I saw Hugh coming out of a dark room, doing up his trousers. No prizes for guessing what he'd been up to.

Sex was all Hugh thought about, and my medication had also been causing libido problems. I just looked at him and carried on walking. Back at the flat, I started packing, and when Hugh came back, we had an almighty row, which became violent. Our friends had to intervene, but not before Hugh had covered me in bruises yet again. His assault left me with injuries which landed me in hospital when I got back to England.

But still I didn't walk away.

Back in Birmingham, Hugh got another job, working in a pub. So we spent less time together. Afterwards, I found out that he became the entertainment when the bar shut. I did kick him out, but he knew I was vulnerable and a soft touch—somehow he managed to worm his way back in. Things continued to go downhill. He would go off to work, resentful that I was lying on the sofa and not understanding just how ill and depressed I was feeling; he made me feel lazy and like I was using him.

Things came to a head in October 1998 when the phone rang and it was an estate agent who revealed that Hugh had bought a house behind my back. It turned out that Hugh hadn't come to see me in the Royal Free because he was supposed to be moving into his new house, but it was a new-build and it had been delayed, so he couldn't do a bunk like he'd hoped. I confronted Hugh about it, and he confessed everything. The only reason he had rekindled our relationship was to buy himself some time until the house was ready for him to move into. I also discovered, to my horror, that he'd been sleeping with my so-called friends, the ones I had been confiding in so trustingly. That was the final straw. I chucked him out, for good this time. I felt desolate and alone: I had been betrayed by the man I had loved and the friends I had trusted.

I soon discovered that Hugh's betrayal was much deeper than I could ever have imagined. The following evening, I went to do my regular shift at the West Midlands Lesbian and Gay Switchboard where I had been volunteering since I moved to Birmingham. As I was leaving at the end of my shift, one of Hugh's friends came out of the pub opposite and said he needed to talk to me. He knew my relationship with Hugh had been playing havoc with my health and he wanted me to know the truth. So he proceeded to fill me in on the full extent of Hugh's betrayal. Apparently, Hugh had been shagging other blokes all the while I was in hospital. In our bed. I'd fallen in love with the local slag.

When I heard this shocking truth, something in me clicked. I decided I needed to get a grip and now my health had settled, the first step towards that was to find a job. I applied for a receptionist's job at The Beeches, a residential management training centre in Bourneville. A beautiful lady called Barbara interviewed me (she reminded me of the wonderful Tricia Hercoe). We got on really well, and it was clear the job was mine if I wanted it, which of course I did. Barbara showed me round the building there and then, introducing me to people who were clearly surprised to see a man in the role of receptionist. 'Yes, he's my toy boy,' twinkled Barbara.

At first, it was great at The Beeches. It had a real family atmosphere, and I was warmly welcomed by the lovely team of women who worked there. Okay, there wasn't an aeroplane in sight, but I was doing what I was good at—working with people and being part of a team. There was only one person who didn't seem quite so keen on me, and that was Doreen, the sour-faced manager. Doreen made her feelings about gays perfectly clear.

Unfortunately, the lovely Barbara left, but she was replaced by another lovely person, who just happened to be gay; Doreen scowled at them too. Then a new supervisor arrived, an Australian called Olivia, who lured me into her confidence. She told me that she had had a friend in Oz with haemophilia, and she was sad because he'd died of AIDS due to the treatment he'd been given.

This was so close to home for me that I—stupidly—told her my whole story. But I also told her that my health was now stable.

The following week, Doreen said she wanted me to clear out a store cupboard rather than work on reception. The girl who was working on reception told me that the cupboard hadn't been used for years and that I should be careful because it was full of things that could fall on me. I told Olivia that I didn't think I would be able to do the job properly because of my arm: because it didn't straighten, I wouldn't be able to lift boxes above my head. As I couldn't do it on my own, she told me to forget it. But after that, I felt as if I was being watched and questioned. They would constantly say to me, 'Are you refusing to do that?'

It's my belief that Doreen felt jealous because I had arrived and immediately got on with everyone, and that she had asked Olivia to get close to me to find out information about me. This may seem paranoid, but it was confirmed by my dad, who had been a union shop steward at the gas board

'They are setting you up. If you refuse to do anything, they will fire you,' he said. 'They are looking to sack you so be really careful what you say. And whatever you do, don't go into any room with them on your own.' I followed his advice.

One day, I received a phone call at work. It was Kevin, a lovely friend I'd made on the gay scene in Birmingham. He was at my house while I had carpets fitted, so he'd been there to take a phone call with the awful news that my nan had been taken into a hospice. After her initial breast cancer diagnosis and mastectomy, Nan Banham had been clear for three years. So I had been devastated when I went to see her one day, and she told me it had come back. Now she was going into a hospice for end-of-life care. 'They're saying you need to go to London immediately,' said Kevin.

I told Olivia I had to go home. Without asking me why, she just said no, I couldn't. 'I'm not arguing with you. My nan is in a hospice, and I think she could be dying,' I said. 'If you want, I am telling you that I am going home sick.'

I went home and grabbed a bag. Kevin was still at my house with another lovely friend called Wayne, and they told me not to worry about the animals because they would look after them. I drove to straight to see Nan in the hospice. I barely recognised her. Then I went to stay with my parents. The following day, I took Mum to the hospice with me. I think she was struggling with the thought of Nan dying, and she'd been planning to go in a couple of days, but something told me that she shouldn't put off her visit. My car had a built-in phone, and while we were driving, we got a call asking for permission to give Nan morphine.

We sat with Nan all day as they upped her morphine. In the evening, I went out to have a cigarette. I could hear the distinct sound of a Concorde, and as I lifted my eyes skyward, there she was, flying across a full moon. I knew that seeing a Concorde was a sign I needed to get back inside as quickly as possible. Nan died ten minutes later as I held her hand. The last thing I said to her was, 'I love you.'

I was inconsolable. But I switched into BA mode—staying calm, controlled and focussed on looking after Mum. It was only when we got back to Mum's, and we sat in the kitchen with a cup of tea, that I started to cry. Dad asked, 'What you crying for?' This is an example of what he could be like. I said, 'I've just watched my nan die!' His reply was, 'Well then, you shouldn't have gone.'

My Nanny Banham had meant the whole world to me. When I was a little boy leaving Nan's after staying with her, I would sit on the back seat, turn around and wave to her. She was always there, waving back. Even when I lived with her and drove away in my own car, I would look at her in my driving mirror and wave. After she died, we went back to Nan's house to organise her things. When we drove away afterwards, I didn't look back. She was gone, and I was heartbroken.

We had to wait three weeks to bury Nan because it was so cold that the ground was frozen. Wayne and Kevin were absolutely wonderful as I continued to stay down south. They reassured me that my three boys were fine and well looked after. I will be eternally grateful to them for lifting that weight from me at a time when I really needed it. My dad told me to get myself signed off sick, which I did; the doctor gave me a few months' sick leave. I sent the note to The Beeches, assuming that it would cover my absence.

On my return, I was called into work to see the managers. I was still covered by my sick note, but I went in to pick up a new uniform because they'd changed it while I was away. My dad had advised me to take a letter of resignation. 'Have it in your pocket because I think you're going to need it,' he said.

Olivia and Doreen were sitting there and told me that it was a disciplinary hearing. 'What for?' I asked.

'You broke the terms of your contract,' said Doreen. 'If you are off sick, you have to phone in every day to update us.'

'Let me get this clear,' I said, trying to keep my emotions in check. 'You wanted me to phone in every day and say, "My nan's still dead, and she's a bit colder today than she was yesterday," while I was in the middle of choosing a box in which to put the person I worshipped?' Then I pulled out the letter. 'You can't actually do this to me, as I'm still signed off. So you're breaking the law. But here's my letter of resignation. You can shove your job up your arses.'

I slammed the door as I left.

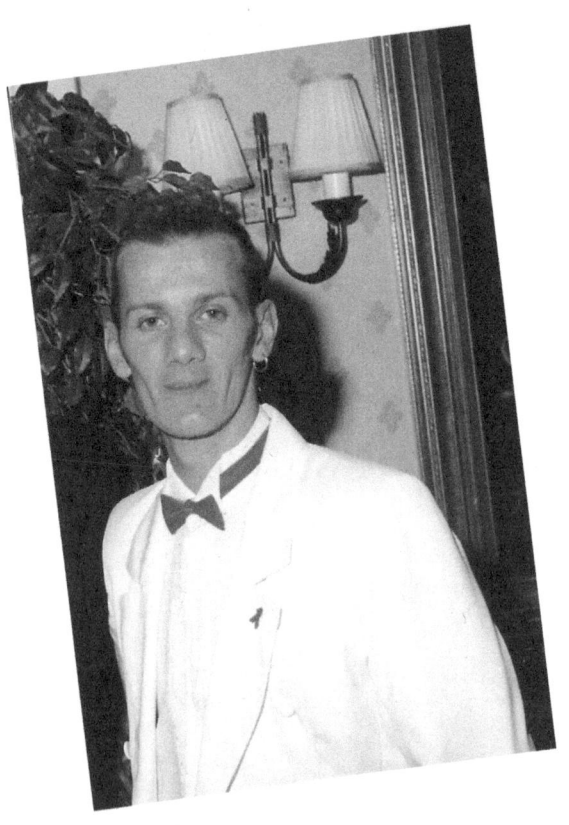

A red tie fundraiser—the last photo I believed I would ever pose for

DARK DAYS

I decided that I wasn't going to settle for any old job and just make do. All my life, I have tried to be the best version of myself, and when it came to work, there was only really one place I wanted to be—in an airport. Lady Luck (or maybe Nanny Banham) must have been smiling down on me because in 2000, I spotted an advert in the paper for passenger service agents at Birmingham airport. I applied and once again breezed through the interview process. I got the job, completed their training and then was back on the check-in desk, boarding planes. I couldn't believe it; I was back in my element and absolutely loving it.

They extended my temporary contract twice, and then I was made permanent. As a result, I was given more responsibility—filling in as a check-in supervisor and occasionally as a duty manager. I was mainly working night shifts; I wanted to work part-time so Ghost, Trojan and Simba weren't left alone at home for too long. This mainly meant a 3am start, working until 7am, after the first flights had boarded at six. I didn't mind the unsociable hours; I was back doing what I loved. But those night shifts sometimes brought more drama than I would have liked...

One morning, I opened up the check-in, and a bloke came wobbling towards me. He was easily ten feet away, but I could smell the booze on him. He was steaming. I went through the whole check-in process and then said, 'Before I go any further, I can tell you have been drinking. When did you last have a drink?' It turned out he had basically come straight from a nightclub to the airport. I advised him to drink as much coffee as he could get down him. 'I am the duty manager, and I will be down at the gate when you board,' I told him. 'If I don't think you are fit to fly, you won't be travelling to Ibiza today.' He promised me that he would drink the coffee. What happened next came totally out of the blue. Going through the usual security questions, I asked him if he had anything sharp in his luggage. 'What, like this?' he asked. To my horror, I saw that he was brandishing a flick knife, which he then held to my throat. My heart was pounding out of my ribs. How could this be happening? I looked around for help, but I was all alone on the check-in because it was so early. Trying not to show my fear, I managed to press the panic button underneath the desk. 'Do you really think you are going to get on board with a weapon?' I said, amazed at how calm my voice sounded. The armed police were there within seconds. I wasn't hurt, but I was badly shaken, and the following day, I just broke down.

For the first time ever, I asked myself, 'What am I doing here?' I had narrowly missed having my throat cut and for what? Minimum wage and a shedload of responsibility.

A couple of weeks later, I was checking in a couple on a Monarch flight. The lady's hand luggage was twelve kilograms—so heavy that, had it fallen out of the overhead locker, it could have killed someone. So I refused to check it in on the basis that, at more than double her five kilogram allowance, it was potentially dangerous. The woman went absolutely ballistic and called me every name under the sun. I tried to help by asking her if she could make it any lighter, but she was having none of it. Eventually, she complained to the Monarch rep, who let her get on the flight because it was the path of least resistance. As a result of this incident, I was hauled in to see the managers, who told me I had done the right thing but perhaps I was a bit harsh. Harsh? I was at the very start of my career when the British Airtours plane, Juliet Lima, exploded on a Manchester runway after catching fire due to poor safety measures—it was a tragedy that stayed with me. Safety has always been paramount to me; it was hard-wired into me. If I found myself in that situation again, there's nothing I would do differently. I couldn't believe that I was being reprimanded for it.

So another little light had gone out; I was gradually falling out of love with a role that had once been my dream job.

The third dimming of the lights occurred not long afterwards. The airport was heaving, and I was helping to check in two flights, one to Palma and the other to Lanzarote. As I looked out at the sea of faces, I saw a couple of men who were much taller than everyone else. One of them had bright blue eyes that reminded me of David. I finally called the owner of those eyes forward to check in. He was absolutely gorgeous. But I was soon swooning for a very different reason. As I bent forward to tag the hand baggage he and his companion had put on the belt, I saw that the bag was open and right there, on top of a towel, was a gun. I surreptitiously pressed the security button, and in the meantime, I carried on 'checking in' the two men, pushing random buttons until the armed police arrived. I said calmly, 'Could you check this passenger's hand baggage? I think there could be something of interest in there.' The two men were quickly taken away. As for me, I told the duty manager what had happened so he could file a report, and then

I had a cigarette and carried on as if it was all in a day's work.

To this day, I don't know whether or not that gun was real and if the whole thing was simply a security test. But for me, it was yet another reason to feel unsafe in my job and to ask myself if it was all worth it. Feeling disillusioned with it all, I wondered if it was finally time to call it a day on my airline career. But in the end, the decision was taken out of my hands.

At this point, my health was stable, and although I was going out in London and Birmingham, I wasn't in self-destruct mode. I had made some nice friends on the gay scene in Brum, including a couple of guys on my team at work, so I felt as though I was part of a community, which was great.

In 2001, a group of about ten of us went to Gran Canaria for some fun. I loved clubbing but as always, I was just there for the laughs and dancing. While my friends were doing their thing, I would happily leave them to it and go home—alone. We had a fabulous time. Then, two days before we were due to come home, I found myself unable to get out of bed. I knew instinctively that it was something serious, so I called my mum. 'Something's wrong, and I don't know what,' I told her. 'Can you call the hospital and tell them to expect me?'

My friends helped me to the airport and onto the plane; in Luton, my parents were waiting. When they got me to the hospital, I collapsed. When I came to, I was in an MRI machine. I couldn't feel my left arm. The news I received couldn't have been worse. They told me I had a lesion on the right motor cortex of my brain that had caused an internal bleed. 'You've had a stroke, Mark,' said the doctor. 'We believe the lesion is the JC virus, which is a brain infection similar to BSE.' He went on to deliver the shattering news that this infection can spread across the brain like cobwebs, shutting it down. So I could suddenly stop breathing or lose my eyesight. Ultimately, as my brain shut down, I would end up as a vegetable on life support. I was told I had weeks, not months, before this happened. 'My advice to you, Mark, is to go home and get your affairs in order.'

I was totally numb. I'd been informed I didn't have long to live on many occasions, but this time it seemed more final. I was absolutely terrified of the darkness that lay ahead. Mum said, 'Don't worry, we'll get this sorted,' as only my mum could do.

She came up to Birmingham with me, and my primary care was transferred from London to the Haemophilia Centre at the QEH. Tests revealed that my blood was so toxic that a lot of my HIV medication had stopped working. Nobody at the Royal Free had bothered to check this, and when my new Birmingham consultant, Dr Wilde, told the Royal Free doctors that my liver function was really bad, they simply said, 'Oh, it's probably his HIV medication.' The Royal Free didn't feel the need to explore any further than that. They kept adding more and more medication to my regime but never took any away unless they absolutely had to. In Birmingham, Dr Wilde stopped all medication so that I could be properly assessed.

When I returned from hospital, there was a letter waiting for me from the Royal Free. It told me that I had been exposed to vCJD (the human form of mad cow disease) because I had received treatment made from the blood of someone who'd died from it. Those infected blood products just kept on giving...

How do you prepare to die? We sold my car, and Mum sorted out my paperwork, but all I really wanted to do was to escape reality by watching telly. I contacted the Macfarlane Trust to see if I could have Sky TV installed, but they told me it was a luxury item, so Mum paid for it. In the meantime, I was being monitored by the hospital, and the regular MRIs finally revealed something miraculous: the lesion was not doing what they said it would. It was not slowly invading my brain, and it was not advancing.

The lesion had not spread.

The QEH was brilliant. I was put under the care of a neurologist who tested me for epilepsy and added some different meds. All of a sudden, everything stabilised, and I was able to use my arm again. It was as if someone had flipped a switch; I felt so much better. After being signed off sick from work for months, I was slowly growing stronger.

By this point, a huge bright light had come into my life. His name was Mark Simmons; he was a social worker connected to the QEH haemophilia unit. He was also gay.

Mark was a real activist and was very proactive in trying to bring about change for our community. He actually went to New York to help out when the AIDS crisis first hit, and he was so clued up about everything related to it. I was totally in awe of him. Mark was able to educate me in a way that doctors had never been able to. He awakened my rebellious side, and I started to fight a little bit more—questioning what the doctors were telling me. Mark also gave me some important practical assistance because he helped me apply for the benefits I was entitled to. 'Even if you die, you've lost nothing,' he said as he sat in my living room. 'Even if you only get fifty pence, it can open doors to get you extra help.' So we applied, and I did receive benefits—just not the right ones. (It would take years and much battling on my part before the DWP corrected their mistake.) Mark also managed to get me a Motability car—because I was able to drive again, having been cleared for epilepsy.

Now that I was feeling so much better, I was desperate to get back to some sort of normality, and I returned to work.

It felt so wonderful to be in the airport after everything that had happened. It gave me a rush of happiness just to hear the noise of the terminal, the flight announcements, and the rumble of the planes. I was home; I was back to life. But my happiness was not to last.

One day at the beginning of 2003, I was checking in a lady; I had just asked her to put her bag on the belt when suddenly I felt very strange and everything around me seemed very indistinct and distant. I heard the lady asking me if I was drunk, then everything went black and I collapsed.

I woke up to find the paramedics all around me. One of them told me I was a lucky man. 'When you fell, you went sideways. Had you gone backwards, you would have fallen on the main luggage belt and been torn apart.' Despite my lucky escape, I felt as if my life were ending. I went to hospital in an ambulance—it was full blues and twos. They weren't too sure what was happening but believed it was something to do with my lesion. I was having spasms in my hand that I couldn't control, and it seemed that my brain was having a crisis.

As I lay in my hospital bed, connected to life support, who should appear but my boss. She was not there to enquire after my health. The purpose of her visit was to fire me on the spot. 'When you go home, call me and I'll come and pick up your uniform so you don't have to trek back in,' she smiled. She genuinely believed she was being helpful.

I was allowed home after a few days; the wonderful Kevin and Wayne had been looking after the animals. When it was clear I would need to go back into hospital, I asked my parents to come and take the boys for me. My dad needed some persuading from Mum, but they finally turned up. Dad refused to come in and eat the food I'd made for them; he just wanted to take the animals and go. I couldn't believe his attitude. *This was cold, even for my dad.* 'What if I die?' I asked him, 'I won't see you again.' But he just told me to bring the boys out so he could get off and avoid the traffic. I suppose this was his way of dealing with feelings he couldn't cope with. But I was so enraged, I threw a punch at him—for the first and last time. He punched me in the ribs, got in the car and drove off—abandoning Mum and me, his dying son.

We didn't speak for five years.

Something changed in Mum that day: it was like she was taking control of her own destiny. She stayed and with a little help from my friends, she looked after the animals and the house, while I was in hospital nursing a cracked rib. When I came out, I was feeling very shitty, and my arm was spasming uncontrollably. Mum would wrap a bandage round it and tie the bandage round my waist to keep my arm down. She had to do everything for me, from cutting up my food to dressing me. I was at a very low ebb, and life seemed to have lost its lustre.

The fight had just gone out of me.

My lowest point came after Mum had gone home because she had to work. After struggling on for a few weeks, I went to my garage and got a rope. I'd had enough. I felt as if I had lost everything and I was going to die anyway, so why prolong the pain?

As I stood on a chair, preparing to hang myself, I looked down, and there were my boys: Simba, Ghost and Trojan sitting, looking at me with their steady, trusting eyes. I didn't care about myself, but I cared about them. Where would they go if I died? It wasn't the first time that I had felt as if my beloved dog, and my beloved cats made life worth living.

There was no way I could leave them.

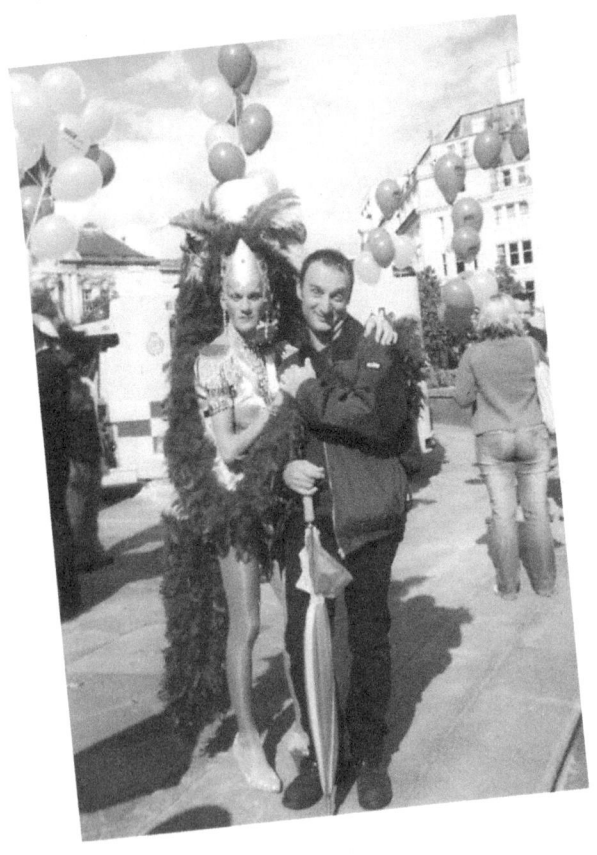

Birmingham Gay Pride 2003—Richard with umbrella at the ready

HIGH ON A HILL
WAS A LONELY GOATHERD

In the summer of 2002, my world shattered when I learned the truth about my HIV status and how I had been infected. Driving my new car, I went to a weekend organised by the Macfarlane Trust, where HIV-infected haemophiliacs and their partners could talk and share information. I met some brilliant people and some very sick people, too; I wasn't expecting the bombshell that was dropped on me that day.

Up until this point, I had always thought that becoming infected with HIV was a terrible accident. But I was told that this was not the case: the pharmaceutical companies and medics had knowledge of these pathogens in the blood products before they gave them to us. Had they tried to do anything to make the products safer, it would have cut down on profits, so they didn't. They were harvesting blood from skid row donors, and it was going straight into the veins of haemophiliacs. We were used for research and weren't protected. Had they put any kind of safety measures in place, then we would not have been infected with AIDS.

It needn't have happened. That's the terrible, unvarnished truth. In the instant I heard this, I went from being a survivor to being a victim.

The only way I can describe how I felt is that it was like

being punched in the face and told that my mum wasn't my mum. Everything you have built your world around is a lie: I was suddenly standing on shifting sand; nothing seemed secure or safe. I just didn't know who or what to believe.

I eventually found out from my medical notes that the Royal Free believed I seroconverted in '82 because that's when most HIV infections took place. I firmly believe it happened when I had my thirteen teeth taken out. As I woke up from the op, something in my care had shifted. Nursing protocol had changed. I was no longer in a normal bed, but in a bed with barriers; I had been put in isolation; the staff were masked and gloved. Why? They must have known that I had been put at risk. And no one had stopped it from happening.

I began to question everything.

Looking back, I wondered if my knee op had simply been research: they knew my HIV status; they knew all about AIDS and the danger I was in, but they did the operation anyway. If I had the choice of getting AIDS and dying, or being in a wheelchair, I would choose the wheelchair. But that choice was taken away from me. I was dying because of what they had done to me.

I struggled with this knowledge for a while, not knowing which way was up, thinking I was going mad. But when I spoke to Mark Simmons about it, he was so understanding and supportive. He did everything in his power to help. That's why he is so beloved within the haemophilia community. He's been a shining light in *my* life, certainly.

Then my body gave me a slap around the face and I was forced to focus: I was rushed to hospital in agony and diagnosed with a kidney stone. It was caused by the HIV medications; once again, my life had been put on the line.

In April 2003, I met another man who was going to light up my life in the most profound way. After recovering from the kidney stone, I went to Gran Canaria with my friend Brian, who had never been before. After all the upset, I was in the mood to just switch off and have fun.

One night, after Brian had been stood up by an Irish guy he'd really liked, I took him to Centre Stage to cheer him up. This was a horseshoe-shaped bar, run by a lovely man called Ralph. He would play clips of musicals on a huge telly, and had an even bigger box of props; everyone in the bar would get dressed up as a character from whichever musical was playing. For example, when Maria gets married in *The Sound of Music*, someone would put on a veil—and then the veil would snake around the bar, until we all had stood beneath it. Of course, we sang along; it was gloriously camp, and great fun.

On this particular night, I was in my element: dressed in a pink bonnet, playing a tambourine, with a cigarette hanging out of my gob and belting at the top of my voice, 'High on a hill was a lonely goatherd.' A class act. Then, as I turned to look down the bar, everyone just seemed to sit back, like in a movie, to reveal this person standing at the opposite end of the bar, under a light. He was laughing his head off. So, class act that I am, I shouted down the bar in my best fishwife's voice, 'Ere, what are you laughing at?'

With that, he came up to me. He looked lovely, and when he put his hand on my back, I swear I felt an electric shock coursing through my whole body. I asked him again what he was laughing at. He just looked at my bonnet and back at me, and then we both burst into laughter.

I already knew, in that moment, that this was someone special.

He told me his name was Richard, and he asked me if I wanted to go outside so we could hear ourselves talk. I will never forget that night, with the low cloud making the surrounding mountains glow yellow. There was something extraordinary in the air, and as we talked, I just opened up my heart to this handsome, kind-eyed stranger. I told Richard everything about my history, about my blood disorder—the whole story. When I had finished, I said he could go running for the hills if he felt like it—he wouldn't be the first. But he didn't run. Instead, Richard kissed me on the lips and said, 'Do you want another drink?'

We talked all night and then went on to the King's Club, where what song should play but Kylie's 'Love at First Sight'. When I listened to the words, it was as if every one of them was being sung to me. Richard and I danced to Kylie that night, 30th April 2003—and that song became our song. I did fall in love with him, and I've loved him a little more every day ever since. We saw one another every evening in Gran Canaria, and I was like a besotted schoolgirl on the last day of my holiday when Richard came to wave us off on the coach.

But I wasn't heartbroken; I knew I was going to be seeing him again.

Back home, I was very involved in Birmingham Pride. Since being fired from the airport job, I had been volunteering with Terrence Higgins Trust and working with a lovely man called Matt. His area of expertise was men's sexual health, and together we worked on our entry into Pride. The theme that year was fantasy, which was right up my street. I came up with a suitably fantastical concept, including silver and purple outfits, unicorns—and not forgetting the Las Vegas showgirls. Richard travelled up from Brighton for it, and I remember being so touched that he walked beside me, and when it threatened to rain on our parade, he held an umbrella over me so that my feathers didn't get damaged.

A man who looks after your feathers is a keeper. Mum thought so, too. She also took part in the march that year, and that's how she met Richard.

I can't describe how much it meant to me to have them both there, walking with me at an event that was so close to my heart. They hit it off straight away, as I knew they would. My mum could see how happy I was: I had emerged from feeling I would die alone and found my joy again. Meeting Richard gave me back my fire: I had a reason to fight, a reason to live.

Then in August that year, I was reminded of how prejudice is never too far away. I went to Jamaica because Brian's mum, Della was getting married out there and I was giving her away. As soon as we arrived, the hostility was palpable; it centred around Brian and me being gay. We would go to a bar and the staff would take great pains to ignore us. People were verbally abusive, and we were even spat at—it was just horrific. If it hadn't been for the wedding, I would have come straight back home. I was glad I was there for Della, and the wedding was lovely, but I will never set foot in Jamaica again. I've been subjected to homophobic abuse on the streets of London, but it was so much worse there—and so constant. It really brought home to me how terrifying it is for many people in the world who can't be themselves.

With Richard, I could wholly be myself, and our love deepened as time went on. With Richard in Brighton and me in Birmingham, it was a long-distance relationship for a while. I had a lovely lodger, Steve, who would look after the animals when I went down south to stay with Richard; having such fabulous friends allowed our relationship to flourish.

As I learnt more about the scale of abuse of contaminated blood products, I had been looking for support from Terrence Higgins Trust—would they help us raise the issue to get answers and justice? But each time I asked, they rebuffed my questions and kept quoting the government line of 'it was an accident'. They even refused to look at some of the documents I had been given. When the office manager called me in and asked me 'not to volunteer as much', it was that extra push we needed.

Richard and I knew we eventually wanted to live together; with Richard in full-time employment and me not working because of my health, it was easier for me to sell my house rather than him sell his flat. So that's what I did. I moved into Richard's Brighton flat in March 2004. The dream was to make a home together, so we started property hunting straight away and found a house just outside Brighton, which we moved into in July.

Now I was living in the South East again, I transferred my care back to the Royal Free: better the devil you know, as Kylie might say; how wrong that proved to be.

Three weeks later, my Nana Ward unexpectedly died. The last of my grandparents was gone. Sadly she didn't get to meet Richard or see our happiness. It really felt as if I'd stepped into a brand-new life. It was wonderful to feel so accepted and so cherished for who I am. He is a truly remarkable man. I finally had some stability, and it felt fantastic. I began to take such joy in simple, everyday things—things that other people might take for granted, such as walking Simba to Brighton pier and back. Suddenly I had my little ready-made family—me and Richard and the boys—and that's how I would sign our Christmas cards.

But as always, my health threatened to pop this bubble of

bliss. My left knee—the one they operated on back in 1984—eventually started playing up again. One day, I was at the beach with Simba, throwing stones so he could chase them, when my leg just gave way. So there I was, stuck on a deserted beach unable to move.

Loyal Simba, who'd been my whole world until I met Richard, stayed with me, and as I crawled my way to the car, he kept me safe, kept circling. I made it home, and a hospital appointment revealed that I needed a total knee replacement. I couldn't afford to fall again, knowing that a bang on the head could be fatal for me. So in January 2005, I had the operation.

It wasn't straightforward: my temperature kept going through the roof. After many tests, it was discovered that I had become resistant to the HIV medication. So they stopped everything for twelve weeks and for a while I felt fantastic, but then they found that my kidneys were severely damaged. My right kidney only functions at sixteen per cent and my left at twenty-three per cent, so I was effectively living in renal failure. This caused me and Mum a great deal of anxiety because Grandad Banham had died from renal failure back in 1977. It had been caused by my medication. And if that wasn't enough, they told me the hepatitis C had caused cirrhosis of the liver. I was also told my highly toxic HIV medication had to be changed due to its impact on my liver and that I needed to be scanned every three months for liver cancer.

Yet again, I seemed to be beating the odds on survival. But with Richard by my side, I now knew there was a life worth fighting for.

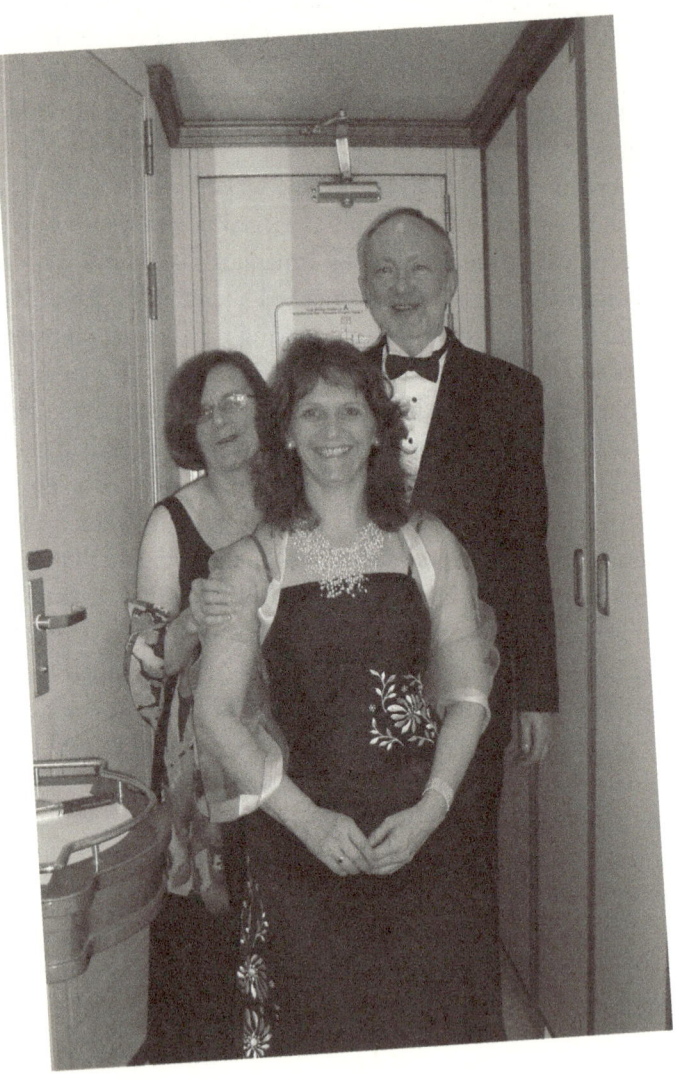

Rose, Louise & Chris—aboard the Sea Princess

ON THE CAMPAIGN TRAIL

After my knee operation in 2005, I was given another regime of medication, which my body seemed to accept. They told me the knee replacement would probably do me for ten years, but that was over twenty years ago, and it has carried me around the world.

Long may it continue to.

At the same time as I was enjoying a period of relative calm health-wise, I was becoming more and more aware of the lies and deceit that many haemophiliacs had been subjected to through the infected blood scandal. As the community stood together and swapped information, I was increasingly shocked by what I discovered. The more I read and investigated, the more questions were raised. The main one was, *how did they let this happen?* Warnings about the treatment had been given by the World Health Organisation and they were ignored. Lives could have been saved, and my multiple infections, which now run into double figures, could have been avoided. I can't begin to describe the range of emotions I have felt over the years as I continue to watch friends die. I have now spent most of my life in a constant grieving cycle. It was time for this deep wrong to be addressed and acknowledged.

We wanted answers.

In 2006, I was asked to join the newly formed campaign group Tainted Blood alongside brothers Gareth and Haydn Lewis, from Cardiff, and their friends Andrew Evans and Sue Threakall.

The aim of the group was to fight for a public enquiry into infected blood so that truth and justice would be served and compensation could be paid in recognition of the real suffering inflicted upon truly vulnerable people. From that moment, my life took another twist because as soon as you raise your head above the parapet and start asking questions, you suddenly have another huge target on your back. But whilst labelled a troublemaker by some, I made friendships with so many more I genuinely love.

We were looking for answers, and we were not going to rest until, one way or another, we found them. Our campaigning wasn't based upon rumour either—it was based on real documents and hard evidence which supported our case that those in charge were aware of the danger they were putting us in. I was shocked to discover that as early as 1974, when little boys were dying, there were already warnings about the blood products' safety. I also discovered that the cryo treatment I had originally been given had not actually been phased out, as the hospital had told me. It is still being used today. So they needn't have swapped me onto Factor 8 in the middle of the night, and I might have potentially been spared AIDS and everything that went along with it.

I was still under the Royal Free, who really didn't like me asking awkward questions. If I asked a direct question, it was often met with a lie or the sort of standard answer that didn't really mean anything. In the waiting room, there seemed to be a concerted effort to keep HIV haemophiliacs apart.

Because of my campaigning work, people would often recognise me from social media, so we might get chatting, only for a nurse to appear and ask one of us if we might prefer to wait in a side room. They didn't want anyone to overhear anything that might pull aside their veil of secrecy and reveal what was really going on.

Each time I visited, I recognised lots of the staff from all the years I had been under the hospital's care, including the nurse who told my parents I was HIV positive. She was now in an admin job and was really friendly to me, always asking how I was—the same stone-faced woman who had delivered my devastating HIV status in such a callous, casual fashion. I was never going to forgive and forget that.

I don't want it to sound as though I was against all the staff at the Royal Free; there were some people I really did like, but it was very hard to like the ones who treated you as if you were unworthy of human kindness, or who seemed to feel it was their duty to constantly forecast your imminent death.

Despite our commitment to exposing the truth about infected blood, taking on the establishment is always an uphill battle that requires all one's energy and fight. In 2006, we discovered that an attempt to take on an American pharmaceutical company had failed. There had been a lot of hope pinned on this effort because it held the promise of huge sums of compensation, so it was a big blow for all concerned.

For me, it was never about the money. I knew that financial compensation was the only fair way to show recognition for the suffering caused, but the money couldn't give me what I had lost. It couldn't un-infect me, and it couldn't take away all those years of fear and suffering. For me, it was always about exposing the truth and getting justice for all those lost little boys who had died unnecessarily. In order to stop the litigation, the Americans had simply changed the law. So they were literally being allowed to get away with murder, despite knowingly sending haemophiliacs for treatment that would infect them. If you can simply change the law when it doesn't suit you, where is the justice? Is there justice?

It felt as though the rug had been pulled from under us, and all the momentum was lost. I took it very hard, and all of a sudden, it came to a head for me. I feared I was on the verge of a breakdown. When I get lost in my own dark thoughts, I know I am capable of some very self-destructive emotions—including the feeling that perhaps everyone would be better off without me. And when I do go to that place, even Richard struggles to bring me back from it.

Richard was, of course, brilliant. When my doctor failed to help me see a counsellor, Richard took me to the Royal Sussex in Brighton. We sat there for hours, only to eventually be told that the psychiatric team weren't even in the hospital that day. So we went home. The following day, I saw a lovely registrar at the Royal Free, who reassured me that he would get it sorted. But once again, I was told there was no counselling help available.

In the end, I contacted Body Positive, an AIDS and HIV support group in Brighton, and through them, I saw a volunteer counsellor called Lynne. The minute I started talking to Lynne, I felt a strong connection to her. She is a very special person, and she totally got me—all of me. I knew I could really let go with her; I could tell her my deepest, darkest secrets without fear of judgement. She has helped me get over some of my trust issues and given me coping mechanisms that I use constantly. She is still my counsellor to this day, and I don't know how I would have coped without her.

After speaking with Lynne, I began to feel able to fight on with our campaign. My campaigning had also made me aware that time is precious: every ninety-six hours, a victim of contaminated blood dies. It's a dwindling community, so every death touches your heart and brings your own death that bit closer.

Richard and I decided that we were going to make the most of whatever time we had left together, to fill it with fantastic experiences, to travel and see as much of the world as we possibly could. Once again, I was choosing to live rather than waiting to die.

In 2004, I was introduced to Richard's mum and stepdad, Rose and Chris, as well as his sister, Louise. We hit it off straight away. Richard's mum was a beautiful lady but sadly, she was diagnosed with MSA in 2006, a rare condition of the nervous system that eventually shuts down the body. After her terminal diagnosis, they moved to Durham, so Richard and I were going up and down the motorway to spend as much time with them as possible. And I arranged a family cruise to the Caribbean in January 2007.

We talked about lovely things we would like to do for his mum to create some wonderful memories, and that's when I had what I thought was a brainwave. Why didn't Richard and I have a civil partnership in Durham—a small exclusive do, so his mum could be part of it? When I put forward my bright idea to Richard, he looked terrified—like a rabbit caught in the headlights. I thought to myself, *Oh, what have I done? Have I messed everything up by pushing Richard too hard?*

I vowed that I would never mention marriage again.

By this time, I was in touch with my own dad. I was sitting in the conservatory one afternoon, doing a puzzle, when the phone rang. He said, 'Mark, it's Dad.' I didn't know what to say—*did I want him back in my life after five years?* But I thought of the pain our separation was causing Mum, so I replied, 'Oh hello Dad, how are you?' And we spoke for a while, then over the next few months, we spoke a little more. And then, when Richard and I were going away for a few days, Mum suggested they come down to look after the boys for us. She said Dad was itching to see the house, and to meet Richard. So come they did! We had two days together before Richard and I flew off. And when we got back, it was like the past five years hadn't happened—we were a family again.

In the meantime, the infected blood campaign had stepped up. Tainted Blood joined in a collective campaign across the country, and in 2007, an independent public enquiry was announced. Chaired by Lord Archer of Sandwell, it was not the full judicial enquiry that we had been calling for because it wouldn't have the same powers, but it was a great start. They couldn't compel witnesses to come forward, but plenty did anyway, and at last, victims had an opportunity to be heard.

I became more and more deeply involved, making frequent trips to parliament, having meetings and helping to write documents to further the cause. One of our allies in all of this was Lord Morris of Manchester, who was president of the Haemophilia Society. He was the most wonderful man and a great character, with no airs and graces. I remember laughing and joking with him about very ordinary, human things. He told us to call him Alf, but that always felt a bit wrong to me, a bit too familiar. Lord Morris always treated us with such kindness and respect, and he taught me so much about how to be a gentleman. He was a great support to us, and I am proud to have called him my friend.

My relationship with the medical profession, meanwhile,

continued to be problematic. In 2007, I was seeing a consultant for my worsening stomach problems and I was asked what treatment I had taken for my hepatitis C. When I replied, 'None,' the doctor said, 'Oh, I suppose it disappeared all by itself, did it?'

Tests revealed that it had indeed disappeared, and after that, everyone at the hospital refused to talk to me about hepatitis C. To this day, no one has explained to me why or how I managed to be virus-free after being chronically infected for so long, nor why the hospital had tried to force Interferon on me when I appeared to have cleared the virus. It's another one of those medical mysteries that the hospital decided I didn't need to know about.

Is it any wonder I have trust issues?

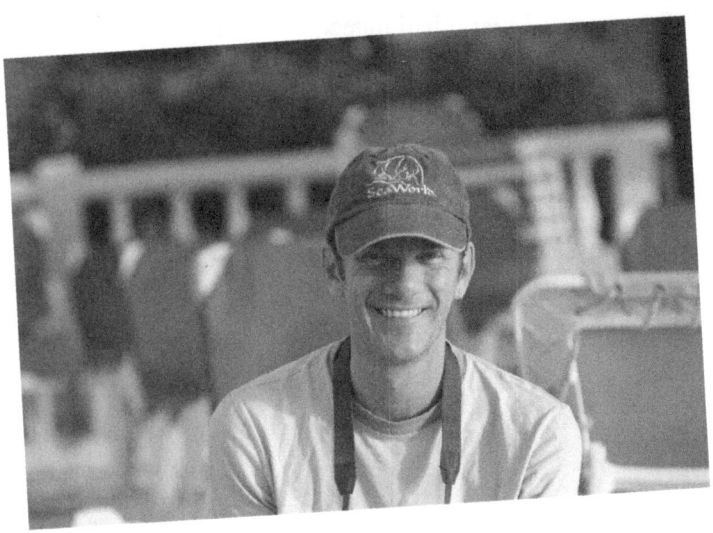

Caribbean Queen

FIGHTING ON

As a gay haemophiliac, I was used to prejudice and false assumptions being made about me: I was HIV+ because of my lifestyle; I was gay because I had been given the blood of gay men; I was different, other, and therefore not 'normal'. You had to cope with this as best you could, but people's thoughtless assumptions could still knock my legs out from under me.

I have always been skinny and had a twenty-six inch waist right up until I was forty. This meant that I was usually a boys' size in clothes. I couldn't get adult trousers to fit me, and my underwear choices were reduced to Spiderman or Batman pants. It drove me mad. I would see something lovely in a shop window, only to find out that the waist size started at thirty inches. One day when I was in my late thirties, I was in a clothes shop in Brighton. I was particularly small at that point because I had lost weight due to illness. So I was in the boys' department looking at jeans, and the underwear beside them. As I browsed, I could feel someone lurking and when I moved away, he followed me. I turned to see who was taking such an interest, and I saw it was the security guard. I thought, *maybe he thinks I'm trying to steal something?* So I picked up a pair of jeans, took them to the counter and asked the shop assistant if I could try them on. She said I couldn't. When I asked why, she replied, 'You've got to go downstairs because people like you aren't allowed in changing rooms near children.'

People. Like. You.

For a second, I was absolutely gobsmacked. Then rage took over, and I flew down the stairs, demanding to speak to the manager. I wiped the floor with him. 'How dare they speak to me like that?' I raged. 'I have a terminal illness, and I have been made to feel like a paedophile. Is that what I look like? A paedophile?' The manager went scarlet. I threw the jeans at him and with a 'you can stick these up your arse!' I stormed out.

Then I burst into tears.

If that wasn't enough, in January 2008 we went with my parents on a cruise in the Caribbean. The itinerary changed and we docked in St Thomas, US Virgin Islands. I was called to the purser's desk, where I was faced by two police officers who took me off the ship, placed me in the back of a police car and took me to the local police station. At that time it was still illegal for HIV+ people to enter the United States. I explained what had happened regarding my infection and was taken back to be placed on the ship as it prepared to depart. I felt like a criminal being punished. Richard, Mum and Dad had been frantic because I'd just disappeared.

Later that year, because of the credit crunch, Richard was made redundant, which gave him the push to go freelance and be his own boss—something he'd wanted to do for a while. His work, which involves big radio broadcasting events, tends to be seasonal, so he works manically throughout the summer, and then it all stops over the winter. That's when we go away to nice warm places to recharge our batteries.

In 2009, not only was I was honoured to represent the haemophilia community—as secretary of Tainted Blood—in the unveiling ceremony of the AIDS memorial in Brighton, but I also turned forty

I never expected to celebrate this milestone birthday, so I booked us on a cruise that travelled from Sydney, up the east coast of Australia, and through Indonesia to Bangkok. It was sixteen nights in all, a wonderful adventure, and with my BA staff travel, not a small fortune. But of course, the downside to staff travel was that you were never guaranteed a seat on any flight; you just hoped there were spaces on the day. It's like a warped version of the *Strictly Come Dancing* results show—you *want* your name to be called out. We had planned to fly to Bangkok to have some suits made, and then we'd fly to Sydney to pick up the cruise. But when we got to Heathrow, the check-in lady told us there were no seats: she recommended that we come back the following day but advised us to go straight through to Sydney. The next day, we left Heathrow in January snow, managing by the skin of our teeth, to get one of the last flights out before the UK was shut down by a massive snowstorm. We flew to Hong Kong and then spent about twelve hours running around trying to get on a flight list for Sydney. Finally, we got seats on a Qantas flight that left at midnight but were told we'd have to run to catch it. So there we were, running hell for leather, me with my dodgy ankle and both of us sweating like a glassblower's backside. We made it in time, only to sit on the tarmac for an hour because of a technical fault.

Still, it gave our hearts a bit of time to calm down.

We had five lovely days in Sydney and then boarded the ship for our cruise. Our last Australian stop was in Darwin, where we gave all of our remaining dollars to the Red Cross to help those affected by the fires that were blazing there.

We had an absolutely amazing time, not least because a group of older gay men took a shine to us and kept inviting us to cocktail parties. Richard and I were thrilled when one of the gentlemen, called Walter, told us he was one of the original Von Trapp boys in *The Sound of Music*. He took us under his wing on the cruise, and over dinner one night, we told him all about how Richard and I had got together, and the part that *The Sound of Music* had played in our meeting. As we were sailing to Singapore, Walter asked if he could take us out to tea once we got there, and we readily agreed.

We had no idea that he was taking us to Raffles! Unfortunately, there had been a downpour, so we sat there looking like drowned rats. Nevertheless we had the most wonderful high tea, all served with white gloves. Walter seemed really grateful for our time, which was so touching, and he, in turn, was touched by the Raffles cufflinks we bought him so he would always think of our time together when he wore them.

It had been the most extraordinary trip, and I couldn't imagine a better way to celebrate the forty years I had been alive.

In early summer that year, I was in the garden dead-heading the fuchsias when I felt my left ankle snap as I stood up to get a drink. I crawled inside and had an injection, and the following day, I went to hospital. The doctor I saw in the haemophilia centre just played it down. She said that if it was broken, I wouldn't be able to walk. But I was forty years old and understood my own body. I knew I had heard and felt my ankle snap. So I went to A&E to have it X-rayed, which revealed that my ankle had collapsed.

I needed an operation, so in May, I returned to the Royal Free—where the nurse in charge of our ward gave me the same feeling I had experienced in Jamaica. He clearly didn't like the fact that I was openly gay, and he was very rude and dismissive towards me. The same attitude seemed to pervade all the team

BLEEDING Fabulous

there, and I woke up from the operation to this couldn't-care-less atmosphere.

It's awful to feel ignored and unvalued at the very time when we need kindness and care. Before long, I started to feel unwell. I had stopped my HIV meds three days before the surgery because they can cause bleeding, but I was beginning to be concerned that it was now six days since I had taken any meds. When I flagged this up to the unfriendly nurse, adding that I thought I had a temperature, he told me that I was a very nice man but that I was an attention seeker. I asked him if he knew what was wrong with me, explaining about my AIDS medication and that without it, my viral load would be building up, which was not a good thing. I asked him to call the HIV team, but he didn't. So I called Richard in tears, and he arranged for an HIV consultant to come and see me, with the hostile nurse glaring in the background. The doctor put me back on the medication and checked my bloods and viral load. Why had it been such a battle to get the treatment I needed?

When I went for an X-ray, I saw with horror that the board at the nurses' station had a red star above my name and, in big letters, 'AT RISK FROM VCJD' so the whole world could see that I was a health risk. On the one hand, the hospital was playing down my viral contamination, and on the other, they were flagging it up for everyone to see. When the consultant came to see me, I told him about the nurses' board. I asked him why there was a big warning there for everyone to read. They didn't even know for sure that I was positive because there was no test for vCJD. (Despite Tainted Blood campaigning hard for a vCJD test, the government refused to fund it.) The consultant said he would look into it. Well, I wasn't going to hold my breath—I was determined to follow this up myself, so

I called Sue at Tainted Blood to see what could be done. Surely, this was a breach of data protection? Sue contacted a solicitor friend, who told me I needed to make a formal complaint and report it to the Data Protection Office. Which I did.

I stayed in that ward for two weeks, and it was a horrible experience. I was vulnerable and helpless, and I was being treated with utter contempt. All I could do was lie there and take it. To add insult to injury, my ankle never fused properly after that operation.

Following a fortnight from hell in the Royal Free, I couldn't wait to get back to Richard and the boys. But that also turned into a bit of a nightmare…

Two weeks after arriving home on crutches, I discovered we had a serious leak in the bathroom wall. We turned all the water off, but further investigation revealed that it had gone under the wall in the living room—as the bricks soaked up the moisture, mould started to appear. The insurance people said that the whole place had to be gutted in order to dry it out. So Richard and I moved out of our house and into a flat in the marina while the workmen moved in.

My parents agreed to take the boys, but then Trojan became very ill. We took him to our vet, and we received the worst possible news. Devastated, we buried our boy in the garden at home before going back to the marina in the driving snow. Was there anything more that could be thrown at us? We finally moved back into our house on 23rd December. My parents spent Christmas with us that year. It was a sad one without our handsome Trojan.

While all this was going on, the Archer Report that we had been waiting for finally came out. Although it was very powerful in what it said, Lord Archer couldn't recommend that the victims receive any compensation. But all was not lost. Our great ally Lord Morris took the report and turned it into a bill in order to get it passed through parliament.

And so the fight would continue.

With the help of Mark Simmons, I had also been doing battle with the Department for Work and Pensions for seven years because they weren't giving me the payment I was entitled to. I didn't like being on benefits; it was yet another stigma I had to deal with. And it wasn't that I didn't want to work: I physically couldn't do it any longer. Having to fight with this cold, faceless institution felt like an insult. I only wanted what was fair and just. I began to despair that it would never be sorted until, in 2010, our MP Simon Kirby got involved.

Richard and I went to see him in his parliamentary chamber about a couple of issues, including my ongoing battle with the DWP. Through the data protection officer, I managed to get hold of my telephone calls to the department—which included someone asking me if I really had AIDS or if it was just HIV—and I sent them to Simon Kirby so he could hear for himself the contemptuous way I had been spoken to. Once Simon got involved, I was finally placed on the right benefit and given a twenty thousand pound back payment. It was wonderful to finally stop living in fear of poverty—dreading those brown envelopes demanding more information and threatening to take away the little money I was receiving.

Then six months later, they made me apply for my benefits all over again, so all that effort had been a complete waste of time. But there was a silver lining, at that time—another special person, Nicola, came into our lives and a fabulous friendship began. I gave some advice to her little boy with mild haemophilia on a coping mechanism I had used when I had a nosebleed and it changed their lives completely.

Meanwhile, Tainted Blood's campaign took a knock when the law changed and we lost our right to legal aid, which we knew would limit our activities substantially. However, where there's a will, there is most certainly a way, and after redoubling our efforts, we secured an important victory in our fight for justice when, in 2010, we won a judicial review. One of our talented Tainted Blood colleagues was the major instigator of this review, which aimed to address the government response to Lord Archer's independent report on NHS supplied contaminated blood and blood products.

It was wonderful that Haydn Lewis got to see this victory just before he died. Like his brother Gareth, who was also part of Tainted Blood, Haydn had been infected with HIV and hepatitis C from contaminated products. Despite becoming very ill, he was there with us in the high court, a dying man still fighting for justice and truth with his last breath. I called him Superman and loved him to bits; I feel I am a better person for having known Haydn. He was such an inspiration, so softly spoken, with a wonderful Welsh accent. The day of his funeral in Cardiff coincided with the funeral in Brighton of Richard's friend Roland. We weren't going to miss either and managed to get to both.

As we tried to pick up the pieces following Haydn's death, Tainted Blood lurched a little. He had been one of our main players, and we felt his loss enormously. But there was still his brother Gareth. A big, loud, rugby-playing alpha male, Gareth was like chalk to Haydn's cheese. They couldn't have been more different, but they both had massive hearts and a fighting spirit. Gareth and I had a great relationship and really respected one another. We also had great fun together. I remember him saying, one night, 'I know Mark's a poof, but I do love him.' I loved him right back.

Sadly, Gareth died in 2010—six months after his brother. The last time I spoke to him was over the phone. We had been discussing the wider Tainted Blood campaign when Gareth said, 'You'll have to do the talking now, I'm in a Little Chef.' Without even thinking, I replied, 'Oh, do I know him?' This was followed by loud guffaws and expletives from Gareth's end. 'You bastard, I nearly choked to death!' he roared. Not long after that, he flew to Spain, and two days later, we received a call saying that he'd died.

We don't know the details, but it was thought he fell over a coffee table and banged his head, which gave him an intercranial bleed that proved fatal. It was a terrible shock and yet another devastating loss. The Macfarlane Trust, which had been set up to help support our community, refused to pay to bring his body home, so his family had to have him cremated in order to get him back. I spoke at his memorial service and told the story of our last conversation. Everybody laughed, which I'm sure Gareth would have loved. It was such a lovely memory to have, but his passing hit me hard.

That November, Richard and I were on holiday in the Caribbean. We were on the beach on World AIDS Day, a date that always makes me reflective. I had taken myself away for a solitary paddle in the sea; when I looked up at the clear blue sky, out of nowhere, a lone cloud appeared in the shape of a giant G. Richard saw it, too. I like to think it was a sign from the universe, almost as though Gareth had popped down and said to me, 'I'm still with you.'

After losing Haydn and Gareth, Tainted Blood lost its way somewhat, until another amazing man stepped into our lives.

Mike Dorricott was such an intelligent, fearless man, who fought hard and tirelessly for our campaign. He had mild haemophilia and underwent two liver transplants, but he never let this stop him from taking on the British government. Everything he did was with such commitment and integrity. It didn't surprise me that he won gold at the World Transplant Games.

Mike's MP was Jeremy Hunt, who was Secretary of State for Health, so Mike was able to see him and bring to his attention all the issues we were fighting for. Jeremy promised all sorts but never delivered, and then Mike died on Richard's birthday in 2015.

Another great man gone too soon—but *he* never let us down.

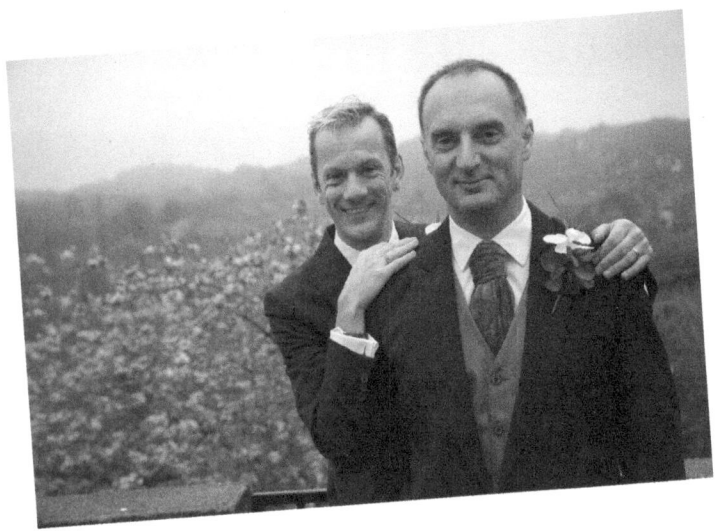

Springtime in Durham—an almost perfect wedding day

PIRATES AND
POPPING THE QUESTION

In 2011, Richard and I booked a Royal Caribbean Cruise, little knowing that it would be filled with thrills that weren't on the itinerary. The cruise was travelling around Oman at the time when Osama Bin Laden was captured, and because of security worries, many passengers had cancelled. So the cruise company had phoned around all their Diamond loyalty scheme members just to put bums on seats (or customers in cabins). As a result, the cruise was only half full, which was brilliant, and there were all these interesting characters, including a senior porn star called Thomas.

To add to the excitement, there was extra security on board because of the prevalence of pirates along our route, and we faced certain restrictions, such as reduced lighting at night-time. We also had to take part in a drill, so we knew what to do in the event of a pirate attack, which it's fair to say, I didn't take too seriously. There was one young officer looking a bit lost, and I said to him, 'Tell me, what does one wear if attacked by pirates? I don't think I have the right outfit for that.' Thankfully, he saw the funny side. For some reason, all these extra measures didn't frighten me at all. In fact, I found it all quite thrilling—especially the hunky security men who were there to protect us. I remember sitting in the pool, listening to Kylie and looking up to see four soldiers jogging round the running track in tiny shorts.

I should be so lucky, indeed.

One day, the captain came on the PA and told us we would be sailing at full speed for the next part of the cruise because we had a military escort. Sure enough, there was an Iranian and a British warship keeping us company. Behind us was an American ship, which we discovered had some very important cargo—the body of Osama Bin Laden. They were rushing us through so that the unloading could take place. And there we were, right in thick of it!

To take our minds off the dramatic events unfolding nearby, a belly flop competition was announced, in which the military took on civilians. I'm proud to say we civvies won, thanks to a late entry from a big guy called Baz, whose belly was perfect for the job! It was all good fun and slightly surreal. And if that weren't over-excitement enough, we also had a medical emergency on board, which meant we had to stop at the entrance to the Suez Canal, where Mossad had a very conspicuous presence.

One way or another, it was an unforgettable trip and lifelong friendships were made.

Then in the September of that year, we had another trip that was unforgettable for a very different reason. Richard and I were in Singapore, watching the Formula One Grand Prix. Although I generally have no interest in sport, I had really got into racing because Richard loves it, and so it was a complete thrill for us to be there to experience it first-hand. After watching the qualifier on the Friday, we were sitting in a restaurant on the Saturday when Richard suddenly said, out of the blue, 'So, if we were to have a civil partnership, you were thinking of a small ceremony up in Durham?'

I nearly fell off my chair. 'Yes…' My face must have been a

picture. After Richard's shocked reaction when I had mentioned the subject before, I had never brought it up again.

'Okay, then,' said Richard.

'Have you just proposed?' I asked.

'Yeah, I suppose I have.'

As soon as we got back to the UK, we drove to Durham to tell Rose and Chris the good news in person. 'It's not a shotgun wedding, is it?' joked Chris, who was always able to make us all laugh. They were delighted for us, and it felt good to be able to give Rose something to look forward to.

We took Rose with us to view venues, and we had decided that we would choose whichever one she liked best. This turned out to be a Marriott hotel in a former coaching house that used to be owned by the Bowes-Lyon family. It was full of history, atmosphere and original features—such as a glorious staircase. It was perfect, and we set the date for April 2012. I ditched my original colour scheme of purple and silver, realising that red, white and blue would be better in such a traditional venue. Also, it meant we could have red and white roses, so Richard's mum would feel part of the ceremony.

Sadly, Rose took a turn for the worse just days before the wedding, and she wasn't able to attend, which was heartbreaking for all of us. But we were determined to include her in our day, so on the morning of the wedding, we popped in. Mum had made Rose a lovely corsage, and we bought her a new duvet set covered in poppies and cornflowers so she could be in our colours. We pinned the corsage to the duvet, and I said to her, 'Next time I see you, you will officially be my mother-in-law,' which raised a little smile.

It was a lovely wedding, and it went by in the blink of an eye. Richard's niece Hazel walked us down the aisle, which was amazing, and we were accompanied by Chris's sisters, who were beautiful in red, white and blue bridesmaid dresses. Richard and I had had our suits made to measure in Singapore. Richard looked *so* handsome; I think I scrubbed up pretty well. My mum was in her element, guiding people to their places, and even Dad behaved.

Phew.

Everyone was terrified of our cake, from Choccywoccydoodah in Brighton—it was ginger and dark chocolate—two big love hearts, a dazzling centrepiece. We had some gorgeous photographs taken in the park, with Durham cathedral in the background, looking in one photo as if it were floating on a cloud of apple blossom. It was a beautiful day, tinged with a touch of sadness for our missing Rose.

We cancelled our honeymoon cruise because we wanted to be there for Rose and Chris, so we went back home after the wedding. It wasn't long before we returned to Durham.

Rose was nearing the end of her life: it was almost as if she had hung on for our special day. Chris had decided to keep her at home; I wasn't too impressed with the carers who came to check on her. When I saw her meds, I was furious. They were giving tablets to a woman who couldn't swallow properly, when she could have had them all in liquid form. After Chris left the room, I wiped the floor with them. It was unforgiveable that they'd not checked the basics to help a woman who couldn't even tell anyone she was in pain.

They changed her medication that day.

The following evening, Richard and I were cooking dinner when Chris came down and said, 'Boys, I think your mum's just died.' More grief. But Rose was at peace.

After Rose's funeral, we cheered ourselves up by going away

on a Mediterranean cruise with my parents. During the trip, I was talking to some officers and told them about our cancelled honeymoon. We couldn't believe it when the purser then told us that, as a goodwill gesture, Royal Caribbean Cruises wanted to offer us a two-week cruise in the Royal Suite at a very reduced price.

We flew home from Malaga, washed and repacked our clothes and then flew out to Palma just two days later to join what was to be our honeymoon cruise.

It was quite a year, 2012, with much joy and sadness. As well as losing Rose, we also lost Simba—my beautiful, faithful canine companion, who had been my comfort and my rock through so many hard times. I can't put into words how much I miss him.

The following year, my fractured relationship with the Royal Free hit a new low. I had been given an appointment for a cystoscopy – quite a daunting procedure involving a camera's insertion into your bladder via your male part. When I went in to see the consultant, he said he was going to give me an intramuscular injection of antibiotics. He clearly hadn't read any of my notes. I told him that I couldn't have an injection in my muscle because I was a severe haemophiliac, so the doctor said he wouldn't bother with antibiotics in that case, despite the fact that a few seconds earlier he'd thought I needed them. I was very alarmed by this. I told him, 'I'm HIV+, and you want to do a procedure without antibiotics? Can't I take a tablet?'

'No,' he replied.

'Why not?'

'Because you can't.'

We were standing there toe to toe, and he was a big bloke, so I felt very threatened. He said, 'If you want to cancel this procedure, the cost will be on you.' I told him I wasn't refusing—*he* was the one refusing to give me antibiotics. I also told him there was an antibiotic I knew I could take orally, which he would also have known if he'd read my notes.

He finally wrote me a prescription and proceeded to do the cystoscopy, very roughly. I felt violated. And afterwards, I went to the haemophilia unit to warn them what had happened in case he tried to give any other haemophiliacs an intramuscular injection. But they didn't want to know. One of the sisters said, 'It's funny how you always find trouble. I think it's about time you found a different hospital.'

And again, I felt threatened. Everything I said was always being questioned. No wonder my stress levels shot through the roof whenever I had any interaction with them. To top it all off, my new haemophilia consultant said she would only see me for fifteen-minute appointments, and I was only to talk about haemophilia, not about viruses or anything else. So I wasn't allowed to discuss any of the things that were continuing to impact on my health. She even said to Richard and me, during a review, that maybe it was time to do the 'Christian' thing—to forgive and forget, and to move on.

The staff at the Royal Free knew what I had gone through since I was put in their care in 1984. They were treating me worse now, than the child I was then. I had spent my life being told by them that I would die 'soon'. I had spent my life preparing for death.

How the hell do you move on from that?

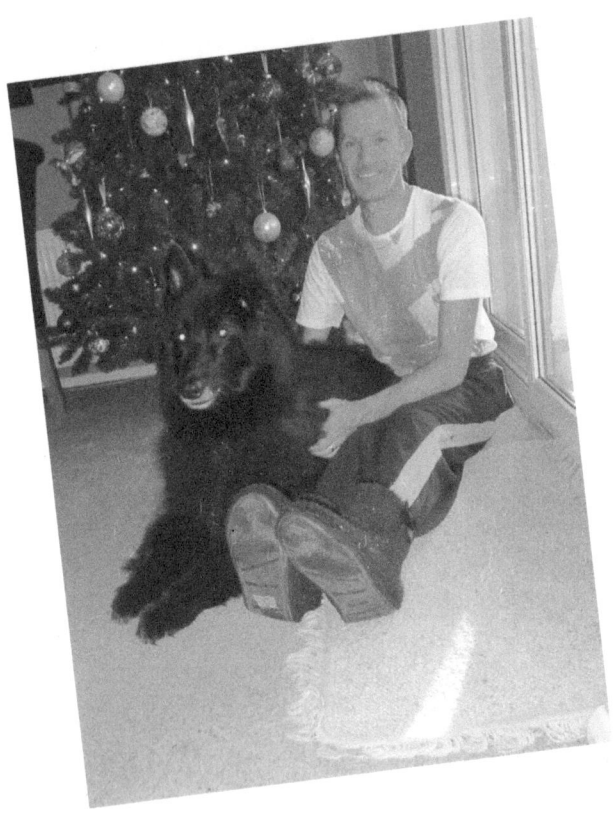

Zena—my pooch princess

DIGGING DEEP

As a proud, openly gay man living with haemophilia, I often felt very alone and unsupported. This was partly due to my treatment by the medical profession, and partly because of the narrative that had been built around my illness—that it was the gay blood that had infected me, that HIV was the gay plague brought on by a certain lifestyle. I didn't want anyone else to feel so alone, and I could see that there was very little help or support for someone like me—just this false belief that there were no gay haemophiliacs.

I tried working with the Haemophilia Society and set up a men's project to raise awareness and offer support. I believe that just knowing someone out there understands can offer some kind of hope, which is so important in anyone's life. But in 2004—at the World Federation of Haemophilia conference in Bangkok—the Haemophilia Society completely dropped the project because they felt it was too explicit; I attempted to keep working with them, but they wouldn't engage with me. So we went through a period of silence. Then in 2011, the Haemophilia Society were contacted by the BBC to give their opinion on gay men being banned from giving blood, but they had no opinion because they refused to engage with the issue. They had put the BBC in touch with me, and I gave my first TV interview, in which I talked about my infections. So now

I was back in touch with the Haemophilia Society, and, I was speaking to them—as was Mark Simmons—about the need to recognise that there are LGBTQ haemophiliacs. I thought we were making progress, but then a change in trustees resulted in the Haemophilia Society refusing to do anything that endorsed homosexuality. Once again, they would not engage with the subjects that were so close to my heart and dropped the projects I was working on. It was at this point that I thought *sod it—I don't need them to be my voice—I don't need them to speak for me.*

So in 2013, I founded Haemosexual with the help of a small team consisting of Dave Allen, Mark Simmons and Georgie Robinson.

Our community-based online information resource promotes equality, sexual health education and acceptance; it also tackles head-on the taboo subject of people with a bleeding disorder who identify as LGBTQ. My hope has always been that, with Haemosexual's support, no one ever needs to experience the isolation I felt for so long.

In 2014, I had to tackle the loneliness I felt on the loss of all my beloved boys. After Simba's death in 2012, we were left with just Ghost, the cat I had watched being born in 1995. Sadly, we lost him in February 2014; he is buried in the garden with Trojan. When Richard next worked away for a few days, I found myself totally alone for the first time since getting Sabre back in 1983.

I hated it.

By the time my birthday came in April, Richard was really busy with work, and my loneliness hadn't subsided. So I looked on the Dogs Trust website and immediately fell in love with Zena—a beautiful, thirteen-year-old, black, long-haired Belgian Shepherd with a wonky ear. I phoned Richard to ask if I could go and see her, which he immediately said yes to, although he was concerned about her age. He knew I would love her unconditionally, and if she died quickly, it would cause me more pain—which was something I could do without.

I told Richard that if I had her for a week, a month or a year then she would be loved, and every day with her would be treasured. But when I called the trust to arrange a visit, they told me she was in a bad way—Shepherds don't cope well in kennels and can deteriorate quickly. They didn't think it would be possible; I asked them to let me know. A couple of days later, the phone rang, and it was the Dogs Trust. Richard was home, and we went over to Shoreham to meet Zena. She looked us up and down and wandered around, not at all fazed by anything. For the next couple of weeks, while Richard went away again, I made the trip daily to build up a relationship with Zena. My mum and dad came down for a couple of weeks to keep me company, and in May, Mum and I went to pick Zena up and bring her home.

Within about five minutes of bringing her home, she walked straight into the pond. She did the same the following day and started to make the place her own. We began a little ritual of sitting down each day for about half an hour so I could brush her gently and make the connection stronger through contact. At night, I would hide a couple of doggie treats upstairs, and then we would play hunt-the-sweetie. Once she found them, she walked to her bed, which was at the foot of our bed, sat down and only when I kissed her on the head and said, 'Sweet dreams,' would she lay down and go straight off to sleep. Like flicking a switch.

Every day, Zena made me laugh out loud. She made me a better person. When she was diagnosed with two antibiotic-resistant infections in her urine, we did everything possible to make her comfortable. Then finally, twenty-two months after bringing her home, the vet came to the house, and Zena went to sleep in my arms.

I ran straight upstairs and booked flights to Thailand for Richard and me; we flew out the following day to grieve. I would have loved more time with her, but I don't regret anything.

I do regret keeping my treatment at the Royal Free. The same year we got Zena, I was subjected to yet another distressing, humiliating experience at the hospital. I had become frightened of attending appointments on my own, so I always took someone with me. This time, Mum had come along for my haemophilia review, and we were sitting in the waiting room when all of a sudden, a security guard appeared. And I just had a feeling about it. I said to Mum, 'He's here for me.' To prove me right, he glared over at me and Mum, and then he proceeded to march up and down the waiting area, not taking his eyes off us for a second. It was very intimidating. I said to Mum, 'If he follows us through to the doctor, I will turn round and walk straight out.'

To my relief, he didn't follow us when we were called in. Before the appointment, I had called and asked that a particularly unpleasant haemophilia nurse not be present because we had history: she was the one who had called me a 'troublemaker' and suggested I go to another hospital, so I had made a formal complaint about her. But there she was, sitting in on my appointment, looking like the cat that got the cream. I knew in that moment that I was being set up. The idea, I suppose, was to provoke me so the security guard had to be called—and I would be thrown out. The doctor, whom I had never met before, did his best to wind me up. The review of my health was more like an interrogation, with this doctor trying to push my buttons. Mum sat beside me with her hand on my back, and each time the doctor verbally attacked, she poked me with her fingers—which was her way of saying 'don't say anything'. No words were needed. The doctor examined my ankle and told me there was nothing wrong with it. He then said to me, 'This is how we do things here; if you aren't happy, I can transfer you to another hospital. I hear Southampton's good.' Well, with no disrespect to Southampton, it did not have a great reputation at that time. So this was clearly a thinly veiled threat: either shut up and put up, or get lost.

I felt as if my world was crashing down around me, and I couldn't do anything to save myself because the people who were meant to be caring for me were the ones inflicting the pain. Mum could see the distress I was in: she had witnessed the way I'd been treated over the years, as well as the impact of their sly remarks and discrimination. Then, I needed my bloods doing; my heart sank when nurse nasty walked in. She was so good at taking blood that she was the one they called when they needed to find a vein in a newborn baby. Yet on this day, she rammed the needle *through* my vein. 'Oh dear, I seem to have missed,' she said. She never missed.

I left the hospital in a state of despair. I felt as if I never ever wanted to go back there, but where else would I get my medication? You can't just switch—you have to make a request and have the centre director's agreement to take on your care. My fear, as a campaigner, was nobody would want a 'troublemaker'. Mum had taken the train north, and I was heading south, towards Brighton; I felt so wretched that, as I stood on the platform, I contemplated throwing myself under the train. I'm not sure what stopped me, but I think it was because I realised that if I took my own life, they would have won.

And then there was my Richard, who had only ever supported

and loved me.

I made an appointment to speak to the hospital's PALS (patient advice and liaison service) about what had happened, and they told me that the reason the security guard had been called in was because they had received intelligence that I had a gun and was going to shoot someone. Me? A gun? I had never heard anything more ridiculous. What kind of person were they making me out to be?

I never went back to the Royal Free, except for one last HIV consultation. I telephoned Tracey Dunkley—one of the most wonderful nurses who ever cared for me, and who was based at the QE in Birmingham with Mark Simmonds. She and Mark made a few calls and got Richard and me an assessment appointment at St Thomas' Hospital. And in October 2014, I transferred there; I have been with them ever since. I had a lovely consultant called Steve Austin, and it's been such a breath of fresh air to be treated like an adult, with respect and compassion. I only wish I had transferred sooner.

I also had my suspicion of being set up for the 'gun' incident confirmed when my security clearance was granted in March 2015. I went to 10 Downing Street, handing in a report for the attention of the Prime Minister. Shortly afterwards, a wish came true for our community when I found myself in parliament with Bruce Norval—my wonderful haemophiliac friend and fellow campaigner—to hear David Cameron, the former PM apologise on behalf of the British government to the victims of the contaminated blood scandal.

A huge milestone for so many people.

In January 2016, I had yet another brush with death. Richard and I went on holiday to Singapore and then Thailand, where I was taken ill. I didn't know it, but I'd had bronchitis that had gone up into my sinuses, which swelled up and caused a bleed in my brain. I was taken to a Thai hospital, and Richard feared that I might never make it home alive: he was even in contact with my consultant at St Thomas' to discuss what he might have to do in order to bring my body back to the UK.

I spent days in bed, and Richard looked after me. One day, he offered to give me a much-needed shower, and he washed my hair and body with a tenderness I will never forget. I also remember that was the day I turned on the TV to hear the terrible news that David Bowie had died.

I was on antibiotics but running out of my treatment. Luckily, I had just enough to last until I was well enough to travel, and Richard managed to get us a flight home in business class so that I could lie flat. When I saw my consultant, he was amazed that I wasn't in intensive care, but all I'd wanted was to be home.

I eventually got better, and I was looking forward to the World Federation of Haemophilia congress that was coming to Glasgow in May. I had been nominated as a 'haemophilia hero' and was supposed to be volunteering at the event. There was even a huge picture of me with a rainbow sash on a big screen in the main hall, along with all the other heroes.

But the day I was supposed to fly up there, I was so sick that I was green, and so sadly, I was unable to go. I ended up in the Royal Sussex hospital on the then-infamous Bristol Ward. It had a reputation for being the worst ward in the whole hospital, and I could see why. In all the years I'd been a patient, I had never seen anything like it. One bloke was threatening the nurses and throwing urine around, and another patient bit one of the sisters—it was horrific. I spent five long days there until I begged to be allowed to go home.

There really is no place like it.

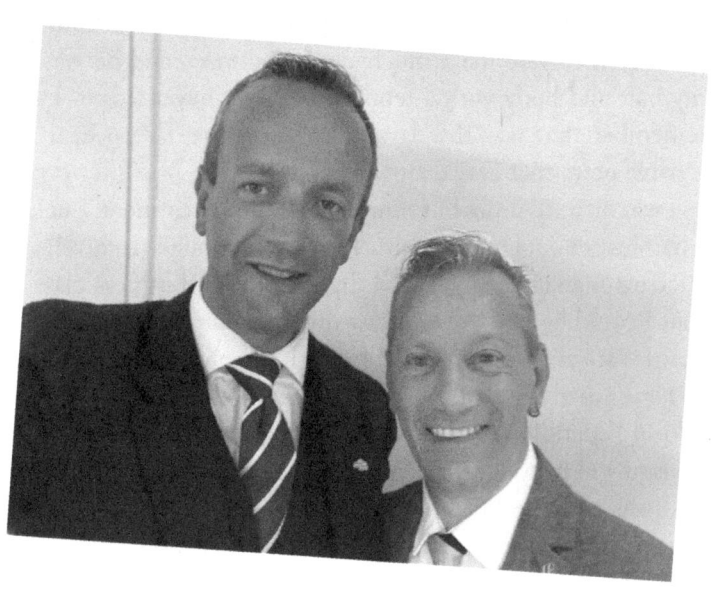

Mr Chairman & his Ambassador—making the fight look fabulous

THE TRUTH, AT LAST

In 2017, those of us who had been fighting hard for justice were delighted to hear that we would have our day of reckoning: Theresa May announced the creation of the Infected Blood Inquiry, and she described what had occurred as 'an appalling tragedy which should simply never have happened'. The inquiry had the power to compel witnesses to attend and for documents to be produced. So there would be no hiding.

In February 2018, it was announced that Sir Brian Langstaff, a former high court judge, would chair the inquiry. Sir Brian said, 'Providing infected blood and plasma products to patients truly deserves to be called a major scandal. I intend through this inquiry to be able to provide both some well-needed answers to the victims and their families, and recommend steps to ensure that its like will never happen again.' We were full of hope that justice would at last be served and that we would at long last get some answers.

As the inquiry got underway, I reached out to many victims around the world, including some in Australia—who invited me out there to help them start their own campaign for justice. Just days before Richard and I were due to go to Oz, Richard's stepdad Chris died. The last time we saw him, he gave us his blessing to go—whatever might happen—because he knew what an important trip it was. I had promised to bring him back a boomerang.

Richard and I arrived in Sydney on Valentine's Day 2018. We were met at the airport by our hotel's driver, a huge ex-Serbian soldier, who pulled up in a blacked-out Range Rover. It was so rock and roll! As we were driving to the hotel, my Australian contact phoned me to say that I was on the cover of the *Sydney Morning Herald*. This contact had been trying to raise awareness of our contaminated blood campaign in the media for ages, but he'd not been listened to. Now, at last, it was getting some publicity with a story about a British campaigner (me!) who was coming over to raise awareness and help Australians with their own campaign. Within an hour of arriving at our hotel room, I was on the phone to ABC.

I had a busy few days ahead but first, Richard and I had to perform our all-important ritual of touching the walls of the Sydney Opera House.

In between my press interviews, we managed to squeeze in some sightseeing. The morning after doing a live radio interview for ABC, Richard and I took a ferry to Manly, a beautiful beachside suburb of Sydney. The next day, I did another live studio interview on a news programme. Then I had a day off, followed by a radio interview with an amazing man called the Reverend Bill Crews, whom I had met in London and am honoured to now call my friend.

It was an action-packed and very fulfilling trip that I like to think helped raise awareness and support for their campaign. We then flew from Sydney to New Zealand, where we spent quality time with some of Richard's family, whose warmth really touched my heart.

But we weren't quite done with Sydney yet.

We returned there to take part in the city's Mardi Gras. This is always a big event in Sydney, but 2018 was a particularly special year. Not only was it the event's 40th anniversary, but it was also the first Mardi Gras since Australia had legalised same-sex marriage. So a double celebration at the biggest gay event on the planet. We expected it to be extraordinary, and it didn't disappoint. We loved every minute of the spectacular celebrations, and we threw ourselves into them, but my ankles felt like hell for days afterwards. I was almost sick with excitement when Cher appeared right in front of us.

After our remarkable time in Australia, we came back to earth with a bang on our return, when we were faced with a round of funerals. Along with Chris's passing, we also lost my dad's sister, Auntie Rose. We had gone to see her before we went to Oz, and just like Chris, I promised her a boomerang as a souvenir. 'But knowing your luck, it will just be a stick that won't come back,' I joked with her. It was the last time I saw her, and so it was good to know that we had parted laughing. Also that year, we lost my lovely friends Keith and Janet, with whom I'd shared some wonderful times in Malaga. I was asked to do a reading at both their funerals, which I was honoured to do. When the vicar told me to 'make it brief'—yes, really—I ignored him and did it my way. Janet would have approved…

For the past two decades, I have devoted a lot of my time to raising awareness of the infected blood scandal, using my knowledge and experience to protect future generations while supporting those who continue to be ignored and do not currently have a voice.

It's not easy to eliminate prejudice, or to change a narrative that has told me I should be ashamed of my illness. What has made everything worse for haemophiliacs is that we're not just up against politicians or the medical profession but also the wider HIV community. Over the years, I have tried to reach out and interact with other HIV organisations, but many haven't wanted to know. There is a lot of 'bad blood' between HIV and haemophilia communities. Gay communities do not like the narrative that the victims of the contaminated blood scandal are seen as 'innocent', which I can understand because it implies that everyone else who has HIV is somehow to blame—having brought this on themselves. As a gay man, I don't like that inference either, but at the same time, we *were* innocent patients harmed by NHS treatments. Becoming infected was something that was done to us—that's a truth that doesn't change. This was recognised when I was asked to join the AIDS Memory UK team, who were lobbying for a permanent memorial for *all* those impacted by HIV/AIDS.

Meanwhile, there is still homophobia within the haemophilia community. I have paid out of my own pocket to attend conferences in order to meet world leaders in haemophilia, only to be treated with distaste. Some victims blame the gay community for their infections because that was the lie we were told. I have been working hard to break down these barriers among communities who really should be supporting one another, and I am cautiously optimistic that progress is being made. My relationship with the Haemophilia Society has now strengthened, and to know they believe in me means the world.

They have recently added 'viruses' to my ambassador role, so I am now the Infected Blood and LGBTQ Ambassador for the Haemophilia Society—the first such ambassador in the world. I am supported by a new team led by Clive Smith, or as I call him, 'Mr Chairman'. This means I can officially go to meetings and say to other communities, 'Don't push us out, and please don't rewrite history.' This is our story. As a little boy, I was held down, and I had viruses injected into me. Repeatedly. Knowingly. By those who were meant to be 'treating' me. Now, how do we work together, find other victims and move forward? How do we combat HIV stigma if organisations are guilty of peddling that stigma?

This all became clear to me when filming with my dear friends who established the National HIV Story Trust. I'd seen something on the internet about a project which aimed to record and preserve the history of those affected by the AIDS epidemic of the 1980s and 90s. From the moment we first met, I knew these people were special. And so is their work. I have the honour of being one of their one hundred interviewees. I believe in everything they do because they understand the genuine need for people's stories to be told, listened too and kept safe. Their work is amazing, and through their teaming up with the London Metropolitan Archive, it will eventually will be available for researchers, historians and the public.

In April 2019, while in Thailand, I celebrated my fiftieth birthday. This was a huge milestone, and it was made even more special when I opened the room door one evening to find Debbie and her partner Paul standing there. Of course, I cried. I always cry—my love for Debbie is so precious to me. This wonderful surprise had been planned by her and Richard, secretly

The past six years, for me, have mainly been about the public inquiry, during which victims have been telling their stories and giving evidence, including Richard and myself. We have watched and listened to all those heart-breaking accounts, and we've also listened to politicians and medical professionals trying to defend the indefensible. Which wasn't easy. But there were also some beautiful people too. The words of Tracey Dunkley prove that: she told me the team at the QE in Birmingham have always said they had the very best of times with the most amazing people in the worst of times.

I felt it was my duty to offer my support to those caught up in this nightmare, and I became the only victim to attend every location across the UK that the inquiry visited. In Belfast, I was approached by a man with haemophilia, who told me he had never met a living HIV+ haemophiliac before. He asked to shake my hand, but me being me, I said, 'well now you have one as a friend,' and we hugged. We now keep in contact via social media.

Once again, I was meeting incredible people and building new bonds.

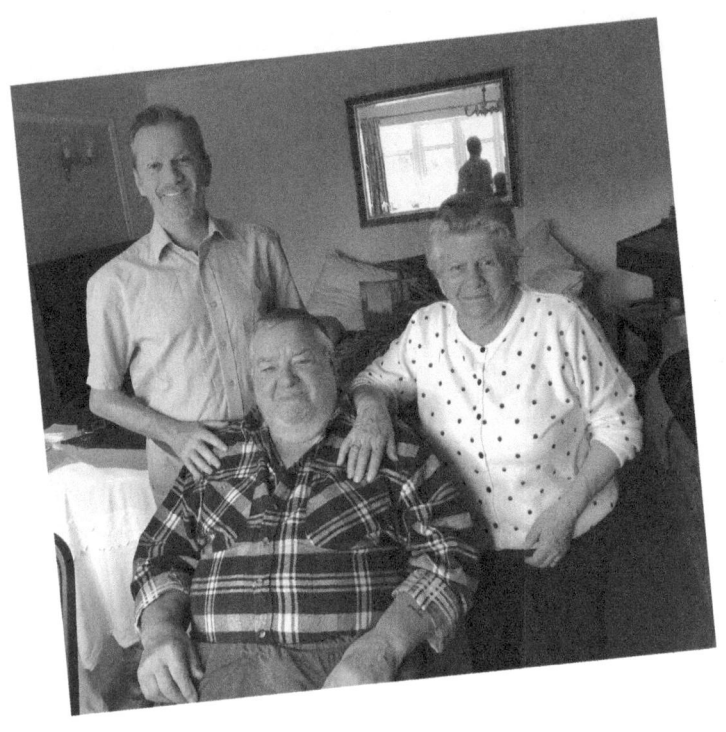

With Mum & Dad—the first post-Covid birthday we could celebrate

THE 'C' WORD

The pandemic brought forty years of psychological trauma and fear rushing back and like many disabled people, I felt abandoned. I went into lockdown in February 2020 because, just having returned from Thailand, we saw what other countries were already doing. It was during the pandemic I set wheels in motion to write this book. Not knowing if I would live to see it published. Once again living in fear of a virus.

The days, then months, and even years rolled past. Ironically, it was the inquiry that kept me going. Sir Brian, his team, our team and all the other incredible people involved just carried on working. I watched via YouTube from home, which proved to be a good idea—I found it hard to control my emotional outbursts and tears. Watching civil servants squirming, and politicians trying to explain why they never bothered to ask the reason that people were dying cannot be called enjoyable—but to me, it had its appeals.

The inquiry hearings also gave rise to some really powerful media coverage, and thanks to marvels of technology like Zoom, I was able to contribute on a regular basis.

Having the vaccine was another huge challenge. I wanted to have it in the hope that Richard and I could move forwards, and not remain trapped in the house. I was terrified, but I can do anything with Richard by my side. The volunteers and staff at the Brighton vaccination centre were so kind and caring. I handed them a letter I'd received from the hospital which gave advice about what people with bleeding disorders should do. They treated me like a rock star and whisked me off through a side door to a quiet area. Richard held my hand as I literally shook with fear and then, in the blink of an eye, it was done. The rush of relief and emotion swept me up; I cried like a baby in Richard's arms.

As things finally calmed down with Covid-19, we returned to the inquiry in person. Kenneth Clarke was giving his evidence. Let's just say that making eye contact with someone who showed so little respect for both the inquiry process and who he was in the room with, was chilling at times.

But because I didn't want to get near crowds, I usually travelled up to the inquiry a little later on the day. Then I could watch a live relay of the hearings from a side room. One day, I was warmly greeted by one of the inquiry officials who said, 'That's fortuitous timing Mark—would you mind just standing there for a moment—we have a guest arriving.' As I stepped to one side, Penny Mordaunt MP walked in and was immediately introduced to me. Without a flicker, my British Airways training kicked in and I greeted the minister in charge of the inquiry with a beaming smile. We spoke for a moment: I thanked her for taking time out of her schedule to attend, as I knew it would mean so much. Afterwards, I told the security guard I loved her coat. It was a gorgeous blue, which I think would have looked fabulous on me too. Shortly afterwards, in her official role as Paymaster General, Penny Mordaunt announced the establishment of a study into a compensation framework which would be conducted by Sir Robert Francis QC.

Was this the beginning of the end?

Another punch-the-air moment for the entire community came when all Health Ministers from across the UK—including Secretary of State for Health and Social Care, Matt Hancock—stated under oath that if compensation was recommended by Sir Brian in his final report then it would be paid. People needed to hear that.

As my campaigning has developed over the years, I've been given more and more opportunities to represent the haemophilia and wider tainted blood community. One such opportunity came when I was contacted by Arlie Adlington, a journalist working on a series of podcasts covering the forty years since the AIDS crisis began; it's entitled 'A Positive Life—HIV from Terrence Higgins to Today,' and it's available on BBC iPlayer, presented by the fabulous Sam Smith.

With that in the can, as they say in the biz, I travelled on Eurostar for the first time—over to Brussels for the rescheduled Thirtieth Anniversary of the EHC (European Haemophilia Consortium). This was now the longest I'd gone without flying on an aeroplane since that first flight back in 1977; I had to make do with a high-speed train.

Part of the delayed celebrations was a project called 'Open Door', which has become very close to my heart. The interviews and pictures form part of a transportable display which relays life stories of people with a bleeding disorder from across Europe through the decades. It was so nice to see familiar faces again. It's become a miniature archive which is designed to be added to. I offered Open Door my assistance, and since coming back to London, most people I've spoken with are really interested in adding their stories. Sadly, I've been told it has now been dropped.

I've been asked why I wanted a public inquiry? In my head, I wanted to literally have my day in court. I wanted to look powerful people in the eyes and hear from those who made those life and death decisions—why did nobody care about so many people dying from NHS treatment? In my dreams, I had hoped for every living Prime Minister to take the stand—like in the Leveson Inquiry. Sir Brian had personally assured me he would 'at the very least get a written statement from each of them' during the early stages of the inquiry. On 27th June 2022, former Prime Minister Sir John Major did appear, and I sat in the main hearing room in front of him, which felt like a huge achievement. That room, and the overspills were packed; gasps rang out when he carelessly claimed people who were infected had been 'unlucky'. Headline news was being made, and after a flurry of interviews with various journalists, I was whisked away in a car to the TalkTV studio.

I was sitting in the green room—after having my make-up done by two lovely ladies—when Jeremy Kyle walked in and said, 'Hello.' Which felt rather surreal. He asked what I was there for and when I told him it was for the contaminated blood story, he kindly shook my hand and said, 'Bless you.' Then he was off in search of a sandwich. Showbiz.

Sitting in a quiet TV studio as people are frantically preparing to go live is a real buzz and, as experienced as I have become, I always think to myself afterwards, *I should have said that*. But it's too late; I always give my best and try to educate those watching.

It was a few days after my appearance on TalkTV when life was tipped upside down again. I tested positive for Covid-19. I'd been extremely careful, so I was angry—as well as frightened, understandably.

The NHS were amazing: when I submitted my positive result, they had treatment to me within an hour because I was in a vulnerable category. It made my clapping for them during lockdown even more heartfelt.

Thankfully, my symptoms were mild and I was able to attend the inquiry to hear evidence from Andy Burnham. He was the only non-infected person to receive a standing ovation from all those attending—which showed how the community feel about him. It meant a lot to me to be there because I had not only spoken to Andy a few years previously, when he was gathering information about the infected blood scandal, but his team had then invited me to speak at the Hillsborough Law Now launch event in Parliament.

The launch had to be transferred to a virtual one for health reasons: the UK was in the grip of the forty-degree heatwave which prevented people from travelling. As always, I spoke from the heart—the little boys and friends no longer with us in mind. Listening to other people who have also suffered tragedies and, like the infected blood community, have had to fight for justice over many years was extremely emotional. Together we are stronger, and maybe I'm not about to hang my campaigning boots up just yet, as I gave them the same promise I gave to my haemophilia friends—whilst I have breath in my body I will fight for justice, for all of us. With such inspirational people joining forces I pity anyone who tries to stand in our way.

Regarding the Infected Blood Inquiry, we are already being vindicated. Documentation has emerged in court, answers have been given and the truth is being seen. That's all I've ever really wanted—to get to the full truth, to have it acknowledged, and to see justice being done.

Sir Robert Francis completed his report in March 2022 and the community waited for a response from government, as promised. Sadly, years of campaigning have made me very cynical, and true to form, the delays began. A written statement to the House of Commons simply thanked Sir Robert Francis KC for his recommendations on compensation and said the government were going to study them. After decades of contempt and trauma, the British government were still going to fight us all the way, playing their usual cruel tactics and using their usual empty words.

We have had to face many false dawns but this felt different—the pressure was on the government to do the right thing. *Dare I hold my breath in the hope that something historic was about to happen?* As the country lurched into a cost of living crisis not seen for a generation, even the (then) Conservative Party leadership candidates Liz Truss MP and Rishi Sunak MP, told the Times newspaper 'Compensation should be paid at once for the years of injustice.'

On 29th July 2022, Sir Brian Langstaff, Chair of the Infected Blood Inquiry announced the publication of an interim report. His conclusion was:

> (1) An interim payment should be made, without delay, to all those infected and all bereaved partners currently registered on UK infected blood support schemes, and those who register between now and the inception of any future scheme;
>
> (2) The amount should be no less than £100,000. As recommended by Sir Robert Francis KC.

And then, late on 16th August 2022, I received a phone call

which took my breath away. I clutched Richard's hand as we sat on the settee together and I relayed the brief conversation I'd just had.

'Tomorrow,' I said. 'They're going to announce a response to Sir Brian's recommendation tomorrow.' This was of course embargoed and strictly confidential; I could not stop thinking about what could be about to happen.

History was made, in a written statement.

The commitment to pay interim compensation met, in full, the recommendations set out by Sir Brian Langstaff in his interim report—that report being built on the study by Sir Robert Francis KC.

Details were announced by Chancellor of the Duchy of Lancaster, Kit Malthouse, who said: 'I am grateful to Sir Brian Langstaff for the work he has done to date on the inquiry, and Sir Robert Francis, for his work on compensation. Of course, no amount of money will compensate for the turmoil victims and their loved ones have faced, but I hope these payments help to show that we are on their side and will do everything in our power to support them.'

Prime Minister Boris Johnson said: 'While nothing can make up for the pain and suffering endured by those affected by this tragic injustice, we are taking action to do right by victims and those who have tragically lost their partners by making sure they receive these interim payments as quickly as possible. We will continue to stand by all those impacted by this horrific tragedy, and I want to personally pay tribute to all those who have so determinedly fought for justice.'

Boris Johnson also made a personal announcement on Twitter, and the interim compensation sum of one hundred thousand pounds was paid in October 2022 to the living infected; it was also extended to bereaved partners.

Su Gorman, the Tainted Blood press officer, lost her husband Steve Dymond in 2018 due to his infection with Hepatitis C through the use of contaminated blood products to treat his mild haemophilia. I first met them both in parliament in 2011, when they joined the campaign; our friendship grew from there, and I came to value both of their opinions immensely.

Following one of my routine haemophilia reviews at St Thomas', I visited Steve who had been admitted to an emergency ward. We chatted about all sorts of things, not just campaigning. As time was getting on, I said I had to go, and Steve got teary because he was so grateful I'd come to visit him. I said to him, 'You know, the real reason I've come to see you today is to see you in your pyjamas.' Su nearly fell off her chair laughing; Steve laughed so much he was crying. I told him from that point on, we were going to refer to him as 'PJ'.

Su was adamant that's Steve's death certificate should include blood products as a contributing factor in the cause of his death. I'd travelled to Maidstone to support Su and give evidence to the coroner; I travelled back to hear the verdict. Su and I sat clutching each other's hands as it was read out; I never doubted that it would go in her favour.

We looked at each other, and Su said, 'We did this for PJ.'

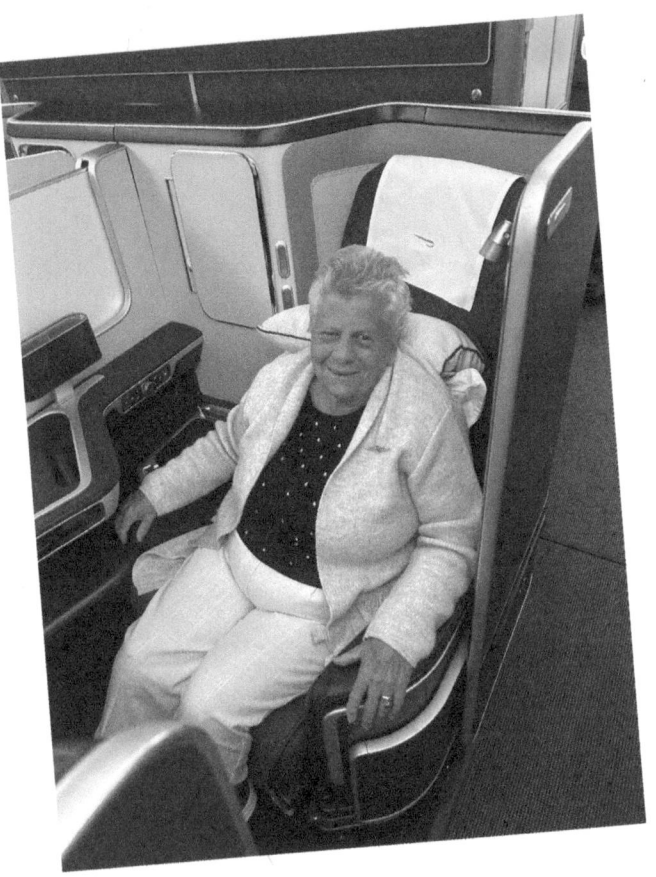

A First Class Mother

A FIRST-CLASS FUTURE

Dad's health continued to deteriorate. His stubbornness made helping him difficult and yet, he needed to be constantly cared for: he couldn't be left alone for more than an hour; popping to the shops and back was all Mum could manage. She felt trapped and it was impacting on her *mental* health. For both their sakes, something had to be done.

I hatched a plan with Mum to get Dad assessed: a doctor came to the house, and when he diagnosed Alzheimer's, we were relieved. We had believed Dad was suffering from the condition, and now it was confirmed, Mum was able to get some extra support. We lurched through the last few months of 2022; Dad had a few falls, which added another layer of anxiety, and then we all spent Christmas together. It felt weirdly like Christmases past—that apprehension that he could kick off at any moment about anything. Still, we managed to have a *fairly* peaceful time.

Six months after we met, Richard and I took our first cruise together, and cruising has become our thing. As retired travel industry staff, I am eligible for special rates on cruises; we had a couple booked when Covid hit and, of course, they had to be rearranged for alternative dates. One was in January 2023. From Sydney. Both Mum and Dad insisted we go ahead with our plans.

I have always spoken to Mum from wherever I am in the world, and Facetime has made that even easier. It was a couple of days after our arrival in Sydney that Mum told us Dad had been rushed into hospital. But she didn't want us to come rushing home: she insisted we enjoyed our holiday. Before we left Sydney, Dad was improving. We wouldn't be able to keep in contact out at sea, but Mum would update us in two days' time when we reached Mystery Island—a beauty-spot in the South Pacific.

Richard and I love to be on deck for departures: it reminds me of old photographs I've seen on the telly where huge crowds are throwing streamers and waving off cruise liners. This time was no different; as the ship pushed off in front of the Sydney Opera House and got closer and closer to the famous harbour bridge, excitement seemed to buzz around the deck. But we had only been one night at sea when there was a medical emergency, and we had to make a detour back towards land so a helicopter could fly out to us: it hovered over the bow of the ship, and we all watched, transfixed, as the injured person was extracted. This had a knock-on effect on the schedule, of course. And later that evening, it got worse.

The captain advised us there was a cyclone heading in our direction and the itinerary had to be changed: instead of docking in Mystery Island and Port Villa, Vanuatu, we would now head for Noumea, New Caledonia. The following day yet another curveball in the form of a second medical emergency: we had to sail full speed towards Noumea so a speedboat could join us and rush the passenger to hospital. But due to the port being full, the rest of us had to spend the night going round the island in circles.

Finally in Noumea, we made our way to the tourist information office where I could use the free Wi-Fi to Facetime Mum. My call woke her up: the time difference was eleven hours. She seemed to be struggling to focus her eyes; I asked if she was alright and she replied, 'Mark, your dad died.'

He had died two days ago. Mum again insisted that we shouldn't change our plans: 'There's nothing you can do right now.' I explained we couldn't get home quickly even if we wanted to because of the cyclone: its predicted path was now directly over Noumea, and the captain had told us we had to sail back to Sydney as fast as possible. All I wanted to do was give Mum a cuddle, and my heart was breaking when I told her it would again be days before I could even speak to her. Of course, she understood and told us to 'take care'.

We set sail, and would you believe it, a day away from reaching Sydney we had a third medical emergency: once again the helicopter came out and did its aerobatics to get the passenger to safety. When we reached port, Richard and I decided our best option was to continue as planned, so we went straight to the airport for our flight to Auckland, New Zealand.

We made it down to Taupo—where Richard's Auntie Susan and Uncle Ted live—but Cyclone 'Gabrielle' had followed us. It slammed into the north, causing devastation, span out to sea, then circled back to give New Zealand another pounding. Thankfully, we were all safe but a state of national emergency was put in place: we were stuck; there was no chance of us getting back to London just yet.

After a couple of days, we drove down towards Wellington to spend some time with Richard's cousin Dawn. We managed to get the date of our flights to London changed, which gave us another five days with Dawn's family—including her son, Henry, with whom I've built up a lovely relationship over the years.

Our long journey from the other side of the world began with a flight back to Auckland, then another to Brisbane—where we spent two nights and had opportunity to meet up with a campaigning friend, Gregg—before flying on to Dubai then London. It ended in Mum's living room: walking in for the first time knowing Dad wouldn't be sitting in his armchair was emotional. We didn't always have the best of relationships, but as I got older, I learnt to see him with more sympathetic eyes.

He had left us strict instructions: he wanted a 'proper London funeral', and he didn't want someone who didn't know him, 'talking about him'. Like they were operating a military manoeuvre, the undertakers arrived bang on time; as I stepped out of the front door, there was the glass carriage carrying Dad's coffin—attached to two enormous black shire horses. They looked beautiful with their feathered plumes and their reins glistening in the March sunshine. At the service, I read Dad's eulogy, finishing with the memory of that oompah night at the Pomme D'or Hotel on Jersey; I told you we never let him forget it.

Mum was now free to do what she wanted, when she wanted; after nearly sixty years of marriage, liberation wasn't going to happen overnight, but she did tell me she was tired of having to say 'no' to things and intended to say 'yes a lot more'. In June we put this to the test: when we asked her to join us on a trip to Lanzarote with our next-door neighbours Juene and Chris, she immediately agreed.

We had a fantastic time: we spent one day whizzing around the local area on mobility scooters, which were available for anyone to hire, and Mum had her first cocktail. Whilst she was a little tiddly on strawberry daiquiri, I asked where she would like to go for her birthday; she told me how much she had missed Thailand. I told her to leave it with me.

Thailand has always been Mum's happy place; in November, we flew to Singapore—where we stayed four days—then on to Phuket to celebrate Mum's birthday with our Thai friends, who are like family. It was so lovely to see Mum relaxed and enjoying herself. Her final treat came on the return journey: back in Singapore airport, we had to check-in with British Airways for our London flight; because the terminal is huge and Mum's mobility isn't as good as it used to be, we had booked assistance; a man whisked us off to the first-class lounge, and Mum twigged then. I had always told her she would fly first class one day.

Whilst Mum was my primary focus at this time, I was also keeping an eye on the Infected Blood Inquiry. In April 2023, Sir Brian published his second interim report, concerning the framework for compensation. In his statement Sir Brian said:

'As you know, the Government has recognised that wrongs were done and that compensation should follow; it made interim payments in October. I believe that the Government was right to accept this recommendation: my conclusion is that wrongs were done at individual, collective and systemic levels. I will set out the detail of what happened and why in my full report, but my judgement is that not only do the infections themselves and their consequences merit compensation, but so too do the wrongs done by authority, whose response served to compound people's suffering. This has been described as the worst treatment disaster in the history of the NHS, and we have much to learn as a nation to help ensure that people never suffer in a similar way again.'

Sadly, it appears this fell on deaf ears at Westminster: our MPs kept pushing for updates and answers, but the government responded with robotic replies, while claiming to be 'working at pace'. Well, not fast enough—in the UK, someone dies every ninety-six hours as a result of contaminated blood. So in July, Sir Brian reconvened the inquiry—summoning Prime Minister Rishi Sunak and other cabinet office officials, including Jeremy Hunt and Penny Mordaunt. And once again, our diminishing community gathered to hear from those in power—those who could easily have ended our suffering long ago.

Of course, my friend the Tainted Blood press officer Su Gorman was there. We couldn't believe how emotionally detached and at times callous the Prime Minister appeared when faced with a room full of dying, grieving and traumatised people. Su said, 'They spoke a lot of words but didn't really say very much.' As usual, she was spot on. I said my goodbyes and gave her a big cuddle, then I had to rush off because Richard and I were again flying to New Zealand.

Henry was about to turn twenty-one, and because I could, I had to be there to give him a hug on his birthday. Cynics will be saying *any excuse to fly on an aeroplane*, and there may be some truth in that, but you should have seen Henry's face light up when Richard and I appeared for his party: he couldn't believe we had flown all that way *for him*.

The highs always come with lows—three days after the party, Richard tested positive for Covid, and I received a shocking message: my dear friend Su Gorman had left the inquiry, travelled home, sat in the chair and died; she wasn't found for some days. Grief is something you never get used to—that punch in the gut, knowing yet another amazing person has left us. Another amazing person has died without seeing justice; Sir Brian's final report had been delayed *again*.

At the beginning of October, I attended the European

Haemophilia Consortium conference, which this year was in the beautiful city of Zagreb, Croatia. In previous years, I had attended to show our LGBT community weren't going to be ignored; I can't explain the feeling of officially being there as LGBT Ambassador. Now, I meet up with friends from across Europe and beyond as one of the family.

The gala dinner is always a fun evening; I let myself go, dancing with a group of Youth Ambassadors like it was nineteen ninety-nine again. In my head I was thinking, *I'll show these young things—this queen's got a lot more life to live.* Of course, I ended up with bleeds in my ankles and had to give myself treatment when I got back to the hotel room. I had changed my haemophilia medication a year earlier for a longer-lasting product, which means I now only have one injection per week. Unless you get what's called a 'breakthrough bleed'—like when you've been giving John Travolta a run for his money. I managed to hobble through the following day and make it back home safely.

The next time we were all together was in April 2024 for the World Federation of Haemophilia Congress in Madrid, which happened to finish on my birthday. The support we give each other is deeply felt: each time one of us made a presentation, the others did their best to attend and provide friendly faces in the audience; you couldn't miss the poster for my presentation: it was rainbow-coloured and stood right out amongst the other black and white ones. The event came to a crescendo the evening before my birthday when seventeen of us went out for dinner: my dessert arrived with a candle in the middle of it as the whole restaurant sang Happy Birthday Mark.

Of course, after the restaurant we had to go to a bar: at midnight, we toasted my fifty-five years with Baileys on ice, and I became the first man Conan, one our Trustees, had ever bought flowers. 'A red rose for our princess', he said in his Northern Irish accent. Being very English, I squirmed at all the love and compliments; I hadn't realised how much of an impact I have had on the community, especially the younger ones. I love my 'bleeding boys and girls', and with such wonderful young people now taking up the reigns—young people who are not afraid to ask questions—I know the future is in good hands.

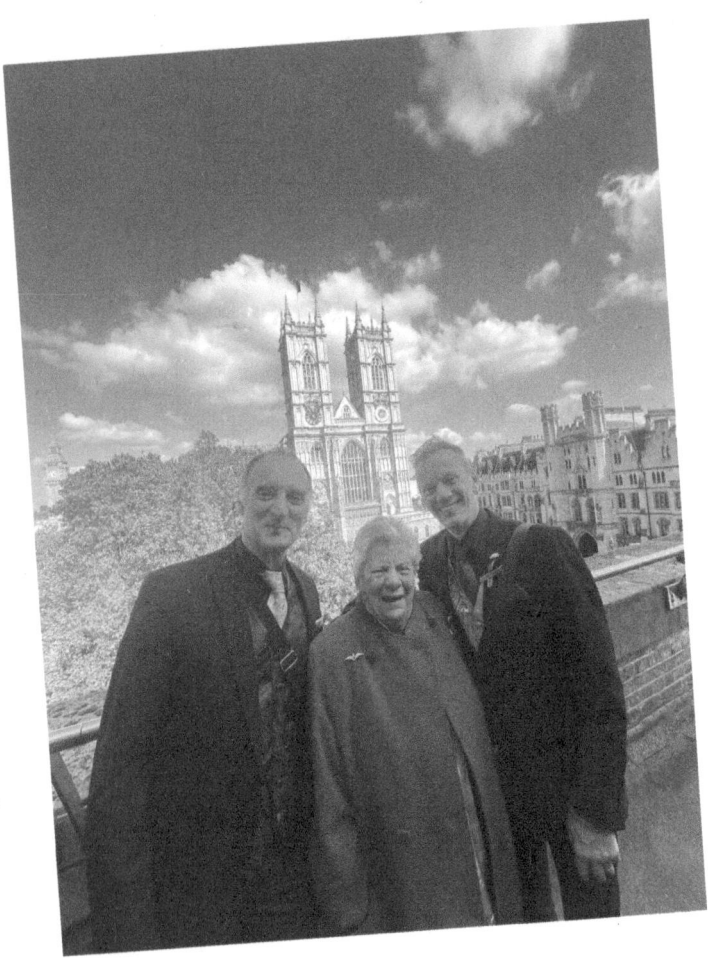

Richard, Mum & me—in matching red, yellow & gold outfits

EPILOGUE

For decades our small, vulnerable community has called for a public inquiry into the contaminated blood scandal. And now the day we had waited a lifetime for was upon us. Although there was a great deal of anxiety across the community, I felt strangely calm as Richard and I travelled up to London on the train. Some were taking part in a protest rally outside Parliament, but we attended an event organised by the Haemophilia Society—afternoon tea and cake for those who wished to simply be with others on the eve of this historic event. It was nice to catch up with the rest of the Haemophilia Society team and with people I'd not seen for years; we shared our hopes for the days ahead. As Richard and I returned to the hotel, I wondered *am I prepared?*

Definitely not.

Monday: At six forty-five, the first taxi of the day was waiting for me; it took me to Millbank for BBC Radio 5 Live, then I was straight into another taxi bound for New Broadcasting House and BBC Radio London. For weeks the media had been planning: I had done a number of pre-recorded interviews with various organisations and I am grateful for all the coverage we received in the build-up to the report, as well as on the day itself. The BBC London team were lovely—they made me feel so welcome and relaxed. I suppose there are times when we all stop to think, *am I really doing this?* Certainly I did as I sat in that studio, headphones on, readying myself to be interviewed. As you wait to go live, you can hear what's being broadcast, and the sports headlines came up—including the winner of the Formula One Grand Prix in Italy, which we had recorded.

Thanks for the spoiler alert, I thought.

Interview in the bag, it was back to the hotel for breakfast. We'd managed to get a bowl of cereal and a few sips of tea down when a call came through from BBC Scotland. I dashed off to find somewhere quiet away from the noise of the dining room. I found a spot by the bar, and Richard followed with a slice of toast, which I tried to force down before going on air.

Then we walked down the road to Westminster Central Hall, where we were greeted by a media scrum. Suddenly being surrounded by journalists whose faces were familiar from our televisions—asking for comment—well, it takes your breath away. In that moment I realised we were part of a massive global news story.

We'd stood back a little, waiting for Mum to join us, when a huge cheer went up from the crowd as Sir Brian Langstaff arrived with his PA, Mary. It was so funny watching him with the media: they wanted to film him approaching from different angles, but all he wanted to do was speak to us, the people. Just as he had from the start of the inquiry, he placed us at the heart of proceedings. Sir Brian spotted Richard and I, smiling, and he came over to shake our hands. He told me he'd seen me on television that morning. 'And I said to my wife, there's a good man.' I nearly burst into tears—such a compliment from such a gentleman. I thanked him and said that his words meant a lot to me. Then he was rushed inside the building.

Mum's train had been delayed, so Richard and I went in to do the formal registration. I was then whisked upstairs to do an interview for ITV Meridian with the lovely Rachel Hepworth, who I have got to know over the years: it was just like talking to a friend; my calmness continued. Thankfully when I finished that interview, Mum had arrived.

In the nick of time.

We were taken up another floor for the live press conference. As we waited to go into the room packed with global journalists, I saw Ben, my solicitor; he, like other legal teams and some journalists, had been locked in a secure room that morning, from seven thirty to twelve thirty to read the report first. From what he had been able to digest, he told me he was happy; he could only give a few key points but said I should feel vindicated.

Then, we took our places for the next part of this historic day. My heart pounded with pride: I felt honoured to represent all those who could not be there. Their faces whirled around my head, and I felt comforted from the other side as Clive Smith, Andrew Evans, and others spoke.

Lunch was as hectic as breakfast, but I did manage to finish a cup of tea before we were escorted to our seats, ready to hear Sir Brian's statement and comments. Somehow I got separated again from Mum and Richard; I sat with my friends, all survivors from Treloars. The room erupted when Sir Brian walked on stage; it was at that moment the calmness left me and I found myself fighting back tears. I don't know why I bothered, because I started sobbing when Sir Brian's words filled the room. All of us hung on every one of them:

'This disaster was not an accident.'

'The government refused to accept that wrong had been

done.'

'They repeatedly maintained that people received the best available treatment and that testing of blood donations began as soon as the technology was available.'

'Both claims were untrue.'

'A level of suffering which is difficult to comprehend, still less understand, has been caused, and this harm has been compounded by the reaction of successive governments, NHS bodies, other public bodies, and the medical profession.'

'I fully expect that the government will wish to apologise in a meaningful way. My principal recommendation remains that a compensation scheme should be set up now.'

After Sir Brian, the memorial event: it began by taking us back to 2018 with a short video of interviews from before the inquiry opened. I was first on screen, and I burst into tears again on hearing my hopes for what the inquiry might do; it all felt a very long time ago. Then there was the choir: it sent shivers down my spine to hear songs I had heard many times before but which seemed, in that moment, to mean so much more. Seeing my fabulous friend Seb Carrington step out to speak made me feel proud to know such amazing people; his heartfelt words—spoken as if by a great leader from a past time—conjured the most wonderful images in my mind. I am grateful to Paul and the technical team who ensured every word was captured and livestreamed, and who have made it possible for anyone to watch it all on the Inquiry's YouTube channel.

As I left the auditorium, two ushers were waiting to take me up to a balcony on the roof for a Channel Five interview with Dan Walker. 'Are you putting me to the test?' I said to one of the team, 'Asking me to keep focus in front of a handsome man like Dan?' She couldn't stop laughing; the interview began, but

I'd barely got further than thanking Dan for the coverage he and the team had given us, when we had to cut away to the House of Commons. And to Prime Minister Rishi Sunak:

'Mr Speaker, Sir Brian Langstaff has today published the final report of the Infected Blood Inquiry. This is a day of shame for the British state. Today's report shows a decades-long moral failure at the heart of our national life. From the National Health Service to the civil service, to ministers in successive governments … at every level, the people and institutions in which we place our trust … failed in the most harrowing and devastating way. They failed the victims and their families—and they failed this country.'

And with that said, it was back to Dan; my interview continued. When we were done, I managed to get a quick photo with him and then it was off downstairs—where I hoped to say goodbye to as many people as possible. We never know if we will meet again. I was able to thank the brilliant legal team who I had the honour to get to know. And yes, of course I got teary. Tears again when Mum announced she had to catch her train. We walked her to the underground and then we walked on to Millbank—for Iain Dale's LBC radio show.

At nine o'clock, we made it back to the hotel. Phew.

Tuesday: The alarm was set for an eight a.m. phone interview on BBC Radio Sussex—which I did from bed. Unlike the previous day, I was determined to get a proper breakfast before setting off for Parliament. My ankles were giving me grief, so we jumped into a taxi. We sat in the back seat, dressed up in black suits with our campaign ribbons and matching ties; the driver turned to us and asked if we were going to 'kick some arse?' I asked if he had heard about the Infected Blood Inquiry on the news. He said he had heard someone on LBC the night before who had been fired by British Airways. I gasped and said. 'That was me! And we're hoping the government are going to announce a decent compensation package today.' When we pulled up outside Parliament, the driver got out, opened our doors for us and gave us both a hug. He said, 'Go get 'em, gentlemen.' And when we tried to pay, he said, 'No charge—this one's on me.' I'm not saying anything about crying—by now, you all know I did. What a kind gesture that was.

Richard and I were met by two Cabinet Office civil servants working for the Paymaster General, who escorted us up to the public gallery to hear John Glenn MP make his 'significant announcement'. The first *punch in the air* moment was the appointment of Sir Robert Francis KC, as chair of the compensation body, called the IBCA. Then when he gave further details, more tears: all those affected are included; this means both Richard and Mum are eligible for their own compensation. I could see my MP, Lloyd Russell-Moyle bobbing to ask a question. It's so funny to watch: MP's have to keep standing up, trying to catch the speakers eye and then sitting back down again. Finally, Lloyd was chosen to ask his question; we knew there were still *lots* of questions that needed to be answered, but the MPs who stopped us to shake our hands as we made our way down to the lobby seemed happy for us.

Lloyd took us for afternoon tea, and then we took off for the train. As it pulled out of Victoria station, I had the first chance to look at my phone: I was shocked to see many missed calls, along with one hundred and twenty-six messages. The community was in emotional turmoil following the government's published tariff levels—and their proposition to stop the support payments we had been told were for life. Money is at the heart of this scandal, and it was tearing people apart still.

BLEEDING *Fabulous*

Wednesday: After a restless night, I once again travelled to London, for a meeting with the All-Party Parliamentary Group on Haemophilia and Contaminated Blood at Portcullis House. Along with friends from the community and Haemophilia Society colleagues, I was asked to give MPs an update on the previous two days from our perspective. This has always been one of the hardest parts of campaigning—trying to explain the genuine fear and pain people are going through. But at least I was in a room with people who wanted to be there. Dame Diana Johnson MP, who chaired the meeting, was joined by other MPs who actually cared about us and were doing everything possible to bring us justice.

Then word went around that Rishi Sunak was about to make another announcement; we watched on an MP's iPad as the Prime Minister walked out of Number Ten into a press throng, and the pouring rain to call a General Election. We couldn't help giggling: this was being broadcast around the world; we live in Britain, where it rains. Did nobody check the weather forecast? We resumed the meeting, and the MPs committed to do everything in their power with the limited time they had left in Parliament. A top priority was to get the Victims and Prisoners Bill passed during what's known as 'wash up'. As we left, I could see the emotion in people's faces: on Monday we thought we had done it; on Wednesday they were shutting Parliament without the law in place to provide compensation.

Thursday: Richard had to go away for work, and as I waved him off, I couldn't help wishing he could stay. The General Election had poured petrol on the fire that was raging across our community. People felt betrayed, yet again, by the British Government, and we all were firefighting the best we could. At Tainted Blood, we had people contacting us talking about suicide, and widows in tears, terrified of losing their homes. A rushed meeting with top civil servants from the Cabinet Office was set up; this 'technical briefing' was originally meant to happen two weeks after the announcement in Parliament. They asked for feedback and, boy, did they get it. To say the meeting was heated is an understatement. The language being thrown around by some from within the contaminated blood community was, at best, embarrassing and, at worst, insulting. There was no respect; I was left feeling worthless and bouncing off the walls with PTSD. I hadn't eaten, but I felt sick. The only place I felt safe was in bed, so I grabbed a pot noodle and shut the world outside.

Friday: The emotional roller-coaster over the past few days had been exhausting, and as I continued to attempt to process all the information thrown at us in such a short space of time, some good news arrived: the Victims and Prisoners Bill had passed into law. When I saw the picture on X of Dame Diana Johnson MP holding the Bill up, I felt as if I could breathe again and carry on fighting. Sir Robert Francis, Chair of the new IBCA, was going to be holding a consultation with the community—in order to present a compensation package to the new government in July. This gave me some reassurance, as Richard and I had spoken to Sir Robert when he was preparing his report: he had listened, and I believe him to be an honourable man.

Compensation won't give me back my life, my career, or even my smile. But compensation seems the only fair way to try to address the wrong that was inflicted on thousands of people. The financial sum also has to be so significant that no future government could ever allow a repeat of this tragedy.

My thoughts go out to those who never lived to see what

has been achieved. It gives me such peace, knowing I kept my promise to those lost little boys, and to all my friends who died. I will be able to hold my head up high and say to those who put obstacles in our way, 'You were on the wrong side of history.'

We little boys were failed, but now everybody knows why.

Thankfully, across the wealthy Western world at least, blood products have been replaced with synthetic ones since the mid-90s, so the risks of the infections that wiped out a whole generation of haemophiliacs have now been dramatically reduced. But I will continue to work hard for safe treatment for *all*, for equality, for recognition, and to educate younger generations of haemophiliacs, as well as others with disabilities to look after their sexual health—in the same way as we all should.

Once this is all over there will be a big void in my life. It has taken up so much of my time and energy. Hopefully, I will get to spend more quality time with my wonderful husband, Richard, whose unfailing support has given me the strength and courage to fight on. We hope to change our civil partnership to marriage, and to start to enjoy the life we should have had twenty years ago. Every moment Richard and I have shared has been overshadowed by my fight for justice, by THE campaign. One thing is sure—however long we have left together, it will be filled with love and new adventure.

I hope this book will assist others when I'm gone. I hope they will read this and see that, no matter how much darkness and pain you have to face, you will find the strength to get through it as long as you have love.

Nothing is more powerful than love.

ACKNOWLEDGMENTS

My journey through life to-date has, let's say, been interesting—filled with darkness, loneliness and, at times, feelings of worthlessness. Who would want a monster in their life by choice? However, my interactions with people all across the world have punctuated that journey with light, with laughter, with nights on the dancefloor, and with love. I've always wanted to make the world a better place, to be more than just a label imposed on me by society. We all have so much to give, and it's because of those who gave to me that I am here today. I now know that I never really walked alone, but was surrounded by amazing people—too many to mention them all—with a few jobsworths and twats thrown in: the lows may have been very low, but the highs have been off the scale.

Many thanks to my wonderful Mum and my husband Richard, and to everyone else whose belief in me has never faltered.

I have come to admire Sir Brian Langstaff and his incredible team at the Infected Blood Inquiry for their compassion and professionalism. For not just supporting, but inspiring people. Those same sentiments are felt for my legal friends, Ben Harrison and Sam Stein KC—whom kindly found the time in his busy schedule to write the preface for this book.

At the time of printing, there is still no national memorial to remember all those touched by the AIDS crisis. With this in mind, my work for equality will continue and I can be contacted via most social media platforms as Haemosexual, or via The Haemophilia Society.

I would also like to give thanks and respect to:

The haemophilia community I am so proud to be part of.

The HIV community.

LGBT campaigners and advocates.

I couldn't have completed this book without Story Terrace and my number one fan in Hastings, you know who you are, thank you. Another friend for life who I've come to love. And thank you to Ash Kotak, for the introduction to Inkandescent.

I hope this book becomes part of a legacy to be proud of. And remember—a man who looks after your feathers is a keeper.

Mark Ward

Special thanks to Bartholomew Bennett for proof-reading the book for us.

Very special thanks to Nick Bailey for his support with marketing and advertising. We are indebted.

Justin David & Nathan Evans—Inkandescent

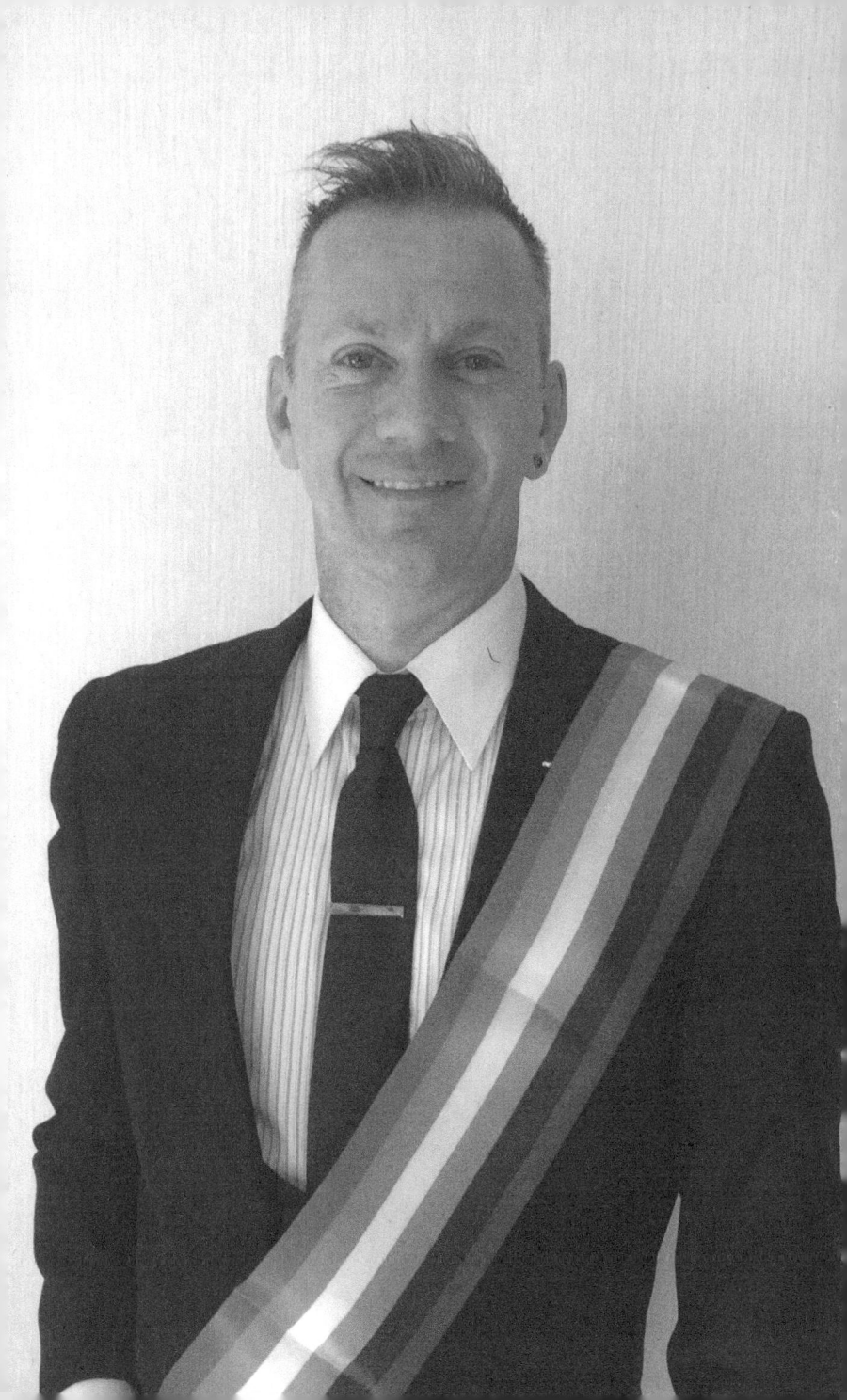

DEDICATED TO

Adrian Goodyear
Adrian M
Alan Burgess
Andrew March
Andy Gunn
Ann Dorricott
April Greenway
Babs Evans
Bev Tumelty
Bill Wright
Carol Grayson
Carol Prior
Charles Loader
Christina Burgess
Clair Walton
Claudette Allen
Colette Wintle
Colin Midgeley
Colin Nicky
Dan Farthing-Sykes
Darren Flack
Dave Allen
Dave Fielding
David & Sharon Tonkin
David Farrugia
Debra Morgan
Denise & Colin Turton
Eileen Anne
Eleanor & Fred Bates
Gary Kelly
Gary Webster
Gaynor Lewis
Georgie Robinson
Graham Manning
Hannah Wilcox
Hassan Efe Hussein
Helen-Marie & Ian Wilcox
HL Campbell
James Hunt
James McSharry
Janet & Colin Smith
Janine & Temple Jones
Jeanne White-Ginder
Joseph Peaty
Kevin Roberts
Kirk Ellis
Lee Brian O'Mahony
Lee Moorey
Lee Stay
Liz Carroll
Liz Green
Lynne Kelly
Marija Nakeska
Martin Haresign
Mary Grindley
Matthew Keogh
Mel Mckay
Melanie Richmond Piesse
Mi Tulip
Michele Digby
Michelle Tolley
Owen Savill
Paul Coleman
Paul Kirkpatrick
Peter Burney
Pip Norris
Richard Warwick
Robert & Alice Mackie
Robert Hodgkins
Rosa
Rosemary Calder
Ryan White
Sandra Molyneux
Sarah & Ellie Dorricott
Sean Cavens
Simon & Nigel Hamilton
Stephen Finney
Steve Bartram
Steve Dymond & Su Gorman
Steve Nicholls
Stuart Mclean & Karen Twomey
Sue Sparkes
Suresh
Susan Daniels
Tony Farrugia
Tracey Dunkley

And so many more inspirational people I hold dear…

HAEMOSEXUAL

Haemosexual is a community-based online support and information resource. We stand for equality, education and better healthcare for everyone with a bleeding disorder, no matter what their sexual orientation.

Sexuality and disability is a subject still not often spoken about, and many people are unfortunately not provided with the support needed from the wider haemophilia professional community. Sometimes this is due to a lack of awareness, information, or someone to confide in, who really understands.

Haemosexual has been designed to offer practical advice and information to patients, medical professionals and other organisations. Our aim is that those who are vulnerable become properly protected, which means communicating with them as people and not a condition.

Alongside the education we have done our best to balance things up with some humour. Fun and laughter really are a powerful medicine.

www.haemosexual.com

Also from Inkandescent

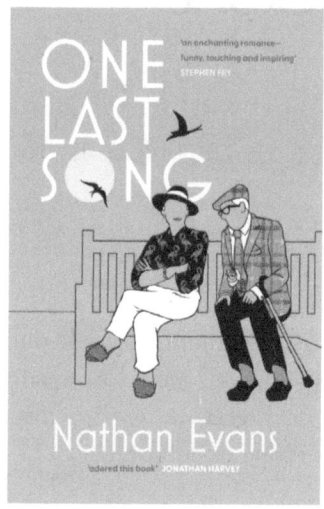

ONE LAST SONG
by Nathan Evans

you're never too old to change your tune

A gentleman called Joan lands up in a care home like a colourful, combustible cocktail... ticking.

A gentleman called Jim doesn't know what's hit him... everything about his new next-door neighbour is triggering.

Battle begins. May the best man win. But beneath antics and antique armour plating, what are both hiding?

Maybe they've more than a wall in common?

Might they even be batting for the same team?

'An enchanting romance - funny, touching and inspiring'
STEPHEN FRY

Also from Inkandescent

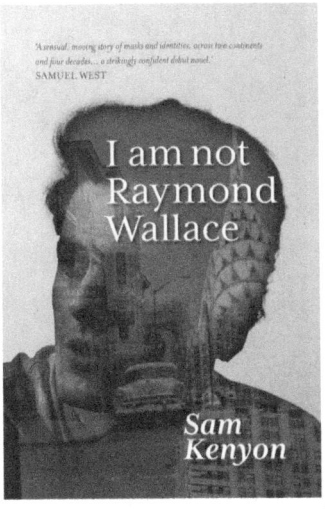

I am not Raymond Wallace
by Sam Kenyon

Manhattan, 1963: weeks before the assassination of President Kennedy, fresh-faced Raymond Wallace lands in the New York Times newsroom on a three-month bursary from Cambridge University. He soon discovers his elusive boss, Bukowski, is being covertly blackmailed by an estranged wife, and that he himself is to assist the straight-laced Doty on an article about the 'explosion of overt homosexuality' in the city. On an undercover assignment, a secret world is revealed to Raymond: a world in which he need no longer pretend to be something or someone he cannot be; a world in which he meets Joey.

Like so many men of his time and of his kind, Raymond faces a choice between conformity, courage and compartmentalisation. The decision he makes will ricochet destructively through lives and decades until—in another time, another city; in Paris, 2003—Raymond's son Joe finally meets Joey. And the healing begins.

'A sensual, moving story of masks and identities, across two continents and four decades... a strikingly confident debut novel.'
SAMUEL WEST

Also from Inkandescent

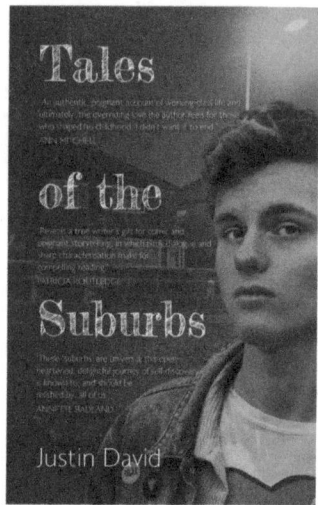

Tales of the Suburbs
by Justin David

Part Two of the Welston World Sagas
First Welston, then the World

As a boy growing up in the Black Country—drained grey by Mrs Thatcher's steely policies—Jamie dreams of escape to a magical metropolis where he can rub shoulders with the mythical creatures who inhabit the pages of his Smash Hits. Though his hometown is not without characters and Jamie's life not without dramas—courtesy of a cast of West Midlands divas led by his mother, Gloria. Her one-liners are as colourful as the mohair cardies she carries off with the panache of a television landlady.

We follow Jamie through secondary school, teenage troubles and away to art school; there he experiences the flush of first love with Billy, and the rush of the big city. But what then? Will he return to the safety of Welston, or risk everything on a new life in London?

These flamboyantly funny stories of self-discovery, set against the shifting social scenery of the 80s and 90s, are for everybody who's ever decided to be the person they are meant to be.

'Poignant storytelling, in which pithy dialogue and sharp characterisation make for compelling reading.'
PATRICIA ROUTLEDGE

Also from Inkandescent

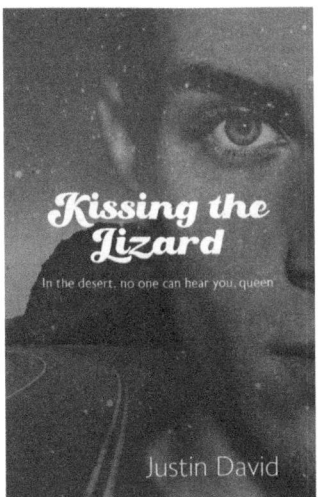

Kissing the Lizard
by Justin David

Part Two of the Welston World Sagas
In the desert, no one can hear you, queen

Justin David's newly-released novella is part creepy coming-of-age story, part black-comedy, set partly in buzzing 1990s London and partly in barren New Mexico wildlands.

When Jamie meets Matthew in Soho, he's drawn to his new-age charms. But when he follows his new friend across the planet to a remote earth-ship in Taos, bizarre incidents begin unfolding and Matthew's real nature reveals itself: he's a manipulative monster at the centre of a strange cult. Jamie finds himself at the centre a disturbing psychological nightmare as they seize the opportunity to recruit a new member. Pushed to his limits, lost in a shifting sagebrush landscape, can Jamie trust anyone to help him? And will he ever see home again?

This evocatively set desert gothic expertly walks the line between macabre humour and terrifying tension.

'There's not much rarer than a working class voice in fiction, except maybe a gay working class voice. We need writers like Justin David.'
PAUL McVEIGH, author of *The Good Son*

Also from Inkandescent

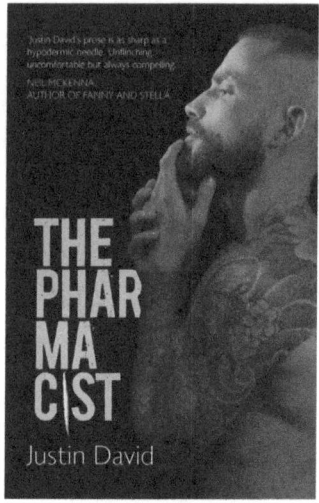

THE PHARMACIST
by Justin David

Part Three of the Welston World Sagas
when love is the drug

Twenty-four-year-old Billy is beautiful and sexy. Albert—The Pharmacist—is a compelling but damaged older man, and a veteran of London's late '90s club scene. After a chance meeting in the heart of London's East End, Billy is seduced into the sphere of Albert. An unconventional friendship develops, fuelled by Albert's queer narratives and an endless supply of narcotics. Alive with the twilight times between day and night, consciousness and unconsciousness, the foundations of Billy's life begin to irrevocably shift and crack, as he fast-tracks toward manhood. This story of lust, love and loss is homoerotic bildungsroman at its finest.

'As lubricious as early Alan Hollinghurst,
The Pharmacist is a welcome reissue from Inkandescent, and the perfect
introduction to a singular voice in gay literature.'
THE TIMES LITERARY SUPPLEMENT

'At the heart of David's The Pharmacist is an oddly touching and bizarre
love story, a modern day Harold and Maude set in the drugged-up
world of pre-gentrification Shoreditch. The dialogue, especially,
bristles with glorious life.'
JONATHAN KEMP

Also from Inkandescent

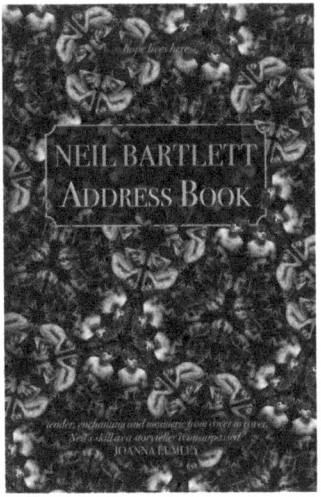

ADDRESS BOOK
Neil Bartlett

'Neil Bartlett is a national treasure. I read everything he writes and am always lifted by his skill, humour, political purpose and elegance.'
DEBORAH LEVY

Address Book is the new work of fiction by the Costa-shortlisted author of Skin Lane. Neil Bartlett's cycle of stories takes us to seven very different times and situations: from a new millennium civil partnership celebration to erotic obsession in a Victorian tenement, from a council-flat bedroom at the height of the AIDS crisis to a doctor's living-room in the midst of the Coronavirus pandemic, they lead us through decades of change to discover hope in the strangest of places.

"Address Book is completely absorbing; tender, enchanting and a mesmeric read from cover to cover. Neil's skill as a story-teller is unsurpassed. This book is something else. I adored it.'
JOANNA LUMLEY

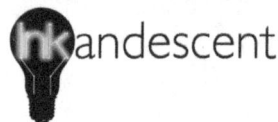

Inkandescent Publishing was created in 2016
by Justin David and Nathan Evans to shine a light on
diverse and distinctive voices.

Sign up to our mailing list to stay informed
about future releases:

www.inkandescent.co.uk

celebrating diversity

follow us on Facebook:

@InkandescentPublishing

and on Twitter:

@InkandescentUK

そして誰もゐなくなる

白石一文

こんなもんかな作戦二つ

昭和五十八年八月十日

　美帆の右の腿の内側には蛇のような形をした赤い大きな痣があった。生まれたときからのものらしく、そのせいで彼女はずっと人前で水に入ることができなかった。母の早苗は言った。「もう少し大きくなったら、その気味の悪い傷をきれいに取ってもらいましょうね。それまでの辛抱よ」。だけど結局、小学校五年の春に手術を受けてのちも、美帆は誰かと一緒に屋外で泳ぐことはしなかった。娘が外で水着姿になるのを早苗が嫌ったためだ。今度の理由は、「せっかくの白い肌が太陽のせいで台無しになってしまうでしょう」。

　ほんとうは美帆はあの太腿の痣を消してしまうのが厭だった。

　自分を生んでくれた母とのたった一つのつながりが失われるのが悲しかった。でも母にそんなことを言うのは子供心にも憚られた。早苗は美帆を我が子のように育ててくれていたし、弟の正也が生まれたあともそれは変わらなかった。

　手術当日の夜、傷の痛みで寝つけないでいる美帆のそばに母は一晩中ずっと寄り添っていた。明け方うとうとして、目が覚めてみると病室はすっかり明るくなっていた。

母が顔を覗き込んでいる。

「おはよう」

目が合うと早苗が言った。

「おはよう」

返したあと、わずかな間を取った。美帆には確かめたい大切なことがあった。

「おかあさん、いつ来たの？」

さり気なく訊ねる。

「ついさっきよ。昨日は痛くなかった？ ちゃんと眠れた？」

「うん。ぜんぜん痛くなかったし、よく眠れたよ」

美帆は答えて、美しい母の安堵の笑顔から視線を逸らした。

目を閉じて、心の中で呟いた。

——おかあさん、ありがとう。

あの日は何て暑かったのだろう。もうどうしようもないくらい暑かった。遮るものも皆無の河原一帯には夏の光が照りつけ放題で、容赦のない陽射しが川面の水をみるみる蒸発させていく。美帆たちが到着した時分には、風はすっかり凪いでしまい、むせ返るような水の匂いだけが周辺に立ち込めていた。

「かたせ桜花園」の子供たちは我先にシャツやズボン、スカートを脱ぎ捨て、下に身につけてきた水着ひとつになって川に駆け込んでいった。子供たちの立てる水音や撒き散らす飛沫のおかげ

4

で幾らか暑熱が薄まるような気がした。ただ、それも束の間のことだった。

桜花園には百五十人近くの児童・生徒たちがいたが、お盆前とあって、大半の子供が里帰りしていた。川遊びに参加したのは、たぶん三、四十人くらいだったと思う。下は三、四歳のちびちゃんから上は高校生まで。といっても幼児や高校生の数は少なく、大半は小学生と、美帆と同年輩の中学生の子たちだった。

指導員のお兄さん、お姉さんも川に入って、子供たちを見守りながらも冷たい水の感触を楽しんでいる。めずらしいことに父の俊彦もサーフパンツにTシャツという姿で正也と共に水に浸かっていた。

美帆一人だけ、河原の大きな石に腰掛けて歓声やはしゃぎ声を上げる人々の愉快そうな姿を眺めていた。

前の晩、どうせ泳げないのだから行きたくない、と早苗に言った。年に一度の発表会を半月後に控え、踊りの稽古に精出していた母は、

「本ばかり読んでいないで、たまには外の風に吹かれるのもいいわよ」

とふだんとは反対のことを言い、

「この前買ったワンピースを着ていけばいいじゃない」

と娘の気持ちをそそってきた。

白い麻地に紫のあじさい柄のノースリーブのワンピースは博多のデパートで何時間もかかって選んだ美帆のお気に入りだった。迷い始めた娘の心を見透かすように早苗は愛用の日傘を持ち出してきた。レースのフリルのついた真っ白な日傘も、一度使ってみたいとかねがね思っていたも

5

のだった。

「あのワンピースにこの日傘をさしていけば、美帆ちゃんに見惚れて、みんな川で泳ぐどころじゃなくなるわよ」

この一言で、美帆は父たちと一緒に片瀬川に出かけることに決めた。

片瀬川は片瀬市の中央を流れる一級河川で、源流をたどれば遠く英彦山に通ずる。町場では穏やかだが、市街地を抜け山岳地帯へとさかのぼっていくにつれ急流へと様変わりする。別名竜神川とも称され、夏場は鮎釣りの漁場として有名だった。といっても鮎が上る渓流は本片瀬と呼ばれる本流の方で、その支流である新片瀬は市内から車で一時間も走ったところにダムが作られ、ダム湖によって川筋は堰き止められていた。

美帆たちが出向いたのは、南片瀬ダムのある新片瀬の方だった。ダム湖の周辺にはキャンプ村が作られ、湖の上流は子供たちにとって恰好の川遊びの場所となっていた。

事件が起きたのは午後のことだった。

園が用意したお弁当をキャンプ村で食べ、一度着替えた子供たちは、ほとんどが昆虫採集や浅瀬での魚獲り、キャンプ場の人に案内されての自然観察ハイキングに回ったが、十人ほどだけは、もう一度水着になって川に戻った。小三の正也も高学年の児童や中学生に混じってふたたび泳ぎ始めた。

午後になるとようやく風も出て、日差しも和み、美帆たちは草の生えた川岸に腰掛けて涼しい川風に当たっていた。

昼の休憩時間、子供たちがひっきりなしにそばに寄ってきてろくろく寛げなかったこともあり、

6

美帆はいつのまにかうとうとしてしまった。

「一人流されたぞー」

という大声が聞こえ、不意に我に返った。隣に座っていた父はすでに立ち上がっていた。美帆も立ってその視線の方角を見ると、わらわらと広い寄洲に人が集まりだしていた。父がそこへ駆け出す。美帆も反射的にあとにつづいた。寄洲の集団が川下へと移動していくのが見える。

「あれは誰やー」

という指導員のお兄さんの甲高い声が響いた。

「小柳君です」

という子供の返事が聞こえる。前を走っていた父が、

「まさやー」

と叫んで全力疾走になる。

父は指導員たちに合流してダム湖方向へと川岸を走り始めた。正也の姿が見えたのは、寄洲が途切れる寸前だった。ちょうど川のカーブが大きくなり、その真ん中を小さな身体が浮き沈みしながら流されていく。

水着姿だった指導員が寄洲の縁から川に入った。ずんずん川中へと進む。水の深さは想像以上だ。あっという間に胸のあたりまで没した。だが、彼は流れに乗ることはせず、そのまま引き返してきてしまった。

「駄目や、流れが速すぎる」

そう言って唇を嚙む。

草の生えた川岸を進みながら父は息子の名前を連呼している。

「おとうさん、早く正也を助けて！」

美帆は背中に何度も呼びかけた。だが、父は大声を出すきりだった。五十メートルも伴走しているうちに正也の動きが鈍くなってきたのが分かった。それまでは平瀬の流木などに何とか掴まろうと手を伸ばしていたが、もう何もしなくなった。

「おとうさん、このままじゃ溺れちゃうよー」

美帆は絶叫した。一緒に走っている大人たちの誰一人として飛び込もうとしない。もがきながら流されていく正也の姿を血走った目で追っているばかりだ。たしかに流れも速く水量も多い。

それでも目の前で九歳の子供が溺れかけているのだ。

そのときだった。後ろからいつの間にか追いついてきた少年が大人たちの人垣を割って一段高くなった土手に立つと、ためらう素振りもなくぽんと頭から川に飛び込んだのだった。

少年はすいすいと抜き手を切って、正也に近づいていった。

大人たちは足を止め、にわかに色めき立った。

「優司、もっと左やぞー」

指導員の一人が手でメガフォンを作って少年に呼びかける。よく聞こえているのか、少年はすぐに進路を左に変える。川の流れに従っているとはいえ素晴らしい泳ぎだった。背中から正也の首の辺りに左腕を回し、今度は流れに逆らってみんなが待っている川岸へと泳ぎ始めた。正也はぐったりとした様子だったが少年に身を任せ、時折、近づいていく岸辺の方へ視線を寄越している。

8

正也を抱えていることもあってか、さすがに少年は泳ぎづらそうだった。

「優司、あとすこしゃ。頑張れ」

大人たちがこぞって岸の土手から励ましている。ずいぶんかかってようやく少年は河岸に到達した。いまや美帆の目にも彼の顔がはっきりと見える。

去年、同じクラスにいた仲間優司だった。

父が草地にひざまずいて二メートルほど下にいる正也に手を伸ばす。優司は空いた右手で土手から飛び出した木の根を摑んで身体を保持すると、首に回していた左腕を正也の脇の下まで慎重にずらし、一気に力を込めて正也の上半身を持ち上げた。

そのとき優司の上腕の筋肉が一瞬紅潮し、たくましく盛り上がるのを、美帆は父の隣で息を詰めて見ていた。

息子の突き出した手に父の手がつながる。正也が岸に上げられると歓声が沸いた。

だが、美帆は弟には一瞥をくれただけで、今度は指導員の一人が差し伸べた手にいましも摑まろうとしている仲間優司を注視していた。

目の前の優司の顔は蒼白で、唇は雨の日のミミズのような紫に変色していたからだ。

「優司、しっかり摑まれよ」

あれはたしか雅光兄さんだったと思う。桜花園で子供たちに一番人気のあった指導員で、美帆も親切な彼のことが好きだった。

仲間優司は伸びてきた大きな手を握り、木の根にかけていた右手も放して雅光兄さんの腕を摑んだ。

9

「よし、引きあげるぞ。その手ば絶対に放すなよ」

兄さんはそう言って中腰の姿勢から上体を反らせた。

優司が土手の土に足を掛けながらゆっくりと上がってくる。

結ばれていた手が切れたのは、あとすこしで優司の顔が土手の際に現れる寸前だった。「あーっ」という雅光兄さんの声と共に優司はふたたび川に落ちていった。仰向けに河水に投げ込まれていく優司の目が食い入るように美帆の瞳を見つめていたのをよく憶えている。

そして、口許にうっすらと笑みを浮かべていたことも。

仲間優司が急流に流されていく場面は、以来、何度も何度も夢に出てきた。その夢を見るたびに美帆の心は凍りついてしまうようだった。

平成十六年三月十七日

処置室からその男女が出てくると、患者たちのあいだに静かな緊張が走るのが分かった。男女も雰囲気を察したのか、細長いベンチが並ぶ待合ロビーの前でしばらく立ち止まり、やがて女が男を引っ張るようにして一列目の誰もいないベンチに陣取った。そこは美帆が腰かけているちょうど斜め前だった。二人が近くに来ると、美帆と同じ列に座っていた数人がじきに席を立った。後方の気配は二人にも分かっているようで、一度女が振り向いて、移動していく子供連れの若い

10

母親をちらりと見た。その瞳には何の色もなかった。きっと慣れっこになっているのだろう。

美帆は俯き加減にしながら、二人の様子を観察していた。他の患者のように席を立つ気は起きなかった。それより両隣にいたマスク姿の中年男性と若い男がいなくなってほっとしていた。少なくとも前の男女はインフルエンザではない。彼らのおかげで感染者たちが消えてくれたのだから感謝したいくらいだった。

昨夜から熱が出て、今日一日実家で寝ていたが熱が下がらなかった。インフルエンザが大流行しているので、もしやと思ってこんな夜更けに救急外来を訪ねたが、さきほどの診察によると、ただの風邪だろうとのことだった。それでも念のためにと唾液を採取され、検査結果が出るのを待っているのだ。

明日は昼前の飛行機で東京に戻り、午後は大事な打ち合わせが入っている。あの超売れっ子の古市先生にまさかインフルエンザをうつすわけにはいかないから、念押しの検査は美帆も望むところだが、病院でウィルスを貰ってしまうのは真っ平御免だ。

ただの風邪ならば薬を飲んでもう一晩眠れば熱も下がるだろう。三十四歳とはいえまだそれくらいの体力は持ち合わせていた。

それにしても大きな男だ。上背はさほどでもないが、胸の厚みや四肢の太さが尋常ではない。外は十分肌寒いというのに半ズボンにTシャツ姿で、首と手首に重そうな金色のチェーンを巻いている。ネックレスもブレスレットも純金製の値打ち物のようだ。アメフトかラグビー選手、またはレスラーとでも言いたいところだが、醸し出す空気がまるで違う。頭は丸坊主で、眉も剃り込んでいる。年齢は二十五、六だろうか。しかめ面の横顔しか見えないので容貌は評しがたいが、

まともな生業（なりわい）の者でないことは明らかだった。

男は左手の指に包帯を巻いていた。その指が痛むのか、体軀に似合わず時折小さな呻き声を上げているのしかめ面もそのせいだ。最初は小指なのかと思ったが、よく観察すると小指ではなく薬指だった。男の小指は第一関節から先がなく、分厚い包帯に隠れて見えなかったのだ。

一緒にいる女はまだ二十歳前だろう。男が呻くたびに心配そうに顔を覗き込み、何か小さな声で囁いている。くしゃくしゃの髪は金髪に近く、ネオンカラーの花柄のワンピースからは細い足が太腿まで露出している。膝の上に置いているのは黒のドレスコート。ピンク色のデニムのバッグはヴィトンのようだが恐ろしくダサい。しかし、厚化粧の下の顔立ちは整っていた。小顔にバランスよく目鼻口が並び、ことに黒目がちの大きな瞳が美しい。美女と野獣とはこのことだ、と美帆は思っていた。

三十分ほどのあいだに三十人近くいた患者たちが半分以下になった。時刻は十二時を回り、新しい患者もやって来ない。

だからその男が救急入口の両開きの自動ドアから入ってきたときは、久しぶりの来院者に皆の視線が集中したのだった。美帆も思わず顔を上げていた。

男は例の二人を見つけると、軽く手を上げて近づいていった。

大男の方は男を認めた瞬間にベンチから立ち上がっていた。隣の女も急いでつづいた。

二人とも直立不動の姿勢で男を出迎えた。

こんな夜更けだというのに男はミラーレンズの嵌（は）まったサングラスをかけている。紺地に細いストライプの入ったスーツを着て、下は白いシャツにノーネクタイだった。髪は大男のような坊主

12

頭ではないが短く刈り込んである。サングラスのせいで顔立ちは判然としない。頬はこけて精悍な感じだ。肌はゴルフ焼けのように浅黒かった。細身だがどこかしら迫力のある体型をしている。引き締まった仕立てのよさそうなスーツが身体に密着しているため両腕や腿の筋肉が窺われる。引き締まったいい肉体だった。よく見ると小さい顔に比べて首がやけに太い。それが、いくぶん肉食恐竜じみた印象を与えていた。

ベンチから離れてしまったうえに声が低いので三人のやりとりは聞き取りづらい。美帆は耳をすます。

「なして、こげんバカなヘマすっとか。親御さんからいただいた大事な身体やろうが」

スーツが大男にやや強い調子で言っている。

「何で俺にすぐ知らせんとか。リリコもリリコやろうも」

スーツの言葉に二人は黙って俯いていた。

「もう二度とすんなよ」

言われて大男が「すんません、兄貴」と頭を下げた。その坊主頭を抱き寄せ、スーツが広い背中を何度か撫ぜてやった。リリコと呼ばれた女の方はいまにも泣き出しそうな表情になっている。

それから三人はスーツを真ん中にベンチに座った。

座る直前、スーツがサングラスを取った。後ろの列にいる美帆と目が合う。向こうが訝しげなまなこになった。美帆の方は何となく諒解していた気がしてそれほどの驚きはない。大きくて切れ長のやさしい目の持ち主だった。だからサングラスなんだ、と美帆は思う。彼のような商売にこんな目は似つかわしくない。

13

どこに行っても見知らぬ男たちにまじまじと見つめられてきたから、ぶしつけなほどの視線にも美帆は動じたりしない。相手を見るでもなく、だが目線はちゃんとスーツの方に向けている。

何か話しかけてくるか、と思ったが、スーツはしばし美帆を見ただけでそのまま背を向けてしまった。

ほどなく診察室に呼ばれた。検査の結果はやはり風邪だった。

看護師から処方箋と診察券を受け取り、薬剤部に向かった。この片瀬市民病院に来たのは数年ぶりだが、ずいぶん立派になっている。新館にある薬剤部の夜間窓口までは長い連絡通路を渡らなくてはならなかった。

薬を受け取り、待合ロビーに戻ってみると、もう三人連れはいなくなっていた。

美帆はほっとした反面、ちょっと肩透かしを食らったような気分でもあった。

会計を済ませて、タクシーを呼ぶために出口そばの公衆電話コーナーに行く。三台並んだうちの真ん中の一台を選び、受話器を耳に当てながらカードを挿し込んだところで背後から肩を叩かれた。びっくりして受話器をそのままに振り返る。

あのスーツが立っていた。

「小柳、久しぶりやな」

仲間優司は言った。

トイレに行っていたという大男たちと病院の玄関で引き合わされ、結局、優司に家まで送ってもらうことになった。

14

病院の駐車場にとまっていた車は黒い大型のベンツだった。助手席に座って優司が運転席に回るのを待っているのを、見送りに来ただけかと思っていた大男とリリコも一緒に後部座席に乗り込んできたので美帆はちょっと意外だった。

「あねさん、すんません」

坊主頭のお辞儀姿がバックミラーに映っている。名前は研一というらしい。「研究の研に一、二の一で研一です」と先ほどかしこまりながら名乗っていた。リリコの方はどういう字を書くのか分からない。本名かどうかも怪しい。

「リリコんちが近所なんだ。悪いけど先に送っていってよかね」

シートに座った優司がエンジンをかけながら言ってきた。

「うん」

美帆は頷く。

かつての同級生といっても仲間優司とは高校二年のあの日以来の再会だった。正確に数えれば十八年ぶり。優司が博多に出てやくざになったという話は小耳に挟んだことがあるが、こうして会ってみると風貌も身なりも雰囲気もまさしくやくざだ。少年時代と変わっていないのはサングラスの下の二つの目だけだった。

そんな男の車にのこのこ乗ってしまうのは不用意と言えば不用意だが、美帆に別段不安はなかった。

研一とリリコの様子を眺めているうちに、何となく今夜この病院に優司がやって来るような気がしていた。やくざ者を目の前にしての単なる連想だったかもしれないが、美帆の場合、そうし

15

た予感は案外現実になる。

「どっか悪かったと?」

車を出してすぐに優司が訊いてきた。

「ただの風邪。もう熱も下がってきたみたい」

たしかに熱も悪寒もいつの間にかおさまっている。

「家は老松のままなんやろ」

「うん」

美帆の実家は老松町という古い住宅街にある。市の中心に建つ市民病院から南に車で二十分ほど行ったところだった。三歳になる前に両親と共に東京から来て、以降、ずっと老松で育った。

むろん家は十年ほど前に建て替えられていた。

優司は黙々と運転する。無口なところは相変わらずのようだ。

市役所や警察署の前を抜けて国道に入る。行き交う車は少なく、明かりのついている建物はコンビニくらい。舗道を歩いている人影もほとんどない。自分はこんな何もない町で十八の歳まで育ったのだ、と思う。もとより故郷への愛惜など彼女にはこれっぽっちもない。

美帆が事務所兼自宅を構えている表参道とは似ても似つかぬ風景だ。

後ろの二人は勝手に喋り合っていた。

「何な、そらあ」

研一が憤慨している。

「俺は昼から何も食っとらんとばい」

16

「そんな急に言われたって、何もないよ」

「何でんよかと。何かあろうも」

「ないよ。うちの冷蔵庫空っぽやけん」

ほどなく研一が身を乗り出してきた。

「兄貴、すんませんけどその先のロイヤルホストで降ろしてくれんですか。俺、腹が減ってたまらんですけん」

「今日は何も口にせんで寝た方がよか。麻酔も打ったっちゃろうが」

優司が言う。

「やけど、この痛みやとどうせ眠れそうになかですけん」

優司が来てからは研一はさすがに呻いたりはしなかった。だが、やっぱり痛いのだろう。眠れないほどの痛みなのに空腹というのも不思議だが、研一の身体だと納得できないこともない。

「兄貴、頼みますけん」

「お昼から何も食べてないなら、食べた方がいいかも」

美帆がつい口を挟む。

優司は何も言わずハンドルを切って左車線に移る。

「あねさん、ありがとうございます」

研一は見かけによらず律儀な男のようだ。リリコは黙っている。

ベンツはロイヤルホストの駐車場に入った。午前一時を回っていたが、数台の車がとまっていた。

優司が車をフラップ板の方へバックさせ始めると、「兄貴、ここでいいですけん」と研一が慌てた口調になる。

「そげんはいかんやろう。お前たち二人だけにしといたら酒まで飲みかねん」

優司はエンジンを切り、キーを抜いた。

「小柳、そういうことやけん店でタクシーば呼ぶよ。送っていけんようなってすまん」

「だったら私も何か食べる」

美帆は咄嗟に口にしていた。なぜそんなことを言ったのか自分でも分からなかった。ただ、優司たちと会ってにわかに元気になったことはたしかだ。それに彼女も今日はろくに食べていなかった。

車を降りて店の出入り口に向かう。研一の後ろ姿を間近に見る。恐ろしく大きい。二の腕だって美帆の腿くらいの太さはあるだろう。ふと振り返ると、リリコは車の正面に佇んだままだった。

「行かないの?」

ベンツのボンネットを見つめているリリコに声を掛けた。

「おねえさん、ほら、ひかりってほんときれいだよね」

うっとりした声でリリコが言う。磨きこまれた車体が店内の明かりにきらきらと輝いていた。

「ひかりって、きれいなものをどんどんきれいにしてくれるよね」

リリコが美帆の方へ顔を向けた。

「あたし、おねえさんみたいにきれいな人に初めて会ったよ。女優さんかと思っちゃった」

18

美帆はいつものように薄い笑みを浮かべる。

「あなたもとてもきれいだわ」

「そうかな」

リリコが嬉しそうな顔をした。

「じゃあ行きましょう」

リリコが頷く。出入り口の方を見ると優司たちが待っていた。

三月十八日

店に入るとすぐ、

「兄貴、焼肉は駄目ですか」

とフロアに飾ってある「九十分食べ放題１９８０円」のポスターを見ながら研一が言い、

「バカ」

と優司に一喝された。四人で窓際の席に案内される。包帯を巻いた研一の左手に気づいたウェートレスがぎょっとした顔になった。

研一がハンバーグ、美帆は真鱈のあんかけ御膳、リリコもエビドリアを注文した。優司はコーヒーだけだ。

「小柳はずっと東京なんやろ」

先に届いたコーヒーを一口飲んで優司が言う。彼はまたサングラスをかけていた。

「うん。お正月は海外に行ってて帰省できなかったから、お彼岸のお墓参りもかねてちょっと戻ってきたの」

「先生たちは元気なんか」

「父は元気だよ。いまは熊本の大学で教えてるから月の半分は単身赴任だけど。母は六年前に胃がんの手術をしたの。でも、もうすっかり元気になったわ」

「そりゃ、大変やったな」

「早期発見だったから。胃も三分の一は残せたし」

美帆と優司が隣同士で座っていた。向かい合わせのリリコが、

「さっき同級生って言ってたけど、高校のですか、中学のですか」

と口を挟んでくる。

「中学よ。片瀬東中」

「じゃあ、やっぱり美帆さんも桜花園にいたんですか」

美帆は優司を見る。表情に変化はない。

「私は違うの。ただ、父が医者をやってて、私が中学の頃は桜花園で働いてたの。だから同級生ってだけじゃなくて、仲間君のことはよく知ってたのよ」

父の俊彦は精神科の医師で、小児精神障害が専門だった。出向のような形で五年ほど現場を経験し、正也が溺れかけた年の翌春、助教授として福岡の大学に戻った。その後は教授、学部長と

20

進んで、六年前に退官。いまは熊本の私大で副学長を務めていた。

「そうなんだ」

リリコは考える顔つきになる。さきほどの美帆の容姿への物言いといい、この子は案外頭がいいのではなかろうか、と美帆は感じた。

料理が届き、三人は食事に取りかかった。優司は、ハンバーグをぱくつく研一をじっと見たり、窓の外の景色を眺めたりしていた。研一は右手でフォークを忙しく動かしながら、治療した左手をテーブルの上に置いたり膝元に戻したりを繰り返している。薬指を落としたのであれば、相当な痛みのはずだが、食事を始めるとすっかり平気な様子になった。

研一は美帆をじろじろ見なかった。そのかわりしょっちゅう隣のリリコの顔を盗み見ていた。そういう男に久しぶりに出会って、リリコがこの男と付き合っている理由がすこしだけ分かった気がした。

優司にしても昔からそうだった。出会ったのは中学に入った年だ。その年の三月に優司は「かたせ桜花園」に入所してきた。彼とは入学式の前に面識があった。四月に入ってすぐに桜花園主催の花見大会が開かれ、美帆は父に連れられて参加した。そこで、同じ歳の新しい園生として紹介された。初対面のときから優司は美帆に対してさしたる関心を示さなかった。中一とはいえクラスの他の男子たちは誰もが美帆に特別な目を向けてきた。そうでなかったのは、もともと無口で独りきりでいることの多かった優司だけだ。

正也の事件のあとは美帆の方が優司を意識するようになった。だが、中三の夏、彼は突然転校

21

していった。高二のとき再会したのは偶然だった。ちゃんと口をきいたのはその一度きりにすぎない。

それでも美帆はいままで優司のことを忘れたことはなかった。

弟の命の恩人ということもある。しかし、それだけではない。

雅光兄さんの手を離れてふたたび川に落ちた優司は、上流からダムへと数百メートル流され、ダム湖で救出されたときはすでに意識不明の重体だった。泳ぎの上手かった彼は溺れてはいなかったが、重度の低体温症に陥っていた。低体温症特有の身体を丸めた姿勢で岸辺にうずくまり、呼吸もほとんど停止していた。駆けつけた救急隊員が腕を持ち上げると元の形に丸めようとしたため、まだ救命の可能性があると判断されたという。

美帆たちが優司を見舞ったのは、その日の夜だった。

意識が回復したという知らせを雅光兄さんから受け、家族四人で市民病院に駆けつけた。病室に入ってみると、目覚めたといっても優司の意識はまだはっきりしていなかった。顔色も土気色だった。早苗が正也の身体を抱きしめ、ベッドに横たわっている優司に泣きながら感謝の言葉を繰り返していたのをよく憶えている。

翌日、塾の夏期講習の帰りに病院に行った。昨夜の病室に入っていくと、付き添いの人も席を外しているのか、優司が一人きりで眠っていた。顔色はだいぶ血の気を取り戻している。しばしベッドサイドに佇み、彼を見つめていた。

不意に優司の目が開いた。

美帆は一瞬おどろいたが目は逸らさなかった。学校でも桜花園でも、すれ違えば会釈くらいは

交わしている。

「昨日も来たんだよ。仲間君、分かってた？」

美帆は何でもない口振りで言った。

優司は大きな瞳を見開いて、こくりと頷いてみせた。素直な反応になぜだか美帆の胸は熱くなった。よく見ると、優司の顔はひどくやつれていた。

「仲間君、ほんとうにありがとう」

美帆が上擦った声で言う。しかし、これには彼は眉一つ動かさなかった。ただじっと大きな瞳で美帆の顔を見上げている。乾いた唇がゆっくりと動く。声は意外なほど明瞭だった。

「俺は、小柳のためならいつでも死んでやる」

優司はそう言った。

研一はハンバーグを食べ終えたあと、ほとんど口をつけていなかったリリコのドリアも平らげ、ようやく人心地ついた風情になった。リリコはいま勤めている店の愚痴を優司にぽつぽつ喋っていたが、研一は「兄貴、ちょっと外でたばこ吸ってきます」と言ってさっさと出ていってしまった。そんな彼の行動にリリコも優司も別段、気にするふうはなかった。美帆は優司の隣でリリコの話を黙って聞いていた。

「会うたびにそげん愚痴るくらいなら、かすみんとこに戻ってくればいいやないか」

しばらくして優司がぽそりと言う。

「あたし、新町で働くのだけは二度とイヤ」

優司はリリコの吐き捨てるような物言いに苦笑してみせる。

「お前みたいな女が中洲の水にどっぷり漬かりよったら、いずれ身体の芯から腐ってくっぞ」

リリコは中洲にある「夢幻」という名前のクラブでホステスをやっているらしい。てっきり十代だと思っていたが、訊いてみると今年二十三になるという。新町というのは片瀬駅前に広がる歓楽街のことで、一年ほど前まで彼女はその新町にある「あかり」という店で働いていたようだった。そこのママが「かすみ」という女性で、どうやら優司と親密な関係であるらしい。

「悪いこと言わんけん、かすみんとこに帰って来い。研一はあげな男やし、いまはまともな事もやりよるが、放っといたらまた何やらかすか分からんぞ」

再度言われて、リリコは黙った。

優司が腕時計を覗く。金色の文字盤のロレックスだった。

「じゃあ、行くか」

サングラスを外すと、伝票を摑んで立ち上がる。

リリコのマンションは、ロイヤルホストから五分足らずの場所だった。一階にローソンが入った割と立派なマンションだ。それにしても、ここから毎日中洲に出勤するのはたいへんだろう。

電車なら一時間弱、車でも四十分はかかる。

研一とリリコが玄関の向こうに消えるのを見届けて優司は車を発進させた。国道に戻り、南へと向かう。老松まで一本道だが、市街地から離れて街灯も間遠になる。すれ違う車も皆無だった。

「こっちで暮らしてるの?」

真っ暗な道を見つめながら美帆が言った。

24

「もう四年になる」

優司が答える。博多でやくざをやっていると聞いていたが、この片瀬に縄張りを移したのだろうか。

「どこに住んでるの?」

「新町」

声に億劫そうな気配が混ざる。

それからは二人とも黙ったままだった。

十五分ほどで美帆の実家の前に到着した。片瀬では一番の御屋敷町だから、午前三時をとっくに回ったこの時間帯、町全体が寝静まっている。小柳の家は中でも豪邸の部類に入る。十年前の新築の際、前後にあった庭を一つにまとめたので、二階建ての母屋の前面に広い芝生が敷き詰められていた。樹齢を重ねた樟、樫、桜の木々が常夜灯の明かりに巨大な影を芝一面に投げている。庭の隅には練習用の大きなゴルフネットがあって、その奥が美帆が寝起きしている離れ家だった。

門の前で車を止め、優司が美帆のシートベルトを外してくれた。

「かえって遅くなって悪かったな」

と言う。

美帆は首を振って、「ありがとう」と言った。助手席側のドアレバーに手をかける。

「近々、東京にしばらく滞在する予定があるんやけど、そのあいだに一度連絡していいやろうか」

優司がくぐもった声で言った。美帆はバッグの中の名刺入れから一枚抜いて差し出した。

「そこが事務所兼自宅だから」

すると優司も背広の内ポケットを探り、名刺の束を取り出した。が、彼はその一枚一枚を吟味

するようにめくったあと、難しい顔を作って再び束をポケットにおさめてしまった。代わりに別

のポケットから紙切れを出すとそこにペンで数字を書き入れて、

「これ、俺の携帯やけん」

と言って突き出してきた。美帆は何も言わずにその紙を受け取り、

「じゃあ、おやすみなさい。送ってくれてありがとう」

もう一度礼を言ってドアを開けた。冷たい夜気が足元から押し寄せてくる。

ドアを閉めると、その途端にベンツはバックのままスピードを上げて離れていった。

ろくに別れの挨拶を交わすでもなく仲間優司は美帆の前から消えた。

三月十九日

髪を洗い終えてシャワーを止めた。

顔の水気を払い、丈二を見る。浴槽のへりに後頭部を載せ、目を閉じていた。水音が絶えてみ

ると微かな寝息が聞こえる。深夜とあって窓の外も無音だった。

丈二は安らかな顔で眠っていた。バスタブは大きめのものを使っているが、それでも上背のあ

26

る彼には窮屈だ。長い足を折って、二つの膝頭がお湯からずいぶん飛び出していた。左右の腕は行儀よく腿のあたりに載っていて、その分、両肩をすくめた恰好になっている。大きな身を縮めて、まるで赤ん坊のように無防備だ。

しばし丈二の姿に目を留める。

このところの彼の消耗ぶりははなはだしい。

今夜もお互い仕事を済ませてから、行きつけの神楽坂の小料理屋で食事の予定だった。美帆は約束通り八時に着いたが、三十分後に丈二から電話が入って中止となった。馴染みの女将さんにお弁当を用意してもらい、それを持って帰宅した。十二時前にようやく丈二がやって来て、二人でお弁当をつついて、それからベッドに入った。

もう午前二時半を回っている。明日は春分の日で、美帆は休みだが、丈二の方は仕事だった。地元入りする堀米幹事長に同行して午前八時半の新幹線で大阪に向かうという。

疲れているときに無理に抱いてくれなくてもいいと思う。丈二は、泊まる日は必ず求めてくる。そのあげく、こうして眠り込まれると、なんだか申し訳ない気分になってしまう。

丈二は浴室で美帆の身体を触るのが昔から好きだった。

いつも浴槽の中で美帆を後ろから抱きかかえて、乳首をいじったり乳房を揉んだり、やがて大きな手で股間をまさぐってきて、ベッドで何度達したあとでも必ずもう一度美帆を上り詰めさせてしまう。

その習癖は、七年ぶりに再会したときも変わっていなかった。

こうして見ると、丈二の身体は若々しい。休日のテニスは最近はさすがに無理のようだが、い

までも寸暇を惜しんでジム通いはつづけている。身長は百八十五センチ。体重は七十五キロ。胸囲は百を超えているがウェストは引き締まっている。腕も腿も胸も学生時代と同様の筋肉を維持している。美帆は百六十三センチだから、決して小柄ではないが、それでも丈二に抱かれればすっぽりと包み込まれてしまう。強く抱きしめられて身動きならなくなると、もうどうでもいいような、どうにでもしてほしいような気分になる。そんな自分が嫌いではない。丈二のたくましい肉体にさんざん翻弄されたあと、そこから再びよみがえってくる感覚が好きだ。抱かれるたびに失われ、そしてまた取り戻す。そうやっていつまでも若々しく生きつづけられたらいい、とたまに思うことがある。

「ジョー」

顔を近づけて細い声で呼んでみた。浴室の中はあたたかい蒸気で靄っている。彫りの深い端整な顔が目の前にある。がっちりした顎と太い眉。閉じられた瞳も大きい。子供の頃、あだ名は「ジョー」のくせに力石徹とそっくりだといつも言われていたらしい。よく見ると黒い長めの髪の中に何本かの白髪があった。

丈二の誕生日は十一月。美帆は十二月。それでも男の三十五と女の三十五はまったく違う。

「ジョー」

ようやく丈二の目が開いた。ぽかんとした顔で美帆を見ている。

その間の抜けた顔を見ながら、一度裏切った人間は、また必ず裏切る、と心の中で思う。私はかつてこの男に何度となくたたかに裏切られた。

「こんなことをいまさら言っても美帆は信じてくれないかもしれないけど、俺はやっぱり美帆じ

28

やなきゃ駄目だって、この七年間ずっと思い続けてきた」

二年前の秋、ワシントンから戻ったばかりの丈二に言われて、美帆は再び付き合うことを決めた。

七年という長い時間、偶然の再会、そして恋人がいない現実。そういうもろもろを考慮した上で、もはや持ち時間は残りわずかなのだからと自らに言い聞かせた。

それでも一年半のあいだ、結婚を口にする丈二に明確な返事は一度も与えていない。美帆が選んだのは避妊をしないということだった。妊娠が分かったらその時は、と思っている。丈二もおそらくそう考えているはずだ。二十歳の年から六年間も付き合い、結婚寸前で別れた二人が、七年の歳月を経てもう一度一緒になるとすれば、そのくらいの根拠は不可欠だろうと美帆は考えている。

だが一方で、きっと自分は妊娠しないという予感もあった。自分はどんなことがあっても母親になんてならない、という確信がある。

丈二のことを愛しているだろうかと自問すれば、頷くしかない。別れてからの七年間も、一度も嫌いになったことはなかった。そうでないならこうして縒りを戻したりするはずもない。だが、丈二でなければどうしても駄目か、と問われれば首を傾げざるを得ない。かつてはそうだった。丈二と結婚すると信じて疑わなかったし、丈二以外の男には眼もくれなかった。そういう自分が丈二の重荷にならないか、嫌われやしないかと毎日が不安だった。

しかし、もうそんな時代は過ぎ去った。

眠っちゃったよ。でも、すんごい気持ちよかった。丈二はそう言って立ち上がる。湯船から出るとき派手な音を立ててお湯がこぼれた。頑丈な身体が美帆の視界をふさいでしまう。男は何で

も女より大きい。身体も声も息遣いも足音も動作も。だが、心は別だ。愛も憎しみも嫉妬も、そして恨みや打算も女の方がずっと深くて大きいに違いない。丈二はしゃがみ込んでボディシャンプーを両手で器用に泡立てると背後から美帆の身体を洗ってくれる。大きな掌が背中に張り付いてずしりと重みを感じる。たまらなく心地よい。

「一人のときは絶対にお風呂で眠っちゃ駄目だよ」

美帆は身をまかせながら、気遣いの言葉を口にする。お風呂で死ぬ人の数って実はすごいんだから……。丈二が浴槽で溺れるなんてこれっぽっちも思っていない。仮に丈二がいま死んだらどうだろう。自分は我を失い、きっと頭がおかしくなるだろう。ただ、そんな悲劇でも起きない限り、丈二が自分の心に決定的な影響を与えることはないような気もする。

母の早苗が言っていたことがある。男の人はね、みんな生命力が弱いの。あの人たちはね、女が子供を産んで生きていくための道具なのよ。男ってほんとに便利よ。上手に使えば何でもしてくれる。なのにいまどきは、男の力なんてあてにしないで生きたいなんて馬鹿なこと言ってる娘がたくさんいるでしょう。そういう子って、自動車もクーラーも洗濯機も冷蔵庫も掃除機もない世界で原始人みたいに暮らしたいって言ってる人と同じよね。せっかく目の前にある便利なものを使わないなんて、損なだけなのに。

丈二はシャワーで丁寧にシャンプーを洗い流してくれる。タオルを取ってきれいに拭いてくれる。美帆はされるがままにしている。

こんなことを幾らされても、昔みたいに嬉しくはないのに、と思う。

30

六時に起きて朝食の支度をした。

七時に丈二を起こし、洗顔や着替えをさせて食卓につかせた。

炊きたてのご飯、豆腐と焼きねぎのお味噌汁、紅鮭の切り身、海苔、刻みオクラ入りの納豆、あとは手製のきゅうりと人参のぬか漬という簡素な食事だったが、丈二はご飯を二膳もお代わりした。

美帆は仕事柄、料理はお手のものだ。揃えている食材や調味料も種類が豊富な分、料理がよほど面倒な作業だと思っているのか、肩代わりするだけで想像以上に感激する。実は、料理なんて簡単だ。基本と段取りさえきちんとマスターすれば誰でも手軽においしいものをこしらえることができる。

おいしいものを作ると男は手放しで喜ぶ。彼らは自分で手を染めたことがない分、料理がよほど面倒な作業だと思っているのか、肩代わりするだけで想像以上に感激する。実は、料理なんて簡単だ。基本と段取りさえきちんとマスターすれば誰でも手軽においしいものをこしらえることができる。

肉を柔らかくするには下味に酢を少々使えばいいし、卵焼きを失敗なく作りたければオーブンで焼けばいい。ガス台のグリルは必ず温めてから魚を入れ、青魚を煮るときは臭みを取ってくれる赤味噌を使う。野菜は茹でずに蒸し、ハンバーグを上手に焼くにはタネの真ん中をへこませるだけでいい。料理本などを見ると「ひと手間かけておいしく」などとよく書いてあるが、美帆は自分の仕事ではそんな言葉は絶対に使わない。そのひと手間が料理の基本なのだし、それを覚え込むのは手間でも何でもない。

31

朝食を済ませると丈二はそそくさと席を立った。玄関先で靴を履いたあと、幾分厳しい表情になって美帆を見た。

「今度、ちょっと相談したいことがあるんだ。大事な話だ」

美帆は「うん」と頷く。何の話だろうと思うが、新幹線の時間があるので引き止めるわけにはいかない。

「じゃあ」

と言って丈二は意気揚々と出て行った。

洗い物をしながら、大事な話とは何だろう、とあらためて考える。思い当たることがなかった。結婚話ならばしょっちゅう出ている。いまさら相談することでもない。

仕事を変わりたいとでも言い出すのだろうか。もともと弁護士になるつもりだった人間だ。大学二年で付き合い始めたとき、東大法学部の学生だった彼は、すでに司法試験の勉強に励んでいた。四年の秋に合格し、卒業後すぐに司法研修所に入った。その丈二が司法修習二年目になって法曹の道に進まないと言い出したときはびっくりした。修習を切り上げ、共同通信社の試験を受け、翌年四月には入社した。

そんな彼だから、もう一度、弁護士を目指したいと言い出す可能性は常にある。ただ、仕事振りを見る限り、現在の職場に不満があるという様子はなかった。ワシントンから帰った当座は、もう少しアメリカにいたかったと愚痴もこぼしていたが、古巣の政治部に戻り、渡米前から昵懇の間柄だった堀米順造が政権党幹事長の要職を占めていることもあり、仕事はやりやすそうだった。大きなスクープも何本か放って、昨年は新聞協会賞の候補にも挙げられている。

32

幾ら考えても、想像がつかない。美帆は考えることをやめた。出がけにみせた丈二の厳しい顔つきからして悪い話ではない。男というのは、嬉しい出来事が起きたり、大きな前進を遂げたときに限って妙にもったいぶった思わせぶりな態度を示す。彼らはいつまでもそういう子供じみた癖を捨てきれない。

どうしても聞き出したいのなら、一緒についていけばよかった。タクシーの中で強くせがめば喋ってくれただろう。そもそも、かつての自分ならば東京駅まで当然のように見送りに行ったはずだ。それがいまは、せいぜい早起きして朝食の支度をするくらいが関の山になっている。これも永すぎた春のなせるわざかもしれないが、丈二との関係においては、あいだに挟まる七年間の冬がすっかり自分を凍えさせてしまい、いまだにその凍傷が癒えていないためだろうと美帆には思える。

五月十八日

広い背中一面を艶々と青黒く光る龍がうねっている。

巨大な龍頭は左脇腹にあり、右前足の三本の鉤爪に握り込まれたピンク色の玉がその頭上、ちょうど肩甲骨の中心で輝いている。太い胴体は首筋へとせり上がり、右肩甲骨の上で左前足を踏ん張らせながら、背筋に沿って一気にすべり降りていく。背骨の真ん中で一重にとぐろを巻き、

血色の赤をてらてらさせていた腹部から青黒くくっきりした鱗に覆われる背部へと文様は逆転する。龍の下半身は腰部全体を埋めるがごとくくねり、尾鰭の付いた刃先のような尻尾は右臀部まで伸びきっていた。

ほんとうに生きているようだった。いましも牙を剥いた大きな口から火の息を吐き出しそうだ。

残忍な眼はじっと美帆を見つめている。機をみて襲いかからんと後ろ足の十本の鋭い爪はいっぱいに広げられていた。

想像していたグロテスクな感じはまったくない。

その一匹の龍は息を呑むほどに美しかった。

美帆は腰から下が痺れたようになって、しばらく身動（みじろ）ぎできなかった。いつの間にか右手だけが持ち上がっている。

「触ってもよかよ」

龍の眼で見たのだろうか、優司が言った。

背筋のあたり、赤く染まった腹の部分におそるおそる手を置く。それから左の龍頭へと掌をゆっくりとすべらせる。優司の肌は冷たかった。女の肌のようにきめが細かい。美帆の手が触れたとたんに龍の前足に握られた玉が赤みを増したような気がした。

「すごい」

思わず美帆は呟く。

「こげんもんをこげん間近で見たのは初めてやろう」

優司が笑いを含んだ声で言う。

34

「うん」

素直に頷いた。

左手も繰り出し、次第に大胆に龍の全体を撫で回す。

「ちょっとこそばゆかな」

それでも優司は黙って触らせてくれる。尻の割れ目までズボンを下ろしている。引き締まった左右の尻の肉に左の後ろ足と尻尾が彫られている。さすがにそこまで掌を下ろすことはためらわれた。

「もうよかやろう」

五分ほど経って、優司が言う。

「ありがとう」

美帆はようやく手を離した。

優司はズボンを上げると、ベッドに脱ぎ捨てていた上着を取り上げて身にまとった。刺青のせいもあるのか、その青いパジャマ姿がまるで本物の囚人を髣髴させてしまう。

「こげんもん背負っとるせいで、個室に一人ぼっちょ」

今日の優司は饒舌だ。慣れない東京で一人きりの病院暮らしだから、本人の言葉どおり、さすがにさみしいのだろう。

優司のはがきが届いたのは昨日だが、聞いてみれば、この病院に入院したのは三月末のことだという。彼はもう一ヵ月半以上も入院しているのだ。

三月に片瀬で再会したとき、近々、東京にしばらく滞在するので連絡してもいいか、と言われ

35

た。それが、何の音沙汰もないので、美帆はずっと怪訝に思っていた。連絡を待っていたわけではないが、といって失念することもなかった。優司は自分に対していい加減なことは言わない、という確信のようなものが美帆にはあった。

昨日のはがきで、だいたいの事情が分かった。

〈前略

　もうしばらくここにいます。よかったら顔を見せてください。その時、見舞いは金も物も一切お断りします。

　信濃町の慶応病院に入院しています。古傷のせいで使えなくなった腎臓を一個切り取りました。いま俺は東京です。

　　　　　　　　　　　平成十六年五月十五日　　仲間優司〉

　この前は、あんなところで会って、家に送るのも遅くなって悪かったです。

　上京の目的が手術のためとは予想だにしていなかった。まして片方の腎臓を摘出するというのは穏やかな話ではない。美帆はあわてて見舞いに駆けつけたのだった。

　新棟七階の優司の病室は個室だった。それほど広くはないがソファも冷蔵庫もある。わざわざ慶応まで来て手術を受けるのも不思議だが、個室というのも意外だ。顔を合わせてすぐに、「どう?」と訊くと、優司は、

「ごめん。さみしか」

　と開口一番言った。

「だったらこんな個室じゃなくて大部屋にすればよかったのに」

36

部屋を見回しながら美帆が呟くと、

「それがそうもいかん」

と、彼は渋い顔で背中の刺青のことを持ち出してきた。

二人で十一階の展望レストランに行った。

手術は一ヵ月前に終わり、傷も塞がって、いまは残った腎臓が正常に機能しているかどうか経過観察中らしい。「来週には退院できるやろう」と優司は言った。顔色もいいし、食欲も旺盛だった。ちょうど昼時とあって一緒に食事したが、彼は生姜焼き定食をあっという間に平らげた。

「そんな脂っこいもの、いいの?」

「全然。腎臓は一個あれば十分なんや。退院を控えて、できるだけ普通の食事をするように先生からも言われとる」

美帆が自分の頼んだサンドイッチを分けてやると、それもきれいに食べてしまう。

「普通に食って、腎臓に問題が出んかったら退院たい」

優司が摘出したのは右の腎臓で、一年も前から機能不全を起こしていたという。

「役に立たんだけなら構わんのやけど、そのうち腹ん中で腐り始めたと」

腐るというのは適切な表現ではないのだろうが、駄目になった腎臓のせいで下腹部の慢性的な痛みや血尿に悩まされていたのだそうだ。

優司が予想もつかないことを言ったのは、「古傷のせいって書いてたけど、どうして右の腎臓が悪くなったの」と何気なく美帆が訊いたときだった。

37

「まだ博多におるとき、組同士の抗争があって、相手方の鉄砲玉にドスで腹ば刺されたんさ。出血がひどうて死にかけたんやけど、そんときのツケが五年も経ってこうして出てきた」

美帆はこの言葉に思わず絶句した。

暴力団同士の抗争劇で組員の一人が襲われ瀕死の重傷を負ったのなら、地元では大きく報じられたに違いない。

「五年前っていつ?」

すこしして美帆は言った。

「九九年の暮れやったなあ。　医者がおらんて言われて病院をたらい回しよ。やくざなんて哀れなもんや」

そうだったのかと美帆は思う。九九年の一月に勤務先の出版社を辞めて片瀬に戻ったが、年の後半はイギリスに遊学した。だから優司の事件を知らないままになったのだ。

優司は当たり前の顔で窓の外を見ている。

信濃町の駅のすぐそばとあって病院の敷地内は花や木々に乏しい。だが、目を三方に転ずれば赤坂御用地、神宮外苑、新宿御苑という都内有数の杜に囲まれている。　時節柄、外苑や御所の緑がみずみずしかった。

やくざなんてやっていたら、そのうち死んでしまうのに、と優司の横顔を眺めながら美帆は思った。そう思うと、さきほど見た一匹龍の刺青が脳裡に浮かび上がってきた。優司が死ねば、あの見事な龍も一緒に死んでしまうのか。それとも優司が死んで、ようやく龍は解き放たれ、天に昇っていくことができるのだろうか。

38

小学校五年生のとき九大病院に入院し、右の太腿の痣を剥ぎ取って、お腹の皮を植えつける手術を受けた。高校になって、痣のあった場所に刺青を入れたいと思った。あの赤い痣と同じ大きさ、色形の刺青を彫りたかった。東京の大学に進学して、彫師のもとへ相談に行こうかと本気で迷った時期もあった。

優司によると、最初に針を刺したのは二十歳のときだったという。その話を病室で聞いて、ちょうど自分も同じ頃に同じことを考えていた、と美帆は思った。

「博多の病院で手術できなかったの」

コーヒーが届いたところで、一番の疑問を口にする。

「ちょっと事情があって、博多には足ば踏み入れんことにしとる」

「そうなの」

「ああ」

事情の中身には優司は言及しなかった。

「でも、どうして慶応にしたの」

「市民病院の先生が紹介してくれたと」

「そう」

頷きながらも釈然としないものが残る。が、それ以上は詮索しないことにした。はがきを貰ったとはいえ、どうして自分がこんなところでこんなやくざ者と時間を過ごしているのか、美帆にはいまひとつ理由が分からない。ただ、優司と一緒にいて恐ろしかったり、気詰まりだったりという感じはなかった。

39

「退院したら、退院祝いにご飯をご馳走してあげる」

はがきに見舞いは不要と書いてあったので、今日は手ぶらだった。それもあって美帆は口にしていた。

「すまんね」

仲間優司はその誘いをすんなり受けた。

五月二十七日

黒川丈二は選ばれた人間なのだそうだ。

彼とは二十歳になった日に付き合い始めた。美帆の誕生日は十二月二十四日、クリスマスイブだが、最初のデートはいまから十五年前、平成元年のイブのことだ。丈二は東大の二年、美帆はお茶の水女子大学文教育学部国文学科の同じく二年生だった。東大、お茶大、日本女子大の合同テニスサークルがあり、二人ともその一員だった。美帆は初めて丈二と顔を合わせた瞬間、強く惹かれるものを感じた。付き合うようになってから確かめると丈二も同様だったというが、美帆の場合は周囲の男性が関心を示すのは当然のことだったから、要は、彼女の感じ方がすべてだった。

美帆は一年半のあいだ慎重に丈二を観察した。その態度、言動、雰囲気などをじっくり見極め、

40

自分がなぜ惹かれるのかという理由を探った。一番の判断材料になったのは、丈二が奈良で大きな建設会社を経営する男の愛人の子供だと知ったことだった。

本妻が亡くなり、丈二が黒川家に母親と共に入ったことは中学三年生の頃だという。そういう話を丈二からあるとき聞かされて、美帆は自分がなぜ彼を選んだのか理解できたような気がした。

小学校五年生の春に全国規模で実施されたIQテストで丈二はトップだった。つまり日本中の十一歳の少年少女の中で彼は知能指数が最も高かった。

「勉強は授業を小耳に挟めばそれですべて分かったし、これはなかなか他人には理解してもらえないんだけど、友達と話していても、その相手が話し出す前にそいつが何を言うのか全部分かってしまうんだ。どうしてこの世界はこんなに超スローなんだろうっていつも思ってた。勉強だって結局は直感だって知ったし、だから、すごい発見や発明をするのがみんな若い連中だってのも、俺には不思議でも何でもなかった」

彼は知り合ってまもないころから、自分は選ばれた人間だと言っていた。「ずっと愛人の子だったからね。それくらい思わないとやってけないよ」と笑っていた。オーナー社長だった父親は羽振りはよかったようだが、愛人である母親に対しては厳しかったという。母子は正妻が死ぬまで奈良市内の小さなアパートで暮らし、母親はずっと青果市場で働いていた。彼の母親は在日朝鮮人だ。

「おやじはよく愛人の子は愛人の子らしく生きろ、と言ってた。肩身の狭い思いをしていればいいんだって。お袋はおやじの本当の気持ちを汲んでたみたいだけど、俺はただ反発するだけだった。本妻が亡くなって、黒川の家に入ってみて、初めておやじのことが分かったよ。要するにお

41

やじは、自分のために用意された苦労はちゃんと真面目に苦労しておけって言いたかったんだ。それが俺のためだって。よくお袋には『あいつは出来が良すぎるから、うんと悔しい思いをさせるしかない』と言ってたらしい。こんな話も俺が大学に入ってから初めて聞かされたんだけどね』

大阪出張から戻ってきた丈二は、七月の参議院選挙に奈良選挙区から出馬するつもりだ、と打ち明けた。相談したい大事な話とはそのことだった。大阪行きも、堀米幹事長と奈良県連幹部との協議の場に出向くのが本当の目的だった。

想像もしていない話で、美帆は心底びっくりした。いままで政治家になりたいなどと、丈二は一度だって口にしたことがなかった。ただ、最初の驚きが過ぎてしまうと、彼が政界に進出したいともくろむのは至極当然のような気がした。幼少期より選ばれた人間だと自任し、出自に抜きがたい負い目を感じている彼は、いわば政治家を目指すにはうってつけの人材かもしれない。彼のような人間が、集団を統率・指導したいと願うのはごく自然なことだ。司法修習を中断すると
き、法を司る者よりも、その法を作る人間の方が社会の上位に立つことにやっと気づいた、と彼は言っていた。官僚ではなく弁護士を目指したのは、「若いうちに組織に頼る術を身に着けてしまった人間は、決して大成できない」という父親の薫陶を受けてのことだった。それが、マスメディアという組織の一員になったときから、すでにこの日のあることを知っていたのだろう。政治記者となることで政権党の幹部たちと誼〔よしみ〕を通じ、いずれは政界に打って出るつもりだったのだ。

「美帆は政治家の女房になるのは嫌か？」

と問われて、何と答えていいか分からなかった。政治家という仕事に興味を持ったことがな

42

ったし、まして政治家と結婚するなど想像したこともない。

「出たら当選できるの？」

美帆はとりあえず訊いた。

奈良は一人区だけど、自民党から出られればまず間違いない」

丈二は言って、選挙区の情勢について詳しく話してくれたが、美帆にはよく理解できない部分もあった。

「もし出馬となれば、美帆との関係もちゃんとしておかなくちゃいけない。急いで結婚するか、せめて婚約くらいはしておきたいんだ」

丈二に言われて、美帆は面食らった。

「別に私は関係ないんじゃない」

「そうもいかないよ。選挙戦となれば候補者のプライバシーだってつつかれるし、当選すれば尚更だからね」

むしろ丈二の方が心外そうな顔をする。

「そうなんだ」

美帆は口を濁したが、自分が選挙のための駒扱いをされているようで内心は不愉快だった。

それから二ヵ月が経ち、公示を一ヵ月後に控えて、丈二の出馬の話は雲行きが怪しくなりはじめていた。党決定による参院比例区での七十歳議員定年制に準じて、三期十八年にわたって務めてきた現職議員が引退の運びとなり、その後継として堀米幹事長の肝煎りで県連に推挙されたのが丈二だった。当初は県連の方でも丈二を公認候補とすることで異論はなかったようだが、先週

43

になって、引退する現職の娘婿で、経済産業省の課長をやっている人物が突然出馬の意向を表明した。この新顔の登場で県連は堀米派と現職派の二派に分裂し、週明けに予定されていた公認決定も急遽延期されてしまった。

公認が下りると同時に会社に辞表を提出し、出馬に向けての本格的な準備に入る予定だった丈二は、すでに社の幹部にも転進の意向を伝え、もう後戻りのできない状況だった。それだけにこの数日の彼はすこぶる機嫌が悪かった。

今日も夜の十二時を過ぎて美帆の部屋にやって来たが、したたかに酔っていた。

「水上のやつ、直接総理に泣きついたらしいよ」

上着を脱ぎ、ネクタイを外して、リビングのソファに座り込むと、美帆が手渡した水を一息で飲み干したあと丈二は吐き捨てるように言う。水上というのが引退する議員の名前だとは分かるが、総理に泣きつくということの意味が美帆には諒解できない。

「そのときの総理の反応が知りたくて、今日一日探ってみたけどいまひとつよく見えない。堀米さんもどうも腰が引けてきてる感じだしな」

そう言うと、「あーあ」と声を上げ、

「こりゃ、ひょっとすると駄目かもしんないな」

と丈二は妙に乾いた口調で言った。

「何かあるんだが、それが見えないんだよなあ」

独りごちている。

かねてから公認が下りなければ出馬しないと言っていた。

44

「お腹すいてる?」

美帆は空になったコップを引き取り、赤ら顔の丈二に言う。

「大体、美帆がはっきりしてないもんな」

丈二は質問には答えず、目の前に立っている美帆を上目遣いに見ながら言った。

「お前が何を考えてるのか、俺にはよく分かんないよ」

最近、酔っ払うとお前呼ばわりしてくる。

「出馬が正式に決まったら、ちゃんと考えるからってずっと言ってるでしょう。もともとそのために形を整えたいってジョーが言い出した話なんだよ」

絡み酒に付き合うのは御免だ。美帆は努めて柔らかな物言いをした。

「俺が言っているのは、そういう理屈じゃないんだよ。流れのことを言ってるんだ」

だが、今夜の丈二は引き下がらなかった。

「流れって?」

「だから、政治っていうのは流れなんだよ。政治だけじゃない、肝心な勝負事ってのは流れが一番大切なんだ。うまくいくときは全部うまくいくし、いかないときは必ずどこかに小さなほころびがある」

「そのほころびを私が作ってるって言うの」

美帆の問いに丈二は答えない。

「私がすんなり結婚を承諾しなかったから、そのせいで公認も貰えなくなったっていうこと?」

たたみかけずにはいられなかった。

45

「そこまでは言っていないだろ。公認だってまだ出ないと決まったわけじゃない」

不貞腐れたような表情を作って丈二が言う。

美帆はグラスを持ってキッチンに行った。水を出してグラスを洗う。気持ちを落ち着けてリビングに戻った。

「だったらいますぐ結婚する。今度のことがあなたにとって一大事だってことくらい私にも分かってる。明日、区役所に行って婚姻届を貰ってくる」

美帆は言った。自棄で口にした部分もあったが、半分は本気だった。こういう成り行きも一つのきっかけだと直感していた。

丈二はソファに座ったまま、感情の乏しい瞳で美帆を見つめる。

「嫌な女だな」

ぽつりと呟くように言う。聞き捨てならない言葉だった。

「何、それ」

「それはこっちのセリフだろ。だったらって何だよ。だったらで俺と結婚すんのかよ」

「ジョーがまるで私のせいでうまくいかないみたいに言うからでしょ。私は、ジョーの人生を邪魔しようなんてこれっぽっちも思ってない。だから言っただけじゃない」

そこで丈二は皮肉っぽい笑みを頬に浮かべた。

「俺にはよく分かってるんだよ。お前は俺のことなんか全然愛していないんだ。九年前のことをいまでも許していないんだ」

この人はどうしてこんなことを言うのだろう。美帆は思った。自分を卑下したいのか、それとも

46

も許しを請いたいのか、はたまたこの場でもっと激しく争うためなのか。

美帆は黙り込む。酔っている男と喧嘩などしても仕方がない。それに、彼の言っていることは間違いじゃない。もちろん全然愛していないわけではない。ただ、昔ほどに愛していないのは事実だ。

美帆は心の中に紡ぎ上げた言葉の織物をじっと眺める。長い長い時間をかけてそれは美帆の中に生まれたものだ。いまや一枚の絵を見るように、一瞬で意識の視野に飛び込んでくる。

そうよ、あなたは私を裏切った。あなたに裏切られて、私は何日も何十日も何百日も考えた。

私のどこがいけなかったのだろう？

何があなたにとって不満だったのだろう？

あなたは私にどうして欲しかったのだろう？

幾ら考えても理由が分からなかった。たしかにお互い社会に出て、学生のときみたいに始終一緒にはいられなくなっていた。擦れ違いの生活がつづいていたし、正也が東京に出て同居するようになってからは、週末に私の部屋で思う存分抱き合うこともできなくなっていた。でも、それでも、私はあなたを心から愛していたし、あなたのことを自分の身体や命よりも大事だと思っていた。

あの頃の私は、誰かのことを信じたかった。私のことを誰かに信じて欲しかった。誰でもよかったのかもしれない。でも、私にはあなただった。私は、あなたと出会って、あなたを信じようと決めた。あなたと私は似た者同士なのだと感じたから。あなたの小さい頃からの苦しみを、私

ならば心から理解してあげることができると思った。

私は、あなたのことだけは裏切らないと誓った。

そして、あなたも私だけは裏切らないと信じた。

愛し方が足りなかったのだろうか？　愛し方が下手だったのだろうか？　それとも、私があなたを愛しすぎたのが重荷だったのか？

あのときの私の苦しみがあなたに分かりますか？　自分が自分でなくなって、胸の奥で、頭の芯で渦巻く醜い感情や嫌悪感に苛まれつづけた。食べることも、眠ることも、笑うこともできなくなった。自分で自分の心を絞め殺したくなって、自分を含めた誰のことも信じられなくなって、どうやってこのさき生きていけばいいのか何も見えなくなった。

あなたなんかにあの苦しみが理解できるはずがない。

言葉で幾ら謝られても、そんなことどうだっていい。私のあのときの気持ちをあなたがほんとうに理解しない限り、あなたには自分がしたことの罪深さは絶対に分からない。

ちょっと他の女に目がいっただけじゃないか。違うセックスもしたかったんだ。まだ俺は若かったんだから。男なんてそんなものだ。それをことさら目くじら立てて、美人だからってプライドだけに振り回されて。お前がもっと大人になればよかったのに。それが女のつとめというものなのに。俺もたしかに悪かった。だけどそんな俺のたった一度の浮気をあそこまで責め立てたお前の心の貧しさにだって問題はあったんじゃないのか。

あなたには分かっていない。私があなたをどれほど愛していたか。私がどんな気持ちであなたと別れたのか。きっといまでもあなたはそう思っている。あなたには分かっていない。私があなたをどれほど

48

そうよ、あなたはいまだって何も分かってはいない。

いつの間にか目の前に丈二が立っていた。顔を上げた瞬間、彼に抱きかかえられ、そのまま無言で寝室へと連れて行かれた。カバーがかかったままのベッドに降ろされ、手荒に服を剥ぎ取られていく。美帆は抵抗するつもりはない。だが、「嫌だ!」、「やめて!」と叫び、全身をばたつかせて精一杯抗ってみせる。丈二が興奮を募らせる。ますます激しく美帆を押さえつけてくる。

レイプ同然の行為。でもそれはレイプとは対極にある行為でもある。

丈二の巨体がのしかかってくる。美帆はその広い背中に腕を回し、尖った爪を立てる。容赦なく皮膚に食い込ませていく。

この人は可哀そうな人なのだ、と思う。そう思うことで美帆の心も身体も何倍にも熱くなっていく。全身が痺れるような快感に包まれていく。

でも……。

ほんとうに、この人は可哀そうな人なのだろうか?

五月二十八日

「米久」の古めかしい硝子戸を引いて外に出ると、優司は何気ない調子で右へと歩きだした。来

49

るときは、反対方向の言問通りでタクシーを降りたのだが、それが分かっているんだか分かって
いないんだか、悠然と歩を進めている。かなり酔っているのはたしかだ。

「久しぶりに酒ば飲んだ」

首を回すようなしぐさをしながら言う。店内では真っ赤だった顔もこうして街灯の下で見れば
それほど目立たない。

浅草名物の牛鍋を大勢の客に混じって広い座敷でつつきながら、ビール三本、日本酒を五合近
く飲んだ。美帆はビールをコップに二杯きりだから素面と変わらなかった。

「酔っ払ったでしょ」

横に並ぶ。

「やっぱうまか」

優司は一人頷いている。

「さすがの仲間君でも、病院では一滴も飲まなかったわけね」

そこで、彼は隣の美帆を見た。にやついている。いわくあり気な表情だった。

「俺、もう五年、酒ば飲んどらんかった」

「えっ」

思わず足を止めてしまった。

「嘘でしょ」

「腐れた腎臓も取ったし、今夜から解禁たい」

優司はますますにやにやしている。

50

「そうだったの」

美帆は呆れてしまう。食事の最中はそんなこと一言も口にしなかった。優司と二人だけで食事をするのも酒を飲むのも初めてだから、食べ物や酒の話も一通りした。

「仲間君は何のためにお酒を飲むの？」

美帆が訊ねたとき、優司は大して考えるでもなく、こう言った。

「俺、酒ば飲まんとうまく笑えん」

小柳なら分かってくれるやろうけど、俺には小さい頃から笑うようなことが何もなかったろう。気づいてみたら笑うことのできん男になっとった。それが、酒ば覚えてからは、酔っ払ったらバカ話もできるし、笑うこともできるごとなった。俺にとって酒は恩人みたいなもんよ。

美帆がその話にしんみりしていると、

「ちょっと泣かせる話やったろ」

優司は笑って、コップ酒をうまそうに飲み干した。

「五年ぶりだっていうのにあんなに飲んでよかったの」

美帆はふたたび歩き始めながら言った。

「全然平気や」

「だけど、顔、真っ赤だったよ」

「もう醒めてきたやろ」

不意に優司の顔が目の前に近づいてきた。酒臭い息がふりかかる。美帆は慌てて後ずさった。なるほど街灯の光に照らされた顔色はもう普通に戻っている。優司の酒は静かな酒だったが、そ

51

れでも表情やしぐさに明るさが生まれている。美帆にはそんな彼の変化が意外でもあり面白くもあった。

ひさご通りを二人で歩く。金曜日の夜とあって商店街は賑わっていた。このまましばらく行けば六区映画街のはずだ。

優司から連絡が来たのは一昨日だった。明日退院すると言われ、約束だから食事をご馳走したいと申し出た。ただし、当日は仕事が入っていたので今日にしてほしいと頼んだ。優司は退院後しばらくは都内の知人宅に世話になるつもりだからいつでも構わないと言った。

「何か食べたいものある?」

訊ねると、

「肉が食いたか。あとは酒があれば他はいらん」

と答えた。そのぶっきらぼうな物言いに美帆は一匹龍を背負った優司の広い背中をなぜか思い浮かべた。

幾つか考えて、「米久」に決めた。優司のようなやくざ者と二人連れなら浅草界隈が一番しっくりくるような気がした。

アーケードを歩いていると男たちが美帆に目を留める。少女時代からそれが普通になっているから気にはならない。ただ、今日はいつもと違った。一人のときや丈二と一緒のときは、往来のほぼ全員が卑猥な色の混じった視線を寄越してくる。だが、いまはちらりと横目に見て擦れ違う者が大半で、中には慌てて目を逸らす者もいた。

美帆は何だか気分がよかった。女優でもモデルでもタレントでも女子アナでもない自分がなぜ

52

じろじろ見られなくてはならないのか。どこか正式に文句が言える場所があれば、すぐにでも訴え出たいといつも思っている。

隣の優司は飄然としている。周囲に睨みをきかせたりしてはいない。それでもその全身から獰猛な気配がうっすらと滲み出ていた。上背は百七十五を超えるくらい。丈二に比べれば小柄だが、横合いから窺う胸板は分厚かった。高二の時、偶然再会した彼は、帯で縛った柔道着を肩に担いでいた。「柔道はずっと続けたの？」美帆が店で訊くと、「あのあとすぐに中退したけんね」と言って笑った。

丈二がどんな獣に譬えられるかはすぐに思いつかないが、優司はまるで豹のようだ。浅黒い精悍な顔からすれば黒豹。もしも上手に飼い馴らすことができれば、どんなにか便利で頼もしい存在だろう。

両脇の店々を冷やかしながら百五十メートルほどの距離をゆっくり歩き、ひさご通りの入口に差しかかったところで仲間優司は立ち止まった。

緑色の日よけがせり出した一軒の居酒屋の前だった。大衆酒蔵と看板にある。優司は何も言わずその店に入って行った。美帆もあとにつづく。まだ時刻は八時を回ったくらいだろう。「米久」に着いたのがちょうど五時だった。

優司は日本酒と、この店の名物らしい牛スジ煮込みを注文した。美帆はウーロン茶にする。店内は人でいっぱいだった。

コップ酒とウーロン茶で乾杯した。

「五年前、酔っ払っとるところを刺されたと。もともと相手の組とは、俺が仕掛けとった競売物

件絡みで半年くらい揉めに揉めとった。中洲の馴染みのクラブを出て、駐車場に待たせた車に乗り込む寸前やった。野郎が陰から飛び出して来た。向こうもビビっとったけん最初の一撃はかろうじてかわせた。手の届く間合いで睨み合った。まだ子供やったよ。短刀を両手で握り締めて真っ青な顔して震えとった。何やと思った。突進してきて、自分では避け切ったつもりやったんやけど、気づいたらこの右っ腹にドスがめり込んどった。アルコールのせいで出血がひどくて、手術室で二度心臓が止まったそうや」

一杯目を舐めるように飲みながら優司は淡々と言う。

「そいで酒もクスリも断った。死ぬ時くらい素面でいたかろ」

そこで一拍置く。

「て言うたらかっこよかけど、本当はいつまた襲われるか分からんと思ったら、怖くて飲めんようになった。飲んでも、笑うどころか冷や汗ばっかりたい」

愉快そうに笑う。

「もう大丈夫なの?」

どこまでが本気でどこからが冗談なのか美帆にはよく分からない。

「どうやら大丈夫のようや。飲んでも怖くならん」

そしてまた笑った。

優司はゆっくりと飲んだ。お代わりしながら美帆の質問にぽつぽつと答える。

中学校三年の時に転校していったのは、福岡市内に住んでいた父方の叔父が彼を引き取ったからだった。当時、それは美帆も聞いていたが、その後については、博多でやくざになったという

54

こと以外は何も知らなかった。

「仲間君、どうして高校辞めちゃったの」

高校二年で再会したとき、優司に退学する気配はまったく感じられなかった。

「叔父貴の借金のカタにマグロ船に売り飛ばされてしまったたい」

「マグロ船?」

突拍子もない話が飛び出して、聞き返す。

「叔父貴がやくざ相手の賭けマージャンで二百万の穴あけて、そのカタに俺ばマグロ船に売っ払ってしまったと。学校辞めさせられて、船に乗せられて、そいで二年近く日本に戻って来られんかった」

「嘘でしょう」

「嘘やない。マグロば追いかけて南極まで行ったばい。何度死にかけたか分からん。航海中に二人死んだ」

それから優司はマグロ船の様子を話してくれた。その詳細な内容からも彼が十八歳で土佐のマグロ船に乗り組み、二十歳になるまでの約二年間、世界の海を渡りながら、死と隣り合わせの過酷なマグロ延縄漁に携わったのは事実のようだった。

「私なんてその頃、東京の大学に行って、学生生活を満喫してたのに」

「それが当たり前やろ。特に小柳は秀才やったけん」

優司が身を乗り出してくる。

「つらか仕事やったけど勉強にもなった。酒も博打も覚えたし、陸(おか)に上がったあと面倒見てくれ

55

た兄貴分とも、この船で知り合ったんや」

兄貴分は、抗争相手の暴力団幹部を銃撃して重傷を負わせ、ほとぼりを冷ますためにマグロ船に乗っていたそうだ。

「ムショに比べれば、これでも天国やぞって兄貴がよう言いよらしたけど、実際、その通りやった」

どうやら優司には服役の経験もあるらしい。刑務所に入った人間と生まれて初めて口をきいた、と美帆は思う。

「酒に博打、それに女もでしょう」

懲役のことには触れず、そう言った。優司は激しく首を振った。

「一ヵ月以上かけて喜望峰回ったら、あとはマグロば追いかけてオーストラリア、インド洋、南極。女っ気なんかあるもんかい」

いかにも心外そうな口振りになっていた。

隅田川沿いの遊歩道をぶらぶら歩いている。遊歩道の一段上に堤があってこんもり葉を茂らせた桜木がずらりと並んでいる。対岸、墨田区側の堤も同様だった。

「ここは都内でも有数の桜の名所なの。墨堤の桜って聞いたことない?」

「あっちが向島やろ」

優司が指差して言う。

「そうそう」

56

「あそこの芸者は年増揃いや」

「そうなの」

「昔の話やけどな」

居酒屋を出たあと、六区から伝法院通りに入り、浅草駅を通り過ぎてそのまま川っぺりに降りた。十時を回って、吹き寄せる川風もすこし冷たくなっている。風の感触が頬や手足に心地よかった。

居酒屋でも三合は飲んだはずだが、優司はすっかり酔い醒めているようだった。足取りもしっかりしているし、次第に無口に戻ってきている。どこに向かうでもなく、いつ帰るでもなく歩いている。先日、慶応病院で会った時に気づいたのだが、美帆は優司と一緒にいても不思議と疲れなかった。億劫でも気詰まりでもない。彼といると何かしら元気が出るような気がする。たとえやくざでも中学からの同級生というのが気安さを生むのかもしれない。恋愛の対象外であることも大きい。

言問橋をくぐって隅田公園の方へ近づいていくと、川沿いにホームレスたちのダンボールハウスが立ち並んでいた。どれも青いビニールシートでしっかりと防水されている。

優司は平気な顔でハウスの前を通り過ぎていく。丈二と一緒にいるときも守られているという感覚はあるが、それとは決定的に異なる色合いがあった。譬えて言えば、格闘家や警察官と付き合っている女性はいつもこんな思いでいられるのかもしれない。きっと暴力というものに対する立ち位置の違いなのだろう。丈二が幾ら屈強でも、彼は暴力の遣い手ではない。彼といる限り、

57

暴力を振るわれる側に身を置かざるを得ない。優司はそうではなかった。彼はそもそも暴力を生業とする人間だ。いわば暴力のプロだった。その点では格闘家や警察官を凌ぐ存在でもある。

美帆はできるだけ寄り添うように歩いた。優司が手を伸ばしてくれれば腕を組んでもいいと思っていた。むろん彼はそんなことはしない。

騒ぎ声を耳にしたのは、ダンボールハウスの団地を五十メートルほど行き過ぎてからだった。左手の隅田公園の中から人の争うような物音が聞こえてきた。何かを乱打する鈍い音、気味悪い哄笑、悲鳴まじりの呻き声。誰かが複数の人間に襲われているのは明らかだった。

悲鳴が届いた瞬間に優司の耳が尖るのがはっきり分かった。直後、右腕を強い力で摑まれた。優司は美帆を引っ張って駆け足で公園の中へと踏み入っていく。まるで目標をすでに捉えているかのように、立ち止まることも速度を緩めることもない。灌木の植わった園内を突き切り、広いグラウンドの隅まで来て、ようやく止まった。

四人の男たちがうずくまった一人を取り囲み、暴行していた。

かわるがわる蹴りつけられているのはホームレスの男のようだ。両腕で頭を抱え、ひぃーひぃーとかすれた叫びを上げていた。四人組の方は少年たちだ。背格好からして高校生くらいだろう。

一人が金属バットを持っていた。

「こら、くず、人間のくず、死ねよ、こら」

けらけら笑いながら男を蹴り上げている。悲鳴が上がるたびに笑い声が高く、大きくなった。少年たちにズボンを剝ぎ取られたのだろう。明かりは遠くの街灯きりだが、どうやらホームレスは下半身裸のようだ。

58

「きたねえチンポしやがってよお。こら。ゴミがいっちょまえにチンポなんかぶらさげてんじゃねえよ」

バットを持った少年がそう言って、バットヘッドをホームレスの股間にねじ込んでいる。

そういう光景を、美帆は一人で見た。というのも、一瞬後にはその光景に音もなく優司の姿が加わったからだ。

優司はバットを持った少年に背後から襲いかかると、あっという間にそれを奪い取った。あと一方的な暴力の嵐が吹き荒れただけだ。優司のバットは情け容赦がなかった。全員が頭をはもう一撃された。頭蓋骨と金属バットがぶつかるゴンという音が静かなグラウンドに響く。ゴン、ゴン、ゴンとリズミカルで小気味よかった。

こんなに残酷な場面に立ち会うのは初めてだったが、なぜか恐怖心は皆無だった。それよりも奇妙な興奮の波が美帆の全身に広がっていた。

少年たちはものの十数秒でその場に昏倒した。

そこからが無残だった。

優司はグリップエンドをハンカチで丁寧に拭うと、バットを静かに地面に置き、頭から血を流して転げまわっている少年一人一人の足を摑んで引きずり回した。腹や顔を何度も踏みつけて弱らせ、傍らにしゃがみ込むと、彼らの右腕の肘を自分の腿に乗せて順番にへし折っていった。骨が折れるバキッという湿った音が四回鳴った。少年たちの絶叫は凄まじかった。

そばに落ちていたズボンを穿かせ、ホームレスの男を背負って、優司が戻って来た。顔色もまったく変わらず、息も上がっていない。それどころか額に汗すら滲ませていなかった。

59

背負われたホームレスは呼吸を荒くしている。だが、見たところどこからも出血はないようだった。とっくに五十は超えている感じだが、意外にこざっぱりした身なりをしていた。着衣は埃だらけだが、髪と爪はきれいに切り揃えられている。顔もすこし腫れていたがそれほど垢じみてはいない。

「おやっさん、どっか痛いとこないか」

優司が足元に目を落としたまま話しかける。

「ない」

男はしっかりした声で答えた。

「兄さんがすぐ来てくれたからな」

つけ加える。

「そうか。そりゃよかった」

優司の声はとても優しい。

「あの子たち、放っておいていいの」

地面に転がったままの少年たちの方を見ながら美帆は言った。頭の方は手加減して殴っといた。携帯使って、ダチ公か救急車くらいそのうち呼べるやろ」

「心配せんでよか。

まあ、自業自得よね、と美帆も思った。手加減したのなら死んだりはしないだろう。

「おやっさん、そこのハウスに住んどるとね」

「ああ」

60

「やったらこのままおんぶしていってやる」

「すまんねぇ」

「よかよか」

川べりの遊歩道を引き返して、男をダンボールハウスの団地まで送っていった。ハウスの中に男を入れて出てくると、優司は足早に街中へと向かう。美帆も黙ってついて行った。時計を見ると、十一時になろうとしていた。

優司は店を見繕って仲見世通りを歩いている。ほとんどがシャッターを下ろしているがまだ開けている所もわずかにあった。一軒の土産物屋に入る。出てきた店員に何か話しかける。奥に引っ込んだ店員がしばらくして戻ってきた。手には一本の棒のようなものを持っていた。優司は包装を断ると、柄の部分を両手で握り込んでまっすぐに構えた。一つ頷いて財布を取り出し、その白木の木刀を買った。

「それどうするの」

美帆は不安になって訊ねた。まさかとは思うが、少年たちをこの木刀でもう一度懲らしめにいくつもりではないのか。

「おやっさんの背中見えたか」

優司はさきほど握った柄の部分をハンカチで拭い、それで柄をくるむ。

「いいえ」

「きれいな観音様ば背負っとらした」

美帆には優司が何を言っているのか分からなかった。

61

「あの人も昔はやくざ者やったんやろ。俺と同類たい」

「じゃあ、その木刀、あのおじさんに渡すの」

優司が口許をわずかに切り上げる。

「今度、連中が来たら、これで一人叩き殺せばよか」

右手に提げた木刀をひょいと持ち上げてみせた。

六月八日

古市珠代は眠らない。

初めて一緒に仕事をしたのは四年前だった。以後は三ヵ月から四ヵ月に一冊のペースで彼女の料理本やムックを作ってきた。多いときは年間で三十冊近い本を出す人だから、料理研究家・古市珠代の全仕事を美帆が独占しているわけではない。

二〇〇〇年、『電子レンジ　目からウロコのクッキング』を美帆は担当した。古市珠代の本を手がけ始めて三冊目だった。これが古市の出世作となった。彼女はテレビの料理番組や女性誌、料理雑誌でひっぱりだことなり、一躍、料理研究家の中でも五指に入る人気者となった。

美帆にとってもこの本の成功は大きかった。前の年に勤めていた出版社を辞め、片瀬に戻ったあとロンドンに半年近く滞在し、二〇〇〇年の年明けとともに再び上京した。母校のお茶の水女

62

子大に聴講生として通いながら臨床心理士を目指すつもりでいたのだが、かつての同僚にぽっぽつ仕事を頼まれるようになり、気楽な学生暮らしとあって、小遣い稼ぎのつもりで手伝っているうちに注文が殺到し始めた。そのきっかけを作ってくれたのが『電子レンジ　目からウロコのクッキング』だった。

カップ一杯の水にかつおぶし一パックを入れて五〇〇Wの電子レンジで一分加熱する。それだけで煮出したものと変わらぬ美味しい出汁が取れる。わたしと種を抜いた四〇〇グラムのかぼちゃは皮を外側にターンテーブルの端に置き、レンジぶたをして五分加熱する。これでどんなに硬いかぼちゃもスイスイ好みのサイズに切り分けられる。熟れていないアボカドやキウィは一個につき一、二分加熱する。あっという間に追熟されて食べごろになる。ピーラーで皮を縞状に剥いたきゅうりを厚さ一・五センチほどの輪切りにし、玉ねぎの薄切りと一緒に耐熱ボウルに移す。一味唐辛子、胡椒を少々振って、きゅうり一本につき市販のすし酢を大さじ三の割合でかけ、オーブンペーパーと皿でおとしぶたをして、二分加熱する。それを冷蔵庫で冷やせばしっかり漬け込んだものと同じ味のピクルスが出来上がる。

いまでは「古市マジック」とまで称されるようになった彼女オリジナルの電子レンジレシピは、一人暮らしのOLや子育てを終えた夫婦、さらにはダイエットや養生のために油分を極力控えたい人などに大歓迎された。家事に追われる主婦たちも、解凍やあたためくらいにしか使ってこなかったレンジの簡単で便利な利用法にいっぺんで魅了された。

二年前には、レンジを使って大幅に発酵時間を短縮し、四十分程度でパンが焼けるという「電子レンジパン」のレシピ集を出版し、古市珠代の名前は一層世間に広まった。この本を一緒に作

63

ったのも美帆だった。

古市珠代は福岡の出身で、いまも福岡市内に立派なキッチンスタジオを備えた自宅兼事務所を構えている。西麻布にも大きなスタジオを持ち、彼女は福岡と東京を往復しながら両方で料理教室を主宰し、テレビ出演、本や雑誌の取材、商品開発、講演などを寸暇もなくこなしつづけていた。

福岡市の隣、片瀬市出身の美帆は同郷でもあった。

今日も午前九時に西麻布のスタジオにスタッフ全員が集合し、撮影に入る前の簡単な打ち合わせを行なった。白のカットソーに白地にベージュのストライプの入ったズボン、いつもの胸当て付きの真っ白なエプロン姿で現れた古市珠代は、相変わらずの溌剌とした生気を発散していた。両腕でたくさんの本を抱えている。

「小柳さん、お元気でしたか?」

三月に料理本を一冊作って以来、二ヵ月半ぶりの再会なので古市は開口一番言ってくる。手の中の本を作業台にどんと積むと、広い台の周囲に腰かけていた今日のスタッフたちにさっそく配り始めた。『古市珠代の英語で上達!日本料理』、『古市珠代の糖尿病に負けない絶品レシピ』、『古市珠代さんちの日替わり季節小鉢』。どれも美帆が他の仕事をしていたあいだに別のフードライターや編集者たちの手で作られた本だった。古市珠代は今年で六十三歳になる。四人の子供を育て上げ、大手鉄鋼メーカーに勤める夫を主婦として支えながら料理の道を究めてきた。本格的に料理研究家としてデビューしたのは、子育てを終え、嫁ぎ先の両親の介護を済ませ、夫が定年で会社を辞めた五十代半ばからだった。

64

〈一年三百六十五日、休みなく毎日二十時間働く〉、〈食事の時間以外に休みは取らない。私の辞書に休憩という文字はない〉と彼女は著書や雑誌のインタビューで公言しているが、そば近くで見てきて、その言葉に嘘偽りはないと美帆は確言できる。

古市珠代はほんとうに眠らない人だった。

「先生、この『英語で上達！日本料理』、とてもいいですね」

〈Mixing tofu in with the meat when making hamburgers lowers the fat and the cholesterol.〉

豆腐入りハンバーグの英文解説を読みながら美帆は言った。

「そうでしょう。ニューヨークでお料理教室を開くとすごい人数が押しかけるんだけど、生徒さんたちが、英語で書かれた日本料理のレシピが全然ないっていうのよ」

欧米でも、より自然に近く、ダイエット効果、制がん効果の高い日本食のニーズはどんどん高まっている。こうした試みには将来性があると美帆は感じた。

「アメリカで発売するものは、もちろん日本語は全部抜いて、英語だけよ」

渡された本には、なるほど〈豆腐を混ぜて作るハンバーグは、低脂肪、低コレステロール。〉といった対訳が付されていた。

他のスタッフは無言で本のページを捲っていた。今日は、婦人誌の料理ページの撮影を行なうが、それとは別に一カットだけ正月号用の大皿メニューも撮ることになっていた。料理ページの方は〈火を使わずにレンジでラク　"チン"　みんな百円台の「居酒屋おかず32」〉という企画だから、ページ全体の構成はちょうどファミレスのメニューのような感じになる。写真はほとんどが切り抜きで使うので、それほど手の込んだ撮影の必要はなかった。ただ、夕方までに三十三品を

65

作ってもらい、それを順次カメラに収めるとなるとスタッフ一同、相当なスピードを要求される。

写真家は人気の料理カメラマン、中村卓也だった。多忙をきわめている上に、こだわりの写真を追求する人だから、本当はこうした数をこなす仕事を頼むのは気が引けるのだが、古市先生の指名とあっては、無理を承知で引っ張り出すしかなかった。

彼はいつものアシスタントの女の子を連れてきている。

あとは婦人誌のフリー編集者の有賀佳恵、器やグラス、クロス、ランチョン、カトラリー類などをそろえてくれるフードスタイリストの杉田潤子、そして美帆の三人だった。有賀も杉田も再三チームを組んできた気心の知れた人たちだ。古市事務所の料理スタッフ三人は、美帆たちが到着した時にはすでに奥のキッチンに入り、今日の料理のための仕込みに余念がなかった。

料理スタッフの一人が出してくれた中国茶を飲みながら打ち合わせを始める。メニューの確認や差し替え、器の選定などは事前に済ませている。七月売りの号なので、古市側から出されたメニューの中の数品を夏野菜を使った料理に変更してもらっていた。それでも一応、この場で最終の確認は取っておく。

古市は一ページ一ページ丁寧に目を通していく。

編集の有賀が大体の構成をレイアウト用紙に手書きしたものを古市に見せる。タイトルやそれぞれの料理のスケッチが上手に描きこまれていた。ページ数は七ページ。

「はい、よろしゅうございます」

古市珠代が大きな声で言い、立ち上がった。それを合図に全員が席を立つ。時刻は九時半ちょ

66

うど。古市はスタジオ中央のオープンキッチンの前に陣取る。料理スタッフが右奥の別のキッチンでレシピ通りに取り揃えた材料を次々に古市のもとへと運び、さっそく調理が始まった。

最初の一品はキムチを使った「韓国豆腐」。一番目が「アボカド納豆のり巻き」。そして「ツナおかきレタス」、「まぐろユッケ」、「簡単つくね」、「むきエビと枝豆の串焼き」、「プチトマトの豚肉巻き」、「コロコロ野菜のチーズフォンデュ」とみるみるうちに料理が出来上がっていく。

美帆はノートに記したレシピに目をやりながら、そばで彼女の手元を注視する。わずかでもレシピと異なる調味料や材料を使ったときは、すぐにその場で確認する。「むきエビと枝豆の串焼き」では、空のボウルにお酒を注ぐと、古市は酒でエビのぬめりを取り始めた。「お酒で洗った

「だって、水がないじゃない」

古市はやや怒気を含んだ口振りで言う。水を張ったボウルを手元に用意しておかなかったスタッフのミスに苛立っているのだ。

「じゃあ、エビは水洗いのままで構いませんね」

「ええ、もちろん」

手を動かしながら古市は顔を上げて笑みを浮かべた。

鶏肉を使った最後の大皿料理の撮影が終わったのが午後六時ちょうどだった。ベテラン揃いのスタッフだから小さなトラブルもなく順調に撮影は進んだ。それでも三十三品を一日で撮り上げるのは大変だった。皆それぞれに疲労の色を滲ませていたが、例によって古市珠代だけは意気軒昂だった。半日のあいだ立ち詰めで三十三種もの料理を作り、他にも全員の昼食用に「ボロネー

方がいいですか?」と美帆は口を挟む。レシピでは「水で洗う」となっているからだ。

67

ゼのマッシュポテト載せ」を大きなバット二つ分オーブンで焼き上げ、撮影終了間際には愛用の

アイスクリームメーカーでこしらえたアイスクリームに手製のクランベリーソースをたっぷりか

けたものを皆に振る舞った。誰よりも疲れているはずの古市が、誰よりも元気だった。

古市は「寝ても醒めても料理のことを考えている」とよく言う。東京―福岡を週に一度は必ず

往復しているが、その移動の機中でも眠ったことなど一度もない。機内誌を見れば、ちょっとし

た記事に料理のヒントを摑み、八百屋やスーパーでかぼちゃ一つ、トマト一個見てもあれこれと

新しい料理のアイデアを考える。彼女が初めて料理に手を染めたのは小学校二年生のときだった。

「料理は際限なく思いつく」と言う。思いつくたびに手近なメモ用紙などにレシピを書きつけて、

それをタイピングする。もうその数だけで十万件を超えている。他にも、若い頃から集めたレシ

ピが山ほどある。雑誌や新聞、料理本の切り抜きやコピーなどだが、その一つ一つが品目別に仕

分けされ、分厚いコクヨのバインダーにファイリングされていた。彼女がそうやって収集したレ

シピはすでに三十万件を突破していた。全国各地での講演や実演が一年に百回以上。東京滞在中

は今日のような撮影を二日に一回はこなし、料理教室も福岡と東京で月に一週間ずつ開いている。

そのうえ、最近は幼児向けの料理教室、ニューヨークでのアメリカ人相手の料理教室なども定期

的に行なっていた。

素早く機材をまとめると、中村たちが真っ先に引きあげていった。それから杉田、有賀も帰っ

ていった。三人の料理スタッフは奥のキッチンで黙々と後片づけをやっている。

「小柳さん、ちょっと二階でお茶でも飲んで行きませんか」

ようやくエプロンを取った古市珠代が誘ってきた。

68

二階の事務所は広いスペースのほとんどが書棚で埋め尽くされているのは四千冊を優に超えるレシピのバインダーだった。入口のドアを開けてすぐ左に作業台があり、壁際に小さなソファが置かれていた。一番奥が秘書の席で、真ん中が古市の席、手前は「フルイチ・アソシエーツ」のもう一人の代表取締役である古市善彦、つまり古市珠代の夫の席だった。善彦は珠代が東京にいるあいだは福岡にいる。珠代が福岡に帰っているときはこの事務所に詰めていることが多い。夫婦はそうやって交互に上京し、スムーズに会社の運営が行なえるよう配慮している。経理関係を含めてフルイチ・アソシエーツの会社業務の全般は善彦が引き受けている。

事務所には誰もいなかった。専属秘書も帰ったのだろう。古市が紅茶を淹れてくれた。作業台に差し向かいで座って、あたたかい紅茶をすする。

「ずいぶんご無沙汰だったけど、元気にしてたの?」

今朝、顔を合わせたときと同じ質問をしてきた。美帆はカップを口許に寄せながら曖昧に頷いた。

「あんまり元気でもないみたいね」

古市が頰笑んだ。

「どうしたの。何か悩みがあるんだったら話してみたら」

美帆は古市珠代を尊敬していた。その徹底した人生には深い敬意を抱いている。ただ、彼女のように生きたいと思ったことはなかった。

「新聞記者の彼氏とうまくいってないの」

69

言われて美帆は頷いた。話してどうなるものでもないし、この程度のことが悩みと言えるかどうかは疑問だが、古市にはこれまでも仕事のことや丈二との関係など、隠さずに打ち明けてきた。

丈二は今回の参議院選挙への出馬を断念した。公認は水上議員の女婿が受けることになった。決まったのは六月に入ってすぐだった。当分はいままで通り、政治記者として活動することになり、堀米幹事長が共同通信の編集局長、政治部長を招いて、直々に丈二の不出馬を伝え、彼の今後の処遇について善処を求めたということだった。

水上側に軍配が上がったのは、総理から直接の要請が堀米幹事長に対して行なわれたからだという。

「水上は郵政省の役人時代に、先代の愛人の面倒をずっと見ていたらしいんだ。堀米さんはそれ以上言わなかったが、他の筋から聞いた話だと、どうやら愛人とのあいだには隠し子がいて、先代が死ぬとき、その隠し子のことも水上は託されていたらしい」

総理の父親は、自民党の副総裁まで上り詰め、郵政族のドンと呼ばれた大物政治家だった。自身の境遇と重なるところがあったためか、一連の経緯を知って、丈二には吹っ切れた感じがあった。しかし、政治家への転身を諦めたわけではなかった。三年後の参議院選挙を睨むのではなく、いずれ行なわれる解散・総選挙に照準を合わせているようだった。

丈二はしきりに結婚したいと言い募っていた。「ちゃんとした形が作りたい。もうあとがないんだ」と美帆の決心を求めてきた。人生の最大のチャンスを失い、喪失感が大きいのだろう。せめて一つくらい結果を出したいと考えているようだった。今度ばかりは適当にはぐらかすわけにもいかない気がしている。

70

「だったら結婚すればいいじゃないの」

美帆の話を聞いて古市はあっさり言った。

「小柳さん、今年でお幾つ?」

と訊いてくる。

「十二月で三十五です」

なあんだ、という顔を古市は作った。

「じゃあ、選択の余地はないわね。その歳だともう子供を産むぎりぎりなのよ。先ずは結婚して、子供を作って、女の人生はそれからよ。私を見ていたら分かるでしょう」

古市の力強い瞳が美帆にはまぶしい。

「前にも話したかもしれないけど、私は二度、この仕事を辞めようと決心したことがあるの。一度は病気。もう一度は夫からあることを言われたとき」

美帆は古市の顔を真っ直ぐに見返した。病気のことは知っていたが、あとの話は初耳だった。

「まだ私が四十代の頃のことよ。全国の料理コンテストでかたっぱしから優勝して、ようやく雑誌や新聞から取材が舞い込み始めたの。私は嬉しくなって、ちょうどその頃は東京住まいだったから婦人誌の料理ページなんかにちょくちょく顔を出すようになってた。そしたら、ある日、夫からものすごい剣幕で叱られたの」

当時、役員就任寸前のところまできていた善彦は、社内で懇意の役員に呼び止められてこう言われた。「きみの奥さんもなかなかご活躍らしいね。家内が雑誌を見て驚いていたよ」。善彦は帰

宅すると血相変えて珠代に抗議した。

「きみが好きなことをやるのは構わない。大いにやればいい。だけど、僕の仕事の邪魔をするのだけは止めてくれ」

それまで聞いたこともないような厳しい口調だった。

「古い体質の会社だったから、どんな仕事だとしても女房を外で働かせてる男は、それだけで役員失格なのよ。夫から、どうして顔や名前をそのまま出すんだ、せめて僕の肩書くらいどうして伏せてくれなかったんだって言われて、私はほんとうに悪かったと思ったの。始めていた料理教室もすぐに畳んで、雑誌の仕事も全部断って、料理のこととはすっぱり諦めた。そのうち夫がまた北九州に赴任することになったから、そのまま私も一緒に福岡に戻ったのよ」

それから夫が退職するまでの十年近く、古市珠代は地元で細々と料理教室を開いてはいたもののメディアに登場することは一切控えた。

「あのとき悔しくなかったと言えば嘘になる。夫のためと割り切ろうとしたけど、簡単に割り切れるものじゃなかった。でも、私は夫や子供のために精一杯のことをやったし、我慢もした。そうやって、できない我慢だってしてきた。そしたら、たいがいのことは我慢できたし、気持ちさえ切り換えられたらいつでも新しくやり直せるってことも分かった。結局、自分が本当に好きなことだったら、いつからだって始められるのよ。結婚や出産、子育てが足かせだなんて思ってる人も多いみたいだけど、言ってみれば、それは全然違う。人間は自分のためだったらどんなことでもできるの。幾ら夫のため、子供のためと力んでみても、自分の命と引き替えっこは絶対にできないでしょう。だから、自分の精一杯を超えて、言ってみれば命と引き替えにできるのって自分のことだけ。だから、自分の

72

夢や希望の実現のためなら、どんな境遇にいたって、そんなの撥ね除けて何でもやれるのよ。それを周りの誰かのせいや環境のせいにするのは、なまけている証拠。たとえ家事や子育てに追われていても、夫も子供も一日数時間は必ず眠る。その時間だけは自分の時間にできる。眠ることさえしなければ、どんなときだって好きなことができるじゃない。一日あたり睡眠時間を三時間削れば、一ヵ月で九十時間。一年で千八十時間。一日の標準労働時間である八時間で割れば、一年で百三十五日分の時間が手に入るのよ。その生活を十年つづければ千三百五十日。つまり四年分近く、夫が会社で働いているのと同じだけの時間が作り出せる。その四年間があれば、やりたいことなんて何だってできるでしょう。人間はそんなに眠らなくていいのよ。一日七、八時間は眠らなきゃ駄目なんて言ってる人は、本当にやりたいことを見つけていないだけ。本当にやりたいことさえ見つけられたら、眠るなんてもったいなくて、誰もそんなことに八時間も使おうなんて思わなくなるものよ」

　古市はいつもの調子で矢継ぎ早に喋った。美帆は黙って拝聴するだけだった。

「とにかくさっさと結婚して赤ちゃんを産みなさい。出産だけはタイムリミットがあるのよ。他のことは幾らだってあとから取り返せるんだから。女は男と違って一つの会社に縛られて、そこでうまくいかなきゃもうおしまいってわけじゃないでしょう。自分の夢を見つける方法なんて幾らでもあるし、何度失敗しても、最後まで探しつづけることもできるじゃない」

　彼女の言うとおりだろうな、と話を聞きながら美帆は思った。いまさら丈二との結婚に躊躇（ためら）う理由などない。二年前に再び付き合おうと決めた瞬間から、こうなることを予期していたし、それが差し迫った現実となると、にわかに迷いが生のように自身を追い込んでもきた。しかし、それが差し迫った現実となると、にわかに迷いが生

73

じてくる。丈二と結婚することによって自分は過去を取り戻せるかもしれない。ただ、その代償としてこれからの未来を失うのではないか。過去を回復することに憂き身をやつしたがゆえに、この九年間で再生させた真実の自己を捨て去ってしまうのではないか。どうしてもその危惧を美帆は拭い去ることができなかった。

さらに、丈二の態度や物言いにも昔と変わらぬ横暴さが窺われた。美帆との結婚などは、それに比べれば添え物程度に過ぎないとでもいうような、そんな傲慢さが透けて見えた。だからこそ、さっさと片づけてしまいたいし、片づけてしまえると思い込んでいるのではないか。

そうした凡庸な相手であれば、古市の言うごとく、存分に割り切って対応すべきなのかもしれない。子供を産み、人生の本当の目的を見つける手段としての結婚でも構わない、と古市は言っていた。

だが、果たしてそれでいいのだろうか。

「あなたは美しすぎるのよね。それがあなたの不幸なのかもしれない。いまだって女優さんになれるくらいきれいだもの」

美帆が物思いに耽っていると、古市珠代がぽつりと言った。

「ほんとうは、もっといい仕事ができる人なのに」

そして、さらに励ますような口調で彼女はつけ加えた。

「美人はなかなか幸福になれないの。それだけは肝に銘じておきなさい」

74

七月十八日

東京は快晴だったが、西に向かうにつれて曇っていった。京都駅のホームに降り立って見上げた空は、いまにも降り出しそうな暗い雲に覆われていた。

奈良行きの近鉄特急に乗り換えるために、構内を歩いているとき、美帆の携帯が鳴った。時刻は十一時半になろうとしていた。

受話口を耳に当てると母の早苗の沈んだ声が聞こえてきた。

「美帆ちゃん、おとうさんが倒れたわ。いま市民病院で緊急手術してるの。脳溢血だって。仕事たいへんだろうけどすぐに帰ってきて」

ディスプレーに母の名前が表示されたときから、きっと父に何か起きたのだろうと感じていたので美帆はさして動揺しなかった。

「容態はどうなの？　危険な状態？」

「分からない。正也に聞いたら、搬送が早かったのなら命に別状はないだろうって」

「いつ倒れたの」

「今朝。朝ご飯食べて、今日は熊本だから八時には出る予定だったの。なかなか書斎から出てこないから行ってみたら倒れてた」

「意識はあったの」

75

「ええ。左の手足が痺れてきてるから脳溢血だっておとうさん本人が言って、それですぐに救急車を呼んだの」

「そう」

「今日、帰って来れる」

「大丈夫よ。いま京都なの。これから急いで新幹線に乗る。正也も戻るんでしょう」

「ええ。病院から大至急羽田に向かうって」

正也は東京医科歯科大の医局に勤めている。医師である彼に母が先に一報したのは当然のことだった。

「じゃあ、直接市民病院に行く。おかあさん、気をしっかり持ってね」

「分かってる」

そう言って母の方から電話は切れた。

携帯をたたんで、父は今年幾つだろうか、と思った。たしか六十六歳だ。まだ死ぬにはすこし早い。

すぐそばにいた丈二が、

「おとうさんが倒れたの」

と確認してきた。

「脳溢血みたい。いま手術中だって」

「こっちのことは気にしなくていい。早く帰ってあげないと。おやじとお袋には俺の方から説明しておくから」

76

丈二はついて行くとは言わなかった。明日十九日は、去る十一日の第二十回参議院選挙で初当選した水上の女婿、青木雄一郎議員の県連主催の祝賀会が奈良市内で開かれる。次期衆議院選挙への出馬をもくろむ丈二としては、いままでの経緯からしても、どうしても顔を出さなくてはならない会だった。

「一緒に行けなくてごめん」

新幹線のホームで電車に乗る直前、丈二は言った。

「私こそほんとうにごめんなさい」

美帆は頭を下げた。丈二の両親に挨拶に赴く当日に倒れるとは、なんて間の悪い父親だろう、と思っていた。

三時半に片瀬市民病院に到着した。手術は終わり、父は集中治療室で眠っていた。医師の説明によれば後遺症の有無はともかく手術自体は成功したとのことだった。ただ、開頭してみると出血の範囲は予想外に大きかったそうだ。

先着していた正也が説明を聞いたという。弟からの報告だったので美帆は一安心した。早苗は家に戻っていた。混乱と憔悴が激しく、正也が言い含めて帰らせたようだった。

「かあさんにはこういうの無理だろ」

と正也は静かに言った。

「麻痺とか残るのかしら」

「分からないな」

「半身不随とかになったら、おとうさん、気が狂うわ」

77

「自殺するだろうな、たぶん」

集中治療室の前の廊下で、長椅子に並んで腰かけて美帆たちは話した。

その日の夕方、父は意識を取り戻した。翌日の昼には個室に移ることができた。丈二からは二度ほど連絡があり、父の容態を伝えた。「とりあえずよかったな」と彼は言い、「うちの親たちも心配してくれてるよ」とつけ加えた。

一体、誰のことを、どう心配しているというの？　と美帆は思った。

十九日は海の日だった。休日の病院は閑散としていた。早苗と正也は昼間から父に付き添っていた。夕方、美帆と交代して二人は引きあげた。

美帆が行ったときは父は眠っていた。昨夜までの顔のむくみもだいぶ取れていた。頭には包帯が巻かれ、左腕からは点滴のラインが伸びていた。父は面高の整った顔立ちをしている。寝顔を見ればまるで外人のようだ。

事実、父の身体にはポーランド人の血が流れていた。父の祖父がフンボルト大学医学部に学び、そのときポーランド系ドイツ人の女性と結婚していた。小柳家はこの曾祖父の代からずっと医者の家だった。祖父も医者だったし、父も医者になった。正也も東京医科歯科大学を卒業し、腫瘍内科医の道を歩んでいる。三年前にニューヨークのスローンケタリング癌研究所に留学し、抗がん剤治療の最先端を学んで、昨秋に東京に戻って来たばかりだった。

父と母とは、父が東京の病院で勤務医をしているときに知り合った。母は精神科の看護婦だった。ベッド数が千を超える大病院だったが、母はその病院で働く看護婦の中で誰よりも美しかったという。

78

確かに母はきれいな人だった。太腿の痣を取るために入院したとき、手術の前の晩に彼女は言った。

「顔と身体は女の武器よ。きれいな女が顔を磨くのは当たり前。胸の大きな女が胸を寄せるのも当たり前。そういうことを軽蔑する女は絶対に幸福にならないわ」

美帆は子供の頃から、母に似ていると言われていた。「やっぱりおかあさんが別嬪やから」といつも言われた。事情を知らない人たちは本当の母子だと信じていた。「あなたは私にそっくりね」とよく言った。その言葉を聞くとまるで本物の子供になれたようで美帆は嬉しかった。だが、もっと嬉しかったこともある。

幼稚園に通っているときだった。クリスマスの発表会で美帆はマリア様の役を演じた。長いブルーのドレスを着て髪には金色のティアラを飾った。舞台を降りると、父が待ち受けていた。父は満面の笑みを浮かべて美帆を抱き上げ、耳元で囁いた。

「お前はかあさんより何倍もきれいだ」

美帆はこの父の言葉を忘れたことはない。

花瓶の水をかえたり、壁際のソファで雑誌に目を通したりして父が目覚めるまで時間を潰した。

一時間ほどして父は目を開けた。

「美帆だけか」

すこししゃがれた声で父が最初に言った。

「うん。おかあさんたちは帰った」

「そうか」

父はほっとしたような小さな息を吐いた。

「どう、つらくない?」

美帆の問いかけに父は返事をしなかった。雑誌をソファの前のテーブルに置いて、美帆はベッドサイドの丸椅子に移動した。顔を覗きこむと父と目が合った。

「おとうさん、大丈夫?」

父は小さく頷いた。そして、

「美帆、かあさんに負けるんじゃないぞ」

ぽつりと言った。

唐突な言葉に何も返せなかった。

「あの人は可哀そうな人だ。あんなふうにしてしまったのはとうさんのせいだ。だが、とうさんだけが悪かったわけじゃない。あの人の一番の間違いは、そのことを決して認めようとしないことだ」

父は淡々と話す。手術の影響で頭が混乱しているわけではなさそうだった。

「スプーンはおかあさんが二階のベランダから投げたんだよ。私、この目で見たの」

美帆は初めて、そのことを口にした。

「そうらしいな」

父は意外なことを言った。

「どうして、おとうさん知ってるの」

「正也から聞いた」

80

「正也が何で知っているの」

そのことは早苗と美帆以外には誰も知らないはずだった。

「正也はかあさんから聞いたそうだ」

どうして？　美帆はすこし当惑した。小さい頃から可愛がっていた飼い猫のスプーンは母から投げ落とされて左の後ろ足が不自由になった。以来、スプーンは死ぬまで早苗に近づこうとはしなかった。

父は女性関係の派手な人だった。結婚したあとも女出入りが絶えず、母は、いつも苛々していた。夫婦喧嘩もしょっちゅうだった。それでも、二人とも子供たちに八つ当たりするようなことは滅多になかった。

だが、母がスプーンにした仕打ちを美帆は決して許していないように。正也が溺れた自分を助けようとしなかった父を決して許せなかった。正也は一度言ったことがある。

「とうさんは僕が死んでもよかったのさ。僕は姉ちゃんと違って、あのかあさんの産んだ子だからね」

彼のこの見方は半分当たっていると美帆も思っていた。

「お前は、結婚したくないのか」

しばしの沈黙のあと父が言った。どうしてこんな話をするのだろう。まるでこれから死んでいく人みたいだ。

「そうじゃないけど」

「無理にすることはないぞ」

「分かってる」

「人間は所詮、一人ぼっちだ。誰かと一緒になって余計そう感じることもある」

「さみしい話ね」

「さみしくなんかないさ」

父の表情は明るかった。大きな荷物を肩から降ろした人のようだった。

「おとうさんはおかあさんより愛した人がいたの」

美帆は訊く。

「いたよ。その人と一緒になればよかったといまでも思っている」

「どうしてそうしなかったの」

「おかあさんがいたからね」

「でも、それなら別れればよかったじゃない」

「そしたら死ぬと言われた。あの人はきっと死んだと思う。まだお前も正也もいないときのことだったから」

「その人はいまどうしてるのかしら」

「もう死んでいた。久しぶりに会って分かったよ」

美帆は父の言うことが理解できなかった。

「昨日、彼女が来てくれたんだ。いろんなことを教えてくれた」

父は目を細めながら言った。

「美帆。私はお前のことを他人と思ったことは一度としてないよ。ほんとうにそう思えなかった。

どうしても自分の娘としか思えなかったんだ」

「おとうさん」

「そんなヘンな顔するな。別に頭がおかしくなったわけじゃないんだから」

そこで父は笑った。

「もし、誰かいい相手が欲しいなら、とうさんがお前に一番似合った人をいずれ見つけてあげるよ」

やっぱりこの人はもうすぐ死ぬのだ、と美帆は思った。

翌朝の午前六時、病院から自宅に電話が入った。父が二度目の脳内出血で息を引き取ったという連絡だった。

七月二十三日

金曜日の晩だというのに「あかり」は空いていた。

優司がドアを開けて入っていくとカウンターのスツールに座っていた女性が出迎えてくれた。

店内はそれほど広くはなかった。左手に七、八人は腰掛けられるカウンターがあり、その右がフロアになっていた。壁に沿って凹型にソファがつづき、手前にはL字型のテーブルと椅子、その先には普通のテーブルと椅子が三セット並んでいた。フロアの席数は全部で二十くらい。カウン

83

ターを入れてもせいぜい三十人も入れば満員の店だった。奥の壁は鏡張りで、右手にはレーザー

カラオケを据えつけた一段高いステージが設けられていた。内装は濃い目のグレーで統一され、

フロアの絨毯だけがベージュだった。客は奥の席に背広姿の三人連れがいるだけで、女の子二人

が相手をしていた。カウンターには若いバーテンが一人。美帆たちに近づいてきた着物姿の女性

は三十歳は過ぎているだろう。なかなかの美人だった。

この人がリリコが言っていた「かすみさん」か、と美帆は思った。

「いらっしゃい」

かすみが優司と美帆の両方に笑顔を向けた。

「彼女がこの前話した、小柳美帆さん。俺の同級生」

優司が照れくさそうに言う。かすみは着物の胸元から名刺を一枚抜いた。

「このたびは御愁傷さまでした。一度だけでしたけど、小柳先生にもお越しいただいたことがあ

るんですよ」

受け取った名刺には「あかり　佐野かすみ」と記されていた。

「そうだったんですか」

「はい」

それからしばしかすみは無言で美帆を見ていた。

「どうしたんや」

優司が言うと、

「美帆さんがあんまりきれいなんで、つい見惚れてしまいました」

84

と真顔で言った。

三人で手前のL字型のテーブル席についた。美帆と優司はソファに座り、かすみは向かい側の椅子に腰掛ける。バーテンがすぐにウィスキーと氷、グラスをトレイに載せて持ってきた。ウィスキーはサントリーの「白州18年」だった。

「水割りでよろしいですか」

かすみに訊かれ、美帆は「ロックでお願いできますか」と言う。優司も「俺もロックにしてくれ」と言った。美帆はバッグから自分の名刺を出してかすみに差し出した。

「わざわざご丁寧に」

かすみは名刺を眺めたあと、押し頂くようなしぐさをして胸元にしまった。

バーテンにボールアイスの入ったロックグラスを持って来させると、優雅な手つきでウィスキーを注ぐ。自分の分は水割りを作った。

「仲間君、ずっとお酒飲んでなかったって言ってるけど、ほんとうなの」

グラスを受け取りながら訊いた。

「そうなんですよ。うちにも滅多に顔出さなかったのが、先月東京から帰って来たら、もう毎晩」

かすみは呆れたような顔を作って優司を見る。

「五年分を取り返すなんて大バカ言ってるんですよ、この人」

優司は何も言い返すずにウィスキーをすすっていた。

「父はいつ頃、こちらに来たの」

かすみは「いつだったかしら」と思案気になり、

「もう三年くらい前じゃないかしら。若くてとってもきれいな方とご一緒でした」

「二人だけで?」

「ええ」

かすみは澄ました顔で頷いた。

「でも、そのときが最初で最後なんですよね」

「ええ」

「じゃあ、その相手の女性は初めてじゃなかったのかしら」

「さあ。そういえば、その前に何度かいらしていたかもしれません」

かすみは言葉を濁す。

女性の身元をもっと訊ねてもよかったが、美帆は深追いしなかった。あの父の女性関係を掘り返したところで、こっちがうんざりするだけだ。

二十日の通夜、一昨日の葬儀の折も、見知らぬ女性が何人も焼香にやって来ていた。正也は「誰にも奪われなかったんだから、まあ、かあさんの勝ちってことなんだろ」と解説していた。予想に反して母はそういう女性を見ても淡然としていた。

通夜の晩は、弔問客が絶えた午後九時頃から雨になった。激しい雨で、雨音が屋内まで響き渡ってきた。

午後十一時。母や正也は控え室に引きあげ、式場には父の妹である叔母と美帆の二人だけだった。その叔母が帰ろうとしていたところへ、喪服の肩口をびしょ濡れにした優司が現れた。外の梅雨の終わりの最後の一雨だった。その叔母が帰ろうとしていたところへ、喪服の肩口をびしょ濡れにした優司が現れた。外の

雨音はますます大きくなっていた。

優司は六月半ば、東京を引きあげるときに一度連絡をくれた。以来、何のやりとりもなかった。

式場に入ってきた仲間優司を一目見た瞬間、美帆は張り詰めていた緊張がいちどきにほどけていくのを感じた。その場に座り込みたいような、もっと言えば、近づいてくる優司にしなだれかかりたいような気分になった。

「大変やったな」

と優司は言った。

祭壇前で焼香してもらい、母たちのところへ案内した。控え室は十畳の和室で、洗面所、バス、トイレの他にキッチンも付いていた。

優司が入っていくと、正也がすぐに気づいて立ち上がった。

「優司兄ちゃん」

と懐かしそうな顔になった。

座卓のそばでうなだれていた早苗も顔を上げて、「仲間君、よく来てくれたわね」と涙ぐんだ。

四人で座卓を囲み、美帆の淹れたお茶を飲んだ。優司は「かたせ桜花園」の本多園長からの電話で俊彦の死を知ったらしかった。

「雅光兄さんが園長先生になってるんだ」

美帆が言うと、

「知らなかったの。もうずいぶん前のことよ」

早苗が言った。

87

早苗は優司の隣にぴったりと寄り添うように座っていた。彼女はにわかに生気を甦らせていた。

去年還暦を迎えたが、喪服の着物姿は歳を思わせぬほどに艶っぽい。反対側に座っている正也も優司の顔を窺いながら、めずらしいほど和やかな表情をしていた。

桜花園時代の思い出話を三十分ほどして、優司は帰っていった。

翌日の葬儀にも彼は顔を見せていたが、たくさんの参列者の最後尾から出棺を見送っていた。

美帆と言葉を交わすこともなかった。

黒川丈二は葬儀に駆けつけてくれた。丈二を母や正也に紹介した。彼は火葬場まで同行し、父の骨を拾ってくれた。葬儀場に取って返しての初七日の法要にも参列し、夕方の飛行機で東京に帰った。

一日置いた今日の昼間、優司から電話が来た。

「先生の弔い酒でもやらんね」

美帆はすぐに承諾した。正也も朝の便で引きあげてしまい、今夜、母と二人きりになるのが気詰まりだった。「夜、ちょっとでかけてきてもいい?」と言うと、母の方もほっとした顔を見せた。

通夜の晩、正也と二人になったときにスプーンのことを訊いた。大怪我をした直後からスプーンが母を避けるようになったことに不審を抱いていた正也は、数年後、彼女を問い詰めた。「簡単に白状したよ。ただ、姉ちゃんにだけは言わないでくれって頼まれたんだ。あの子に知られるのは怖いって。僕もそうした方がいいと思った」。正也はそう言ってから「ずっと黙っていて、ごめん」と謝った。美帆は自分が最初から知っていたことは伏せたまま、「いいのよ。私、知っ

88

たら何をしたか分からないし」と言った。

だが、早苗は美帆が目撃していたのは百も承知だった。庭にいた美帆が絶叫しながら庭池のそばにうずくまるスプーンに駆け寄るのを彼女は無言で見下ろしていた。美帆が猫を抱きしめ、怒りの視線を遠くベランダに向けると、

「さっさと那須田さんのところへ連れて行きなさい」

早苗はそれだけ言って平然と部屋の中へ戻っていった。　那須田さんとはかかりつけの獣医の名前だった。

正也は言っていた。スプーンは俊彦が知人から譲り受けた猫だったが、きっとその知り合いというのが愛人の一人だったのだろう。

「それに気づいて、かあさんはあんなことしたんだ」

しかし、美帆はそんな話ではない気がした。母は、あのとき、何かひどく苛々して、ただ衝動的に猫を二階から放り捨てたのだ。それまでも濡れた洗濯物にちょっかいを出すスプーンをよく叱りつけていた。

美帆には分かっていた。女出入りの止まない父を母は心から軽蔑していた。だが、そういう夫にしがみつくことでしか生きていけない自分はその何倍も恥じていた。母の終わることなき嫉妬と焦燥は、母自身の耐え難いほどの自己嫌悪から生まれていたのに違いない。浅草のときのようにアルコールを胃袋に流し込むといった感じではなかった。ほとんど口もきかず、静かに飲んでいた。

優司はゆっくりとグラスを傾けていた。

美帆はかすみと話した。

89

「仲間君って、高校を中退したあとマグロ船に乗ってたのね」
と言うと、
「優ちゃんのマグロ船の話は面白いですよ。もちろんすごい大変なこともたくさんあったみたい
ですけど」
とかすみは言った。
「マグロ船のお昼ご飯はマグロの刺身って決まってるんですって。船員さんたちはマグロにマヨ
ネーズつけて食べるんだそうです。それが一番美味しい食べ方なんですって」
「そうなんだ」
「ええ」
「あとね、魚はやっぱり冷凍より生の方がおいしいじゃないですか。だけど、マグロだけは一度
冷凍したほうが身が締まって美味しいって。その話聞いてからは、私、マグロ買うときは必ず冷
凍マグロにしています」
「それも初耳」
二杯目を空にしたくらいから美帆はくつろげるようになってきた。かすみがきれいな標準語を
喋るのが好ましかった。自分の方が歳上というのも気安い。
「かすみさん、東京の人？」
美帆は訊いた。
「はい」
と頷く。

90

「じゃあ、いつこっちに？」

「結婚して、それで博多に来たんです」

美帆はやや面食らう。

「いろいろあって別れたんですけど」

かすみは言い添えた。

「東京には戻らなかったんだ」

「いまさら帰れるような身の上でもなかったから」

かすみは古風な物言いをした。やくざの情婦になったのだから、帰る実家も失ったということだろうか。

「優ちゃんに助けてもらったんです。優ちゃんがいなかったら、私、破滅してたと思います」

かすみは優司の方へ流し目を送りながら言う。

「大袈裟なことば言うな」

優司がぼそりと言った。

「ほんとなんですよ。だから私、優ちゃんのためなら何でもするし、してあげたいんだけど、この人、何も言わない人だから」

「助けてもらったって？」

美帆が訊く。

「ここじゃ、ちょっと。これでもお仕事中ですから、私」

かすみは笑みを浮かべてかわした。彼女の瞳の中に刺すような光が一瞬灯ったのを美帆は見逃

さなかった。

飲み始めて一時間ほど過ぎると、ようやく優司がぽつぽつ口を利くようになった。酒が回って気分の下地が明るんだのだろう。

「俺が桜花園ば出て行くとき、小柳先生がわざわざ訪ねて来てくれたと」と優司は言った。

「そうだったの」

美帆はびっくりした。当時、父はすでに大学に戻っていた。

「叔父さんの家に行っても、困ったときはいつでも訪ねて来てくれって言うてくれた。俺はそんとき生まれて初めて名刺いうもんを貰った。裏には老松の自宅の住所と電話番号も書いてくれとった」

優司はグラスに残っていたウィスキーを飲み干し、かすみにお代わりを頼んだ。

「マグロ船に乗せられると分かったとき、よっぽど先生んとこに相談に行こうかと思うた」

「どうして来なかったの。二百万の借金くらい父は喜んで肩代わりしたと思うよ」

そうすれば高校を中退することもなく、やくざになることもなかったのにと美帆は思った。

「身内の恥やったからな。俺が自分で借金作ったんなら頭の下げようもあるけどな。叔父貴の恥で俺が頭下げるのは筋違いやろ」

それに、と優司は言った。

「先生は言ったんよ。きみのためならお金でも何でも出すよって。そう言われたら、そのまんま金の話を持ち込むわけにもいかんしな。いま思えば、とにかく相談に行っときゃよかったかな、とは思う。子供やったんやな」

興味深そうに聞いていたかすみが口を挟んだ。

「お金でも何でもって、他に何を出すつもりだったんだろ」

優司は反応しなかった。美帆は、この優司の話を聞いて、父のことを幾分見直した気がした。

いずれ正也にも伝えなくては、と思っていた。

十一時を回った頃、リリコが店にやって来た。

優司や美帆を見てリリコは嬉しそうな顔になった。「なんで、なんで」と言いながらかすみの

横に座った。

かすみが美帆の父の死を告げると、リリコは「お姉さん」といって涙ぐんでしまった。今日で

二度目の対面だったが、美帆も久しぶりに会ったリリコが、ずっと昔からの親友のように思える。

四人であらためて飲み直すことにした。リリコが生ビールのグラスで乾杯しようとして、慌て

て手を引っ込めた。

「リリちゃん、今日はお店は？」

しばらくして、かすみが言った。

ビールグラスに口をつけながら、「休み、休み」とリリコは言い、

「研ちゃんが昨日から落ち込んでるから、独りきりにできなくってさ」

とつけ足した。

「だったら何で出て来れたのよ」

「なんかもう大丈夫そうだから」

この言葉にかすみは眉間に皺を寄せた。

93

「あんた、まだ研ちゃんにクスリやらせてんの」

ビールを一気飲みしていたリリコに厳しい口調で言った。

「やらせてなんかいないよ」

リリコは心外そうに言い返した。

「嘘でしょ。クスリあげたんでしょ。だから出てきたのね」

かすみの突然の剣幕にリリコは下を向いた。優司は何も言わない。

「あんたも勝手な夢を追いかける前に、ちゃんと足元見直しなさいよ。研ちゃん、ちゃんと

クスリやめてないんでしょ。そのままにしてたらいずれ大事になるわよ」

リリコはむずっと黙り込んでしまった。空のビールグラスをじっと見ていた。

「ねえ、リリちゃん、分かってるの」

「それくらい分かってるよ」

「だったら、研ちゃんにどんなにねだられてもクスリあげちゃ駄目だよ」

美帆は二人のやりとりを聞きながら、クスリというのは覚醒剤か麻薬のことなのだろうかと思

った。そんな話を平気でしている二人が違う世界の住人に見えた。

「リリコ」

ようやく優司が口を開く。

「ケンとは早く手を切れ。あいつは長生きできる男じゃないぞ」

「ママだって同じだったんじゃない。研ちゃんのこと責める資格なんてないよ」

リリコは優司の方へ顔を上げて訴えるように言った。

94

「かすみはクスリとはすっぱり手を切っとろうが」

優司がドスのきいた物言いになった。

「ママは他人が幸せになるのが好かんだけなんよ」

不貞腐れた口調でリリコが言い返した。

「いい加減にせんか、こら！」

突然、優司の怒声が店内に響き渡った。

一瞬で美帆は身が竦んでしまった。奥の客たちが驚いた顔でこちらを見ている。正面のかすみも、その隣のリリコも怯えきった姿で凍りついていた。

「かすみはお前とケンのことば思って言いよるだけやろうが。自分がクスリで苦労したけん尚更、悲惨な目にお前たちをあわせたくなかったい。こんとこケンが店ばバイトに任して、妙なことに手ば出しよるんを俺が知らんとでも思うとっとか。今度、俺に隠れて何か悪さばしたらケンはもうおしまいぞ。リリコもそれくらいよう知っとけ」

かすみが彼女の肩を抱こうと手を伸ばすと、そのまま自分の身を任せた。

リリコは半泣きの形相で頷いた。かすみが彼女の肩を抱こうと手を伸ばすと、そのまま自分の身を任せた。

十月五日

とても気味の悪い夢を見て、目覚めた。

部屋のベランダに干しておいたシーツを取り込んでいた。薄いブルーのシーツは夏の風にあおられ、顔に覆いかぶさってくる。それを両手でたくしこんで物干し竿から引き摺り下ろした。太陽にぬくもったシーツが半袖の腕に熱いほどだった。丸めたシーツをとりあえず寝室のベッドの上に置いた。生地が冷めたら畳むつもりだった。

寝室を出ようとすると、背後で甲高い振動音のようなものが聴こえた。振り返る。止んでいた音が再び立った。丸まったシーツの中からだった。

ブーンという耳障りな音とガサゴソと蠢くような音が交互に聴こえた。シーツに何かがとまっていたなんて。背筋に冷たいものが走った。まったく気づかなかった。

美帆はおそるおそるシーツに近づいた。一歩ごとに不気味な音が立った。真上から見下ろしても分からない。中に隠れている。両端からそっと中味をこぼさないように丸めて抱える。そのままベランダの手すりまで走っていって、強い風にまかせるようにシーツを一気に拡げた。

何もいなかった。蜂もコガネムシも、ナナフシも。

虫、だろう。それも大きな。

知らぬうちに飛び去ったのかもしれない。だが、あれだけの音を立てていた虫だ。気づかないことがあるだろうか。

怪訝な気分のままベランダから部屋に戻った。

窓を閉めた途端だった。ものすごい羽音がした。真っ黒い巨大なものが目の前を掠めるように飛び去った。羽音が止む。

思わず瞑ってしまった目を開けた。ゆっくりと部屋の中を見回す。ふと気配を感じて天井に視線をのばした。

美帆は鋭い叫びを上げた。

そこで目が覚めたのだった。天井にぶら下がっていた巨大な物体のディテールはもう忘れていた。赤と黒の奇怪な固まりであったことだけは憶えていた。

午前十一時を回っていた。今朝の五時過ぎまで原稿を書いていた。シャワーも浴びずに眠ってしまった。ベッドから降りるとまっすぐに浴室へ向かった。

髪を乾かしながらコーヒーを淹れた。マグカップになみなみ注いでリビングのテーブルに置く。椅子に座って一口すすったあとテレビのスイッチを入れた。

昼のニュースをやっている時間だ。

画面に現れた映像に目を奪われた。音量を上げてナレーションを聞きやすくする。

「現場は、隅田公園そばの川沿いで、近年、この一帯にはホームレスの人たちのダンボールハウスが立ち並び、昨夜も数十人のホームレスがハウスの中で眠りについていたといいます。殺害された二人の少年を含む六人は、深夜午前二時頃、バットやバール、灯油の入ったポリタンクなど

97

を持って隅田公園に集合。その足で現場に向かい、灯油をばら撒いてダンボールハウスに火をつけて回ったと見られています」

マイクを持った男性レポーターがカメラを連れて走っていた。彼が走っているのは、およそ四ヵ月前に優司と二人で歩いた隅田川沿いの遊歩道に間違いなかった。カメラが止まった。

「この警察ロープの向こうに焼け落ちたダンボールハウスの残骸が積み重なっているのが見えるでしょうか」

「ああ、見えます見えます。真っ黒なゴミの山みたいなあれですよね」

「そうです、そうです。現在、警察と消防の現場検証が続いている模様ですが、ここから見ましても数十はあったと思われるハウスのほとんどが焼失してしまっています。こうやって近くにいますとビニールが焼け焦げたようなつんとくる臭いがまだ漂っているのが分かります」

レポーターとスタジオのキャスターとがやりとりしているあいだも、カメラは規制線の奥をきれいに映し出していた。制服姿の人間がうようよしている。景色に明らかに見覚えがあった。優司が元やくざの男を背負って連れ帰ったダンボールハウスはたしかにあのあたりだ。

「昨夜二時半頃、火事に気づいたダンボールハウスの住人たちが外に飛び出し、火をつけていた少年たちと乱闘になったのです。現場にいたホームレスの一人の話では、慌てて外に出ると、バットやバールを振りかざした少年たちが襲い掛かってきたといいます。逮捕された海江田茂樹容疑者もこのハウスの住人の一人で、彼は以前、やはり少年たちにリンチにあったこともあって所持していた木刀で応戦。二人の少年の頭部を木刀で殴り、結果的に殺害してしまったのです」

「じゃあ、海江田容疑者をリンチにかけた少年たちと、今回の少年たちとは同一犯と見ていいん

98

ですか」

「はい。昼前の警察の発表では、どうやら少年たちの一部は同一だったと見られています。六人の少年たちは、二人が殺され、残りの四人も重傷を負っているので、調べは進んでいないようですが、その中の一人の少年の供述によれば、今年の五月下旬に彼らのうちの四人が海江田容疑者を襲い、そのとき、たまたまそばを通りかかった男に逆に半殺しの目にあったことを恨んで、今回、いわば仕返しのために、他の二人にも声を掛けて現場に乗り込んだようです」

「しかし、五月というのはずいぶん前の話ですね」

「はい。ただ、この五月のときに四人とも右腕を折られてしまっていて、その右腕がようやく回復したということで今回の犯行に及んだと見られています。詳細は、今後の捜査を待たなくてはならないんですが」

スタジオではゲスト解説者の一人が「その五月にそばを通りかかった男というのは、一体何者なんでしょうね」と疑問を投げかけていた。「いきなりリンチの場面に遭遇して、少年とはいえ四人もの相手の右手を全部へし折るなんて、通常だと考えられないですね。格闘家か何かなら別ですが」。もう一人のゲストも、通りがかりの謎の男の存在に興味をそそられているようだった。

「引き続き、今後の捜査の行方を見守っていくことにしましょう」

キャスターが締めくくって画面はコマーシャルに切り替わった。

それから美帆はチャンネルを次々に切りかえて、各局のワイドショーをチェックしていった。

事件のあらましは、最初の番組でおおかた足りていた。

昨夜、隅田公園そばのダンボールハウスの団地を襲ったのは六人。四人は中学時代からの同級

99

生で、現役の高校二年生と中退組が二人ずつ。あとの二人は、一人が十九歳の大学生、一人は無職の十八歳の男だった。十八歳の男が主犯格だったようだが、彼は海江田容疑者に殺されてしまった。もう一人の犠牲者は中退組の一人。残りも海江田の奮戦を見て乱闘に加わった二十数人のホームレスたちによって大怪我を負わされていた。逮捕者は海江田を含めて八人にのぼり、少年たちへの暴行がどのような形で行なわれたかはいまだ不明だった。ただ、逮捕されなかったホームレスの証言などから、少なくとも大学生殺害の実行犯が海江田容疑者であることは確かなようだった。「バールを振り回して暴れてたのがリーダー格みたいだったけど、そいつは木刀持った男に頭を割られて、あっという間に死んじまったよ」とカメラの前で語るホームレスもいた。殺されなかった方も、高校二年生の一人は意識不明の重体。他の三人も重傷と報じられていた。警察の尋問に答えているのは十八歳の無職の男で、この男だけがどうやら口がきける状態であるらしかった。五月のリンチ事件で海江田容疑者を助けた通りすがりの男については、どの局でも伝えていたが、内容は最初の番組と大差なかった。

ホームレス狩りの少年たちが返り討ちにあい、逆に二人が殺害されたというこのショッキングなニュースは、新聞、テレビで大々的に報道されていた。

美帆はテレビとパソコンの前に釘付けの状態だった。風呂上りに淹れたコーヒーを口にしたほかは飲まず食わずで、一心不乱にワイドショーやニュース、インターネットを見つづけた。

ふと気づいてみると夕方になっていた。

テレビを消し、パソコンの電源を落として、美帆は息をついた。部屋の中は薄暗くなっていた。半開きにしてあったリビングのカーテンを思い切り引いて、天井の明かりを点けた。外はまだ夕

100

暮れ時には間があるようだった。掛け時計の針は五時を回っていた。

すこし頭痛がした。テレビやディスプレーを見過ぎたせいだろう。右の後頭部から目の奥にか

けて鈍い痛みがあった。薬を飲む前に何か食べなくてはと思うが、食欲はまったくなかった。ロ

キソニンを一錠飲んで、ソファに横になった。

ひどく静かだった。

三年前に買ったこのマンションは、表参道の裏手に位置する。昨年、同潤会アパートが取り壊

され、跡地の再開発が始まっているが、その建築現場と神宮前小学校のあいだの道を入って数分

歩くとたどり着く。原宿駅へも十分とかからなかった。人波であふれる表参道からは想像もつか

ないが、一帯は閑静な住宅地だ。下見を一度したきりで即座に購入を決めたのも、その喧騒と静

寂とのコントラストに惹かれたからだった。三年住んでみて、ますますここでの暮らしが気に入

っている。

もちろん築二十年の中古物件だった。2LDK、六十五平米と決して広くはなかった。価格は

七千万円。知り合いの不動産関係者に探してもらったので、それでも格安の物件だった。月々の

ローンは相当だが、美帆の収入であれば賄えない額ではなかった。

今日は、その静けさが不安な心地をあおっていた。

少年二人を撲殺した海江田茂樹は、五月二十八日の晩に優司が助けたホームレスの男に違いな

かった。彼が殺人に使った凶器が、優司が仲見世通りの土産物屋で買って届けた木刀であること

も確実だった。あの木刀を買ったとき、男に渡すのかと美帆は訊ねた。優司は、連中が仕返しに

来たらこれで一人叩き殺せばいいんだ、と薄笑いを浮かべていた。そして、海江田は優司の言っ

た通り、再びやって来た少年を叩き殺した。しかも二人も。

凶器を渡しただけではない。少年たちが復讐心を滾らせたのは、優司が彼らの右腕をへし折っ
たからだった。同じ痛めつけるにしても、優司のやり方は度を越していた。

地面に転がってうめく少年たちに、優司が執拗に暴力を振るうのを自分は黙認した。制止しよ
うなどとは露ほども思わず、むしろ彼らの腕が順々にへし折られる様を間近で見て、奇妙な快感
に身を震わせていたのだった。

そして、あの過剰な暴力の直接的結果として、昨夜、二人の少年が死んだ。

どうして木刀を渡すのを止めなかったのだろう。どうして優司があれ以上暴力に走るのを止め
なかったのだろう。　腕を折られて泣き叫んでいる少年たちを、自分はどうしてそのまま放置して
しまったのだろう。

美帆は考えているうちに息苦しくなってきた。

テレビやネットを見ている間も、これが重大な事態だということは感じていた。ただ、そこか
ら先は考えなかった。事実確認の作業に没頭することで気を逸らしていた。

二人の人間が殺されたのだ。その殺人に自分たちは手を貸してしまったのだ。

美帆は顔を両手で覆って、何度か深呼吸した。

警察に知られてしまう。　最も考えたくないのはそのことだった。

胸の中で呟いた。

警察の捜査がどういうものか分からないが、凶器の出所というのは真っ先に特定すべき事項に
違いない。海江田は木刀の入手経路を厳しく追及されるだろう。もちろん五月のリンチ事件の詳

102

細についてもだ。闇夜とはいえ街灯の明かりはあった。そのあとおぶってハウスまで送り、あげくもう一度引き返して木刀を渡した。海江田は優司の顔も、一緒にいた美帆の顔もはっきり憶えているはずだ。

名前も素性も言わなかった。だが、海江田の記憶からモンタージュでも作られたらどうする。浅草界隈の店を片っ端から警察が聞きこみに回れば、優司と美帆が米久で食事をしたことが露見する。当日の予約台帳から美帆の連絡先が割れるのは時間の問題だ。

警察が来たらどうすればいい。知らぬ存ぜぬでその場を切り抜けたとしても、美帆の周辺を調べればいずれ優司の存在が浮かび上がる。優司は前科者だ。指紋も写真も警察は握っている。

喋れるようになった少年たちに優司の写真を見せるだろう。彼らは口を揃えて「この男が俺たちを半殺しの目にあわせた。こいつに仕返ししたくてホームレスを襲ったんだ」と供述する。

メディアは五月のリンチ事件の折、偶然通りがかった謎の男に依然興味を持っている。その男が特定されるのだ。しかも、当の男は福岡のやくざ。書き得とばかりに週刊誌も群がってくる。

そして、そのやくざ者と一緒にいた女。腕を折られて転げまわっていた少年たちを置き去りにし、二人を殺すことになる木刀をやくざ者と共に容疑者に渡した女……。

美帆は思わずソファから飛び起きた。頭の痛みは一向におさまらない。息苦しさはさきほどよりひどくなっていた。何気なく額に手を当てる。ひどく熱い。風呂上りの薄着のままずっとテレビを見ていた。風邪を引いたのかもしれない。

どうしよう。そんなことになれば破滅だ。

立ち上がってキッチンに行く。冷蔵庫から缶ビールを取り出した。プルトップを開けて、一気

103

に喉に流し込む。冷たいビールの感触が食道から胃へと降りていく。飲み干した缶を調理台に置いてリビングに戻った。窓をいっぱいに開けた。涼しい風が入ってきた。風を顔に受けて外を見た。街並みの向こうに赤く染まった太陽があった。

それはそれでいい。こんな人生、どうなろうと別に構やしない。

美帆は思った。

自分なんてどうだっていい――美帆は肝心なときは必ずそう思う。意志の力によってではなく、ごく自然に思える。胸の芯に巣食う投げやりな心が、いつか人生を台無しにしてしまいそうでたまに恐ろしくなる。一方で、それが自分のほんとうの強さのような気がするときもあった。

夕食を終えて、明け方にまとめた原稿の手直しをしていた。

九時のNHK、十時のテレビ朝日のニュース番組を見てから仕事部屋にしている玄関脇の八畳間に入った。両局とも事件はトップ扱いだったが新しい情報はほとんどなかった。意識不明の重体だった少年が一命を取り留めそうだということくらいだった。

玄関のチャイムが鳴った。美帆は時間を確かめる。十一時十五分。

一体、こんな時間に誰？　丈二のはずはなかった。彼は昨日からベトナムに出張していた。ハノイで開かれるASEM（アジア欧州会合）首脳会合を取材するため、昨日からベトナムに出張していた。

まさかもう警察が？　玄関に出て美帆は緊張した。

ドアスコープを覗くと仲間優司が立っていた。

慌ててドアを開ける。

104

「どうしたの?」

美帆は素っ頓狂な声を上げた。

「忙しいとこすまんな」

優司は申し訳なさそうな顔になった。

「ちょっとそのへんでビールでも飲まんか」

と言う。まるで近所に住んでいる友人がぶらっと訪ねてきたような物言いだった。夕方の飛行機で来た。名刺の住所を頼りに表参道の駅で降りたまではよかったが、それから美帆のマンションを探し出すのに三十分以上かかった。

「東京の道はいっちょん分からんばい」

歩きながら優司はぼやいた。

表参道に出てから246方向に五分ほど歩いた。一軒の店の前で立ち止まると、さっさとドアを開けて入っていく。扉には「ONE PENNY」と記されていた。ギネスの看板も出ていた。アイリッシュパブのようだった。

店内はそこそこの混み具合だった。出てきたボーイを無視して優司は一番奥のテーブル席へと向かう。サングラスはしていなかったが、ボーイは何も言わずについてきた。

「ここ、いいかな」

優司が言うと、ボーイは直立して「はい」と返事した。

美帆が革のシートに座り、優司が手前の木製の椅子に腰掛けた。

「小柳んちまで行く途中で、この店ば見つけたんよ」

105

メニューを開きながら、優司が笑みを浮かべた。優司はギネスの一パイント、美帆はキルケニ

ーのハーフパイントをオーダーした。つまみはフィッシュ・アンド・チップスだけ。

「お腹空いてないの」

美帆が訊くと、

「俺はビールだけでよか」

と優司は言った。

グラスが届き、乾杯する。クリーミーな泡が舌に心地よい。冷やし方も程よかった。

「ニュース見たやろ」

三分の一ほど飲んだグラスを置いて、優司が言った。美帆は黙って頷いた。

「忘れろ」

あっさり言った。

「小柳にはショックかもしれんけど、大したことやない」

美帆は優司の顔を注視する。切れ長の目が大きくて優しげだ。やっぱりこの人はやくざには向

かないと思った。

「それを言いにわざわざ来たの」

美帆は声を落として言った。

「おう。小柳がビビってサツにでも駆け込んだらわややろ。俺たちは何も悪いことしとらんが、

罪をでっちあげるのはサツの専売特許やからな」

「私を黙らせに来たのね」

106

「まあな」

優司は笑った。

美帆はその笑顔を見て無性にむかっ腹が立ってきた。

「ごめんなさいくらい言いなさいよ」

「何で」

「私をこんなことに巻き込んで」

「俺は何も悪いことはしとらん」

優司は顔色も変えずに言う。

「あんなにひどい目にあわせなくってもよかったじゃない」

「あんときはああするしかなかったろうも。そうせんとあの晩に連中はハウスに火ばつけにいっとる」

「そうかしら」

「そりゃそうやろ」

「どうしてそんなこと分かるの」

そこで優司は怪訝な顔になった。

「あいつらポリタンクば持ってきとったろうが。あの油ばぶん撒いて火をつける気やったに決まっとる」

「ポリタンク?」

意外な言葉に美帆は聞き返した。

「二つ地面に置いてあったろうが。すぐそばに。小柳、見とらんかったとか」

さすがに優司が呆れた声を出した。

「おやっさんにも、いずれあいつらが火つけに来るぞて言うといた」

美帆は予想外の話に多少面食らってしまっていた。

「だから、仲間君、あいつらの腕を折ったの」

「そりゃそうやろ。そうやなければ警察に届けるべきだったと思う。ポリタンクがあったのなら警察だって放っておかないはずよ」

優司はビールを飲み干し、もう一杯ギネスをオーダーした。ギネスとフィッシュ・アンド・チップスが届いた。

「だったら警察に届けるべきだったと思う。ポリタンクがあったのなら警察だって放っておかないはずよ」

美帆はしばらく考えてから言った。

「サツが何ばしてくれっとか。まして未成年やろ。保護はできても逮捕はできんとばい。公園のトイレで見つけたホームレスば血祭りに上げて、そいで景気つけてからダンボールハウスば焼き払いに行くつもりやったんぞ。そげんやつらば許せっかい。おやっさんのちんちん見たかい。バットで小突かれて竿も玉も青黒く腫れあがっとったばい」

優司はきつい目で美帆を見た。そんな目を見るのは初めてのような気がした。

「そげなやつら、腕の骨ば折ったくらいで何が悪いとか。そげなやつらば、お前、本気で許せるとか」

108

「だけど、二人も亡くなったのよ。だったら二人は死んで当たり前だったの。仲間君があんなこ
としなきゃ、ホームレスの人に木刀渡したりしなきゃ、こんなことになってなかったかもしれな
いじゃない。そのせいで、私だっていつ警察に呼び出されるか分からないし、仲間君だってそれ
が心配で来たんでしょう」

「俺はサツが怖くて来たんやない」

優司がぼそりと言った。

「だってそう言ったじゃない。私に警察へ行かれたら困るからって」

優司は黙った。もどかしげな表情で美帆を見る。

「小柳」

優司は言った。

「小柳、人間の生き死には一つ事て。殺されることもあれば殺すこともあると。やけん大事なん
は、そこに生きるべき義、死すべき義があるかどうかたい。今度のことは、おやっさんたちの方
に明らかに義があるやろ。やったらそれに手ば貸した俺たちも何一つ恥じることはなか。おやっ
さんが俺たちのことばチクることは千パーセントなかし、たとえ警察の手が伸びてきたとしても、
一体俺たちに何の罪があるとね。あの状況で木刀一本おやっさんに渡しておくのは人の情やろう
も。それに、俺が腕ばへし折った連中やって被害届なんか出しとらんよ。幾らサツでもどうやっ
たら俺たちば引っ張れるとね。小柳。あのガキたちがやったことは戦争よ。戦争やったら死ぬの
は覚悟やろ。誰のことも責められん。小柳も自分のことば責める必要はなかと。そいができんな
ら、全部俺のせいにすればよか」

そこまで喋って優司はビールを飲んだ。

「俺はガキん頃から、不良も年少上がりも嫌というほど見てきた。やつは、あげな弱い者いじめは絶対にせん。ああいうガキどもは生まれついての外道よ。小さかときから犬や猫ばいたぶって殺すような変態野郎たい。世間の片隅で細々と生きとる人たちのことば虫けら扱いして、面白半分に焼き殺そうとする奴らが死ぬのは当たり前やろ。どうせあげな腐れたことする連中は、このさき生きてもろくなことはせん。そいだけは俺は断言できるばい」

店を出たのは二時過ぎだった。優司はギネスばかりを十杯近く飲んだ。美帆もつられてかなり飲んだ。

「送っていっちゃる」

優司は先に歩き始めた。美帆が追いついて並んだ。さすがに人通りはまばらになっていた。夜風が火照った顔に気持ちよかった。二人とも無言だった。マンションの前まで来て、

「仲間君、これからどうするの」

美帆は訊いた。

「そのへんのネットカフェで時間潰して、一番の飛行機に乗る」

優司の口からネットカフェという言葉が出たのがちょっと不思議だった。

「何ならうちに泊まっていく？　ソファで仮眠くらいできるよ」

「よかよか」

慌てたように優司は手を横に振ってみせた。

「じゃあな」

110

そう言うと、彼は背中を向け、早足で美帆の前から立ち去った。

十一月七日

ふかひれの姿煮が終わって、鮑とつぶ貝の季節野菜炒めが出された。ウェーターが取り分けて四人それぞれの前に皿を置く。

ずっと丈二が政局の今後の見通しについて喋っていた。

七月の参議院選挙で敗北を喫したものの、非改選議席を合わせ過半数を維持した首相はその責任を取ることなく続投を表明した。九月には内閣改造、党役員人事が行なわれ、党三役は堀米幹事長を除く二役なりと了承された。有力な後継候補がいないこともあって、これは与党内ですんが交代し、首相の宿願といわれる郵政民営化に賛意を示す人材で内閣と党の主要ポストを固めるという露骨な郵政民営化シフトが敷かれた。

「党内はまだ半信半疑な人や、そんな無茶をするなら倒閣だと言いつつも、幾らなんでもできないだろうと高をくくっている議員がほとんどだよ。しかし、総理の郵政民営化にかける決意はなみなみならぬものがある。改造前、訪米中にニューヨークでやった記者懇に出たけど、民営化については凄まじかったよ。『民営化を進めていく決意に変わりはない。これが分かってない人は駄目だ』というコメントしかどこの社も書かなかったけど、ほんとうはそんな生易しい表現じゃ

111

なかったからね」

丈二の話に父親の庸一も母親のみどりも熱心に耳を傾けていた。美帆は彼らの箸の進み具合を観察しつつ料理を口に運んでいた。

「来年の夏にかけて政局は一気に動くよ。総理は何が何でも郵政民営化法案を通すつもりだから、官邸が本気だと分かった段階で党内は二分されて大騒ぎになる。下手をすると党が割れる可能性もあるし、そうなったら総理は政権の命運を賭けて解散総選挙に打って出るかもしれない。堀米さんなんかは、すごい危機感だよ。常識的には分裂選挙になったら敗北は必至だからね」

丈二はまだ残っていたふかひれにようやく箸をつけた。

「お前はどうするんだ」

紹興酒で頬を染めている庸一が言った。七十間近の年齢だがとてもそうは見えない。黒々とした髪はてっきり染めているのだろうと思っていたが、違うらしかった。丈二と同様に立派な体軀の持ち主だ。顔もよく似ていた。

「解散はチャンスだよ。郵政民営化が争点になれば、反対派は公認から外されるだろうし、新人がつけいる隙が出てくる。やってやれないことはないよ」

丈二も紹興酒を飲んでいた。みどりがウーロン茶なので美帆はお酒は控えていた。みどりは早苗と変わらぬ年回りだった。細身で目立たない風情なので早苗のような華やかさはなかったが、顔立ちは整っていた。

「児玉先生はどっちなんだ」

児玉というのは丈二の地元、奈良一区選出の衆議院議員のことだった。一区は奈良市のほとん

112

どを選挙区としていた。

「あの人はガリガリの反対論者だよ」

「郵政大臣を務めたしな」

「そうそう」

「となると、お前と児玉先生の一騎打ちもあり得るわけか」

庸一が難しい顔を作った。八月に初めて丈二と二人で奈良を訪れた折も、父子で同じような話をしていた。児玉代議士を支援している桐山組は黒川建設と県内を二分する建設会社で、社長の桐山貞行と庸一とは長年の盟友関係にあった。もしも丈二が一区に出馬となれば、その関係にひびが入るのは避けられない。

丈二はお盆のお参りのために片瀬をふたたび訪ねてくれた。そこで早苗や正也ともじっくり話をしていた。四十九日前のお盆とあって、あとは身内しか招かなかった。だから優司が姿を見せることはなかった。

東京に帰る途中、美帆は丈二の実家に出向き、庸一とみどりと対面した。庸一とはそれ以来だったが、みどりとは九月にも会っていた。所用で上京して来て、五日間ほど高輪の丈二のマンションに泊まったのだ。美帆も一日、料理を作りに行って夕食を共にした。そんな中で、みどりが外見とは裏腹にひどく勝気な女性であることを知った。初対面のときから苦手だと感じたが、この九月の再会で尚更その思いを強くしたのだった。

北京ダックと湯葉の揚げ物が出てきた。北京ダックは丈二の好物なので美帆が自分の分を彼の

113

皿に移すと、

「まあ、仲がいいのね」

とみどりが笑みを浮かべて言った。赤ら顔の庸一は大きな身体を美帆の方に向けると、

「美帆さんは養子だそうだね」

と言った。九月にみどりと会った折、自らの出自についても詳しく話した。

相手の顔を見て、

「はい」

と美帆は答えた。

庸一の背後には都心の夜景が広がっている。四人がいるのはホテルニューオータニ二十六階にある「大観苑」の個室だった。丈二が目指す国会や首相官邸もすぐ目と鼻の先にある。

「実のご両親のことは何も憶えていないんだそうだね」

「はい。二歳で施設に預けられて、それからすぐに養子になりましたから。いまの両親に引き取られたときの記憶は鮮明なんですが、その前のことは全然憶えていないんです」

両親、と言いながら父はもういないのだ、と美帆は思った。俊彦の死が初めて少し哀しく思われた。

「他に身寄りは誰も？」

みどりが言う。

「叔父が一人いたそうです」

114

「その叔父さんは？」

ふたたび庸一が訊く。

「憶えていないんです。父や母の話では、その叔父も私を預けたあと行方不明になってしまったみたいで」

庸一は釈然としない顔つきをしていた。

「戸籍を調べれば本当のご両親のことは分かるでしょう」

「だと思います。だけど調べたいと思ったこともないし、父と母に訊ねたこともないんです」

これにはみどりも怪訝そうな表情になった。

「やっぱり本当のご両親のことを知りたいんじゃなくて」

「母はたぶん亡くなっていると思います」

美帆は言った。このことは丈二にも話したことはなかった。

「どうして？」

庸一が言う。

「何となくです」

「何となく？」

「はい」

答えながら、腿の痣を取るための手術を受けた晩のことを久々に思い出していた。

「きっとお美しいお母さまでしたでしょうね」

みどりが言った。

115

「さあ」

美帆は首を傾げるしかなかった。

「いまのお母さんもすごくきれいな人だよ」

と丈二が言った。

美帆は、亡くなる前の晩の父の美しい寝顔を思い浮かべた。同時に父があのとき語った言葉を反芻した。父は、かつて誰よりも愛した人がすでに死んでいることを、その人と久しぶりに会って知らされたと言った。その人が来てくれて、ほかにもいろんなことを教えてくれたと言っていた。

「だけど、美帆さんのようにきれいな方がよくいままでお独りでいたわね」初めて会ったときも、九月に会ったときもみどりは同じことを言った。「あなただったら世界中の男性が言い寄ってくるでしょうに」と言われたこともあった。

「だから、その話はしたじゃないか。僕が悪かったんだ。僕のせいで美帆は男性不信になってしまったんだ」

これも丈二が毎回説明していることだった。

そして、そのたびにみどりは嬉々とした表情になる。今日もそうだった。

要するに、この母親はそんな息子が自慢なのだ。これほどの美女を男性不信に陥れ、七年も袖にしてあげくに再度ものにした。そういう息子の手腕と魅力がどうしようもなく誇らしいのだ、と美帆は思った。

「あんまりきれいだとか美人だとかおっしゃらないでください」

美帆は言った。

「あら、どうして」

みどりが意外そうな声を出す。

「美帆さんは、そういうことに飽き飽きしてるんだろう」

父親が笑った。

「だけど、他人が褒めるのとはわけが違うでしょう。私が言っているんだからお世辞なんかじゃないわ」

みどりはわずかに色をなした様子で言った。

「お母さまに言われると、何だか顔がきれいなだけの空っぽの女だと言われているような気がします」

この美帆の一言にみどりはさっと顔色を変えた。隣の丈二も啞然とした顔で美帆を見た。

円卓に四人で座っていた。左が丈二、右が庸一、正面がみどりだった。

美帆はかねがね思っていたことを口にしたに過ぎなかった。

「何言ってるの。美帆さんはお料理だってとても上手だし、お仕事もすごく頑張っているんでしょう」

美帆は謝った。

「すみません、失礼なこと言ってしまって」

「もう、いいじゃないか」

庸一がとりなすように言う。椅子に座りなおして、彼は改まった口調でつづけた。

117

「丈二が出馬ということになれば仕事を辞めなくてはならないのかな。さっきの話だと、早ければ来年夏頃には選挙ということになりそうだし、そうなると二人の結婚も少し急がなくてはならないが」

美帆が喪中でもあり、結納は年明け、挙式は来年の六月くらいにという話になっていた。

「それはこの前、お話ししたとおりです」

と美帆は言った。八月に奈良を訪ねたとき、丈二が当選した場合は仕事を辞めて家庭に入ると約束した。選挙期間中はもちろん選挙活動に専念するつもりだともつけ加えておいた。

「選挙のときはよろしく頼みますよ。あなたほどの美人ならば身内や後援会は大喜びだが、一般の有権者はとにかく嫉妬深いものです。一段下げる頭を二段、二段下げる頭を三段下げる心がけでやってください」

庸一が家長としての威厳を示すかのように、鷹揚な口振りで言う。

「大丈夫。私、もうおばさんですから」

美帆は言った。

どういうわけか、気持ちがぐらぐらしていた。この場の雰囲気に耐えられなくなってきている自分を唐突に感じた。

「あら、そんなふうに言わないで。結婚する丈二が可哀そうじゃない」

すかさず、みどりが棘のある言葉を繰り出す。

「ですが、選挙のためにはおばさんくらいでちょうどいいんじゃないですか。お父様がおっしゃっておられるのも、そういうことだと思いますけど」

118

「主人が言っているのは、自分が美人だからって鼻にかけてはいけないということよ。何もプライドまで捨てろと言っているわけじゃないでしょう。代議士の妻になるべき人は常に毅然としていなくては駄目よ」

「私は、そんなことを鼻にかけたことありませんよ」

「だから、そういう思い込みが他人の誤解を招くのよ。もっと謙虚にならないと。主人が言っているのはそういうこと」

みどりは押さえ込むように言い切った。

美帆は俯いた。丈二も庸一も固唾を飲むような雰囲気で黙り込んでいた。

ずいぶん長いこと沈黙がつづいたような気がした。

美帆は一度小さく息をついた。そしてお腹に力を込めた。奥歯を一回ぎゅっと嚙み締めた。

ゆっくり顔を上げて目の前の丈二の母親を見た。

今日、このときのために丈二と縒りを戻したのだ、という気がした。

「もう、あなたたちにはうんざりです」

美帆ははっきりと言った。

ぽかんとした顔の三人を順繰りに眺めてから、言葉を継いだ。

「初めて会ったときから、『きれいだ、きれいだ』ばっかりで、いい加減イヤになりました。あなたたちは自分の息子の婚約者に対して、何か語るべき他の言葉を持ち合わせていないんですか。あ会えば二言目には、きれいだ、美人だ、これならどこに出しても恥ずかしくない。一体いままであなたたちは何を学んで生きてきたのですか。私がきれいだというだけで、どうして息子の嫁と

して恥ずかしくないのか、私にはまったく理解できない。美人だから何だっていうんですか。私
は努力してこの顔に生まれたわけじゃないし、別にきれいに生まれたいと望んだ覚えもありませ
ん。ただ、人より多少整った顔に生まれてしまった。それだけのことです。そこには私の意志も
努力もこれっぽっちも反映されていない。私に言わせれば、私がきれいだなんてことはどうでも
いい。そんなこと知ったことじゃないんです。自分自身がひとかけらも関心を持っていないこと
であれこれ言われるのは、たとえそれが褒め言葉だったとしても、うんざりなんです。不愉快な
んですよ。大体、一人前の大人に向かって外見だけの賛美を繰り返すなんて、およそまともに頭
を使っている人間のすることではないし、下品です。

　私は、これまでこの容姿で得をしたことも何度となくありますが、それ以上に損もしてきたん
です。だから、私は顔だけでちやほやされ、容姿が衰えた途端に使い捨てにされるような仕事に
は見向きもしませんでした。なろうと思えばモデルにもアナウンサーにも女優にだってなれまし
た。街を歩けば、必ず毎日何人かのスカウトに声を掛けられたし、写真家や映画監督、ディレク
ターに誘われた回数なんて数え切れません。若い頃から誰でも彼でも、男だけじゃなくてあなた
みたいな女までが、女といえば顔だ、若さだ、とまるで物扱いしてくる。そうやって物扱いする
ことで、自分が優位に立った気になって、実のところ嫉妬してるだけなんです。それともあなた
たちは、顔の整った人間は美しくない人よりも人間的に優れているとでも本気で考えているんで
すか。そういう下品な考え方にももう飽き飽きです。ただ面倒くさい。それだけなんです」

　美帆は言い終えると、膝の上のテーブルナプキンを静かに円卓に置き、椅子を引いて立ち上が
った。

120

「今日はこれで失礼させていただきます」

部屋の隅のコートハンガーに掛けておいたバッグを取ると、振り返ることなく部屋を出た。黒川家の面々は誰も追ってこようとはしなかった。

十一月八日

美帆は若い頃から、男女の肉体関係は神聖なものだと考えていた。その考えはいまも変わっていない。二十歳の誕生日から黒川丈二と付き合うようになったが、美帆にとって丈二は初めての男だった。丈二と再会するまでの七年間、美帆が真剣に交際した男性は一人きりだった。その人とは二十八歳のときに知り合った。

丈二との破局のあと美帆は仕事に没頭した。ちょうど新しい女性誌の創刊メンバーに選ばれていたので、寝る間も惜しんで働くにはうってつけの職場でもあった。あるとき、たまの休みに海にでも出たい、という理由だけでクルーザーを衝動買いした。クルーザーといってもたまの小さなものだったが、編集部の友人と二人で船舶免許を取得し、月に一度か二度は東京湾に出ていた。そこでその人と知り合った。彼は三千万円クラスの船を何艘も持つ人で、一度船上パーティーに招かれ、親しくなった。それからは友だちと二人で操船のコツを学んだり、東京湾内、湾外の安全なルートを教えてもらったりした。

彼は不動産会社とホテルを経営する実業家で、当時四十五歳。一度結婚に失敗していた。

すでに丈二と別れて二年半ほどが過ぎていたので、一晩中泣きつづけたり、その後の丈二の消息を偶然耳にして過呼吸に陥るといったことはなくなっていた。それでも夢に丈二が出てくることはあった。丈二が隣にいて、安心しきった自分が心から幸福を感じているという夢。決まって明け方で、仕事が忙しいときに見た。そんな夢を見たあとは必ず泣いた。

実業家の彼は親切で優しかった。ある晩、船の上で食べたカキに当たって美帆が寝込んでしまったことがあった。彼は友人の医者を船に呼んでくれ、一晩中面倒を見てくれた。丈二以外の男性にそこまで手厚くされたのは初めてだった。一月ほどして身体の関係を結んだ。

男性の生理については分からない。男は誰とでも寝ることができるのかもしれない。だが、女はそうではないと美帆は思う。すくなくとも自分は、心を開かないかぎりは、相手とベッドを共にすることは絶対にできない。

丈二と付き合い始めたときも、彼にはかつて恋人がいて、その人とも寝ていたと聞かされ、内心激しいショックを受けた。丈二が記者になり、出張で同行した代議士連中に誘われ、どうしても断りきれずにモスクワの娼婦と一晩を過ごした、とのちのち聞かされたときも二ヵ月のあいだ顔を合わせなかった。いま思えば、あの出来事のあとから、二人の関係はわずかずつ変わっていった気がする。正也が東京に進学してきて、それまでの半同棲生活ができなくなった時期とも重なっていた。丈二がテレビ局に勤める後輩の女性記者と深い仲になってしまったのは、その翌年だった。

交際を始めて半年後に彼に結婚を申し込まれた。すこし考えさせて欲しいと言って、その晩は

122

別れた。帰り道、途中でタクシーを降りて、当時住んでいた碑文谷のマンションまでのゆるやかな坂道をのぼった。東京にしてはめずらしいきれいな星空だった。

プロポーズを受けようと思った。明日にはきちんと返事をさせてもらおうと決めて部屋に戻った。十一時過ぎだったが、留守番電話に母の声が吹き込まれていた。「今日、市民病院に行って検査を受けました。胃がんだそうです」という重苦しい声だった。

翌日、美帆は片瀬に帰った。それからしばらくは母の入院、手術、退院で瞬く間に時間が過ぎていった。

二ヵ月後、美帆は正式にプロポーズを断った。彼のことを丈二ほど好きになる自信がどうしても持てなかった。

「きみは、着陸できなくなった飛行機のようだ」

最後にそう言われた。

美帆が会社を辞めたのは、その人との別れも大きな原因の一つだった。

ニューオータニを出るとまっすぐ羽田に向かった。せいせいした気分だった。何一つ後悔はなかった。丈二も含めて、あんな家族とは付き合っていられない。もともと美帆は家族など信じていなかった。幼い時に親に捨てられた人間が、家族を信ずるなんてナンセンスだ。美帆にしてみれば、それはまるで奴隷が主人の娘に恋するようなものだった。そんなことをすれば自分を失うだけだ。丈二と別れてからは、特にそう考えるようになった。結局、人間なんて誰も信用できない。

123

丈二が今夜、神宮前のマンションを訪ねてくるのは目に見えていた。家に戻るわけにはいかなかった。都内のホテルに泊まるくらいだったら、いっそ片瀬に帰ろうと美帆は思った。

ふと仲間優司に会いたくなったのだ。

一ヵ月前は優司が突然やって来た。今度は自分が不意打ちを食らわせてもいいような気がした。

八時発の全日空福岡行き最終便にぎりぎり間に合った。

福岡空港に着いたのは午後十時過ぎ。

空港でタクシーを拾って片瀬駅前まで行った。新町の「あかり」のドアを引いたのは十一時ちょうどのことだった。

あかりは前回とちがって混みあっていた。急な来訪にもかすみはそれほど驚いた顔は見せず、とりあえずカウンターの隅に美帆を座らせ、若いバーテンに隣の席には誰も入れないよう指示して客たちのところへ戻っていった。それからは三十分置きくらいに声を掛けにきた。美帆はカクテルをいろいろ作ってもらいながら、バーテンとお喋りしていた。

十二時を過ぎて女の子たちが引きあげると、客たちも次々に帰っていった。

「もうすぐ看板にするから、二人で飲み直しましょうね」

かすみはそう言い残して、お客を店の外まで何度も見送りに出た。テーブル席に移ってかすみと隣同士で座った。閉店後のスナックで飲むのは初めてだ。さきほどまでの喧騒が嘘のような静けさだった。

バーテンも引きあげ、二人きりになったのは一時過ぎだった。

「お疲れさま」

と言い合ってビールで乾杯した。

「お久しぶりですね」

かすみが微笑みかけてくる。

「ごめんなさいね。急に押しかけてしまって」

「そんなあ。美帆さんみたいなきれいな方とまた会えて光栄です」

かすみは今夜は着物ではなくドレスを着ていた。襟ぐりが大きくカットされた黒のミディアムドレスだ。胸の谷間は深かった。

「福岡でお仕事だったんですか？」

空になったグラスにビールを注いでくれながら言う。

「ちょっとむしゃくしゃすることがあって、さっき、衝動的に飛行機に乗っちゃったのよ」

酔いも手伝って美帆は正直に話した。

「じゃあ、東京から」

「うん。片瀬駅まで来たら、何だかここに来たくなったの」

美帆は冗談めかした口調で言った。優司に会いたかったからとは言わなかった。

「ありがとうございます」

かすみはグラスを持ち上げて、小首をかしげるしぐさをした。

「だけど、へんよね。この街が小さい頃から大嫌いなのに」

呟くように美帆が言った。

「故郷なんてそんなものなんじゃないですか。あった方がいいか、ない方がいいかで投票したら

125

ちょうど半々みたいな感じ」

「そうかもね」

面白い言い方をする。

美帆は頷いた。

「私ね、貰いっ子なのよ。本当の娘じゃないの」

「そうだったんですか」

「もともとの生まれは東京。かすみさんと同じ」

「私は違いますよ。千葉だから」

「そう言われると、私もはっきりした記憶はないわ。都内の施設に預けられてたってだけだか
ら」

「じゃあ、優ちゃんと同じなんですね」

かすみの口から優司の名前が出た。

「そうね。でも仲間君は養子に出たりはしてないものね。まあ、それが良かったかどうか分から
ないけど。私みたいにお金のある家に貰われてれば、やくざなんかにならなくてもすんだかもし
れないし」

そう言いながら、優司の場合はきっとそうだったろうと思った。

ビールが一本空くと「美帆さん、何にしますか」と言いながらかすみは席を離れ、カウンター
の中へ入った。カウンターの向こうの彼女はさすがに様になっている。

「かっこいいわね」

美帆が言う。かすみは訝しげな顔をした。

「なんだか、そうやってるとママさんって感じ。颯爽としてる」

「そうですか」

かすみは語尾を上げるように言った。

水割りを二つ持って戻ってきた。座りなおした途端に、

「でも、四年前に優ちゃん、きっぱり足を洗ったから」

とかすみが言った。

グラスに伸ばしていた美帆の手が止まった。

「え」

つい声を上げていた。

「それ、どういうこと」

言葉が詰まる。今度はかすみが不思議そうな目になった。

「美帆さん、知らなかったんですか？」

何度も首を縦に振った。

「五年前に、優ちゃんが刺されて死にかけたのは知ってます？」

無言で頷く。

「そのあと、優ちゃん、やくざの世界から足洗ったんです。一家名乗り直前で、若い衆も集めたし、足抜けするとなれば世話になった親分さんの顔をつぶすことにもなるんで、きっと大変だったと思います。私には何も言わなかったけど、お金も相当使ったはずですよ。結局、向こう十

年間、博多の町には一歩も足を踏み入れないという一札を入れて、きれいさっぱり組とは縁を切ったんです。まあ、そんな誓約も半分は親分さんの温情だったって優ちゃんは言ってますけど」

美帆はかすみの話を耳に入れながら、半ば唖然としていた。

まさか優司がやくざ稼業から足を洗っているなどとは想像もしていなかった。

「だから、いまの優ちゃんは正真正銘の堅気ですよ」

かすみがちょっと自慢げにつけ足した。

ホームレスの男を助けたときの「あの人も昔はやくざ者やったんやろ。俺と同類たい」という優司の言葉が脳裡に甦る。あれは言葉通りの意味合いだったということか。

「じゃあ、彼、いまは何しているの?」

かすみは幾分、呆れ気味の風情だった。

「優ちゃん、この駅の裏で焼き鳥屋やってるんですよ。繁盛していて、もう市内に支店が三つもあるんです」

「焼き鳥屋?」

思わず聞き返してしまう。

「はい。『焼鳥の富士本』っていうんです。といっても、優ちゃんはもう店には出てませんけど。支店が増えてきて、裏方に回るようになったから。そうそうリリコの彼氏の研ちゃんが二号店の店長ですよ。あの人、もともと優ちゃんの弟分だったんですけど、優ちゃんが片瀬に引っ込んだときに一緒についてきたんです」

128

あの研一が焼き鳥屋の店長？　そういえば、七月にここでみんなで飲んだとき、店をバイトに任せきりにして研一が妙なことに手を出している、と優司がリリコをたしなめていた。その物言いには美帆もすこしひっかかった覚えがあった。

「研ちゃんって左手の小指を詰めてるよね」

美帆は訊いた。

「ええ」

「この三月にもう一本詰めたんじゃない？　となりの薬指」

「そんなことないですよ。研ちゃんも組とはとっくに切れてるから」

急に何を言い出すのだ、とかすみの表情が物語っていた。

じゃあ、あれは単なる指の怪我に過ぎなかったということか。包帯にくるまれた薬指の先が欠けているかどうか、この目で確かめたわけではなかった。

「そうだったんだ」

美帆はそれ以上、口がきけなくなった。それならそうと、どうして優司は言ってくれなかったのだろう。しかし、考えてみれば、美帆が思い込んでいただけで優司は別に隠すつもりなどなかったのかもしれない。

優司が足を洗っていたとなれば、いままでの彼の言動がまったく異なった色調で思い出されてくる。

死ぬ時くらい素面でいたいから酒もクスリも止めたと言っていた。刺されたあとは、いつまた襲われるかと思うと恐ろしくて飲めなくなったと言っていた。生死は一つの事だが、そこには生

129

きる義、死ぬ義が必要なのだと言っていた。

慶応病院の病室で背中の一匹龍を見せながら、

「こげんもん背負っとるせいで、個室に一人ぽっちよ」

とぼやいてもいた。

「美帆さん」

ぽうっとしていたのだろう。かすみが声を掛けてきた。

「かすみさん、仲間君のこと詳しいのね。彼とはどうやって知り合ったの」

自分の気持ちの動揺を見透かされたくなくて、美帆は質問した。彼女の話ぶりだと二人はかなり古い付き合いに違いない。むろん男女の関係でもあるのだろう。

「この前も話しましたけど、優ちゃんは私の命の恩人なんです」

かすみには前回よりも打ち解けた感じがあった。美帆が優司とそれほど親しい間柄でないと知って一安心なのだろう。

「私、二十二のときに結婚して、福岡にやって来たんです」

かすみは水割りを一口すすって話し始めた。

短大時代に知り合った二つ年長の夫は博多の出身だった。彼は大学院を出ると中学教師の職を見つけ、郷里に戻ることになった。かすみはこれを機に、二年間勤めていた都内の会社を辞めて彼と一緒に博多に行く決心をしたのだった。

「学校が始まる直前の三月末に、慌てて福岡市内で結婚式を挙げたんです」

翌年には長女が生まれた。この子は今年で小学校三年生になっているはずだという。名前はあ

130

かり。ちょうどあかりを産んだ頃に夫が心臓病で倒れた。それまで何の兆候もなかったのが、ある日、いきなり発作を起こして倒れたのだった。病院で調べてもらうと重度の心筋症と診断された。

夫は何とか教壇には立ち続けることができたが、激しい運動は禁じられた。セックスも厳禁と医師に宣告された。

それでもお互いに我慢できずに一度だけしたことがあった。案の定、夫はひどい発作を起こしてしまい、救急車を呼ぶような騒ぎになった。

博多に来て三年経った二十五歳のとき、思い余ってかすみは出会い系サイトに手を出してしまった。月に一度か二度、後腐れのないセックスができればそれでいいと思った。

三人目の男がやくざだった。

最初のセックスから覚醒剤の水溶液を膣に塗り込まれた。男が恐ろしくて抵抗などできなかった。

二度、三度と呼び出されているうちにクスリの力に引き込まれていった。やがて家事も育児も手につかなくなり、半年もすると夫の両親にも勘づかれていた。もうその頃にはいっぱしのシャブ中になっていた。

またたく間に離婚され、病院に放り込まれた。

男の手引きで病院から脱走した。シャブがやれないなら死んだ方がましだった。自分にはもはや何も失うものはないと思っていた。

中洲に連れて行かれ、男の言いなりに風俗で働くようになった。お決まりのコースだった。

131

一年も経たずに、男が大きな借金を作って姿をくらました。ある朝、住んでいたマンションにやくざたちが押しかけてきた。部屋にはかすみ一人だった。やくざたちはかすみの判子が押された借用書を広げてみせると、逃げた男の代わりにたっぷり稼いで貰うからな、とすごんでみせた。

そして、連れて行かれたのが優司がいる組事務所だった。

優司はかすみを一目見るなり、「もう二度とシャブには手を出すな」と言った。

それから時間をかけてかすみの身の上を聞いた。

昼になるとすしの出前を取ってくれて、彼が淹れてくれたお茶を飲んだ。そのお茶があまりに美味しいのでかすみはびっくりした。すしを食べ終わると、車に乗せられ、とあるマンションに運ばれた。

殺されるとは思わなかったが、ここで毎日何十人という客を取らされるのだろうと思った。だが、そんなことよりもクスリを切られることの方が怖かった。

「そこは、優ちゃんの自宅だったんです。いきなり部屋に連れ込まれると両手両足を縛られて、ああ、この人はきっと変態なんだ、これから私をいたぶりながら犯して楽しむつもりなんだって思いました」

かすみは笑いながら言った。

それから丸四ヵ月のあいだ、優司はかすみを自室に半ば監禁して、彼女の身体の中の覚醒剤を一滴残らず抜いたのだ。

「最後は幻覚で半狂乱になるんです。汚い話だけど、オシッコもウンチも垂れ流し状態。なのに優ちゃんは、私が暴れているあいだ、一晩でも二晩でも一睡もしないで世話をしてくれたんで

132

す」

きれいな身体になって外に出てみると、薄汚れた街の景色でさえ「輝いて見えた」という。結局、彼女は優司の紹介で中洲のクラブで働き始めた。いつの間にか前の男の借金は消えていた。

「だけど、どうして仲間君はあなたのためにそこまでしてくれたのかしら」

話を聞いていて、その点が美帆には一番ひっかかった。

「私も、ずっとその理由が分からなかったんです。中洲の店で一年くらい働いて、そしたら年の暮れに優ちゃんが刺されてしまって。そのとき初めて、優ちゃんがどうしてあそこまでしてくれたのか何となく分かった気がしたんです」

美帆は手にしていたグラスをテーブルに戻した。

「優ちゃんが入院しているとき、ある女性がお見舞いに来たんです。私、たまたま病室にいて顔を合わせたんですけど、その人と私がすごくよく似ていて、まるで姉妹じゃないかっていうくらいだったんです。きっと向こうもそう感じたと思います。で、私、ピンときたんです」

かすみの言わんとするところが美帆にもすぐ了解できた。

「その人はどういう人なの」

「詳しくは分からないし、私も優ちゃんには何も訊いてません。ただ、名前は富士本美由紀と名乗っていました」

「富士本……」

美帆は独りごちた。

「優ちゃんが足を洗っていまの店を始めるとき、屋号に富士本ってつけたんで、私は、やっぱり

133

なって思いました」

退院した優司は組を離れることになり、かすみは彼について片瀬まで来た。新町のバーでさらに二年勤め、必死で貯めたお金でこの店を居抜きで買ったのが一昨年の春だったという。

「優ちゃん、そんなこと一言も言わないけど、あの富士本美由紀という人とのあいだにはきっと深い事情があるに違いないって、私は睨んでいます」

かすみはそう言って、小さなため息をついてみせた。

カウンターに置かれた携帯電話が鳴ったのは、かすみがグラスを洗っている最中だった。美帆はテーブルを拭いていた。

時刻は二時半を回っていた。

水を止めたかすみが手を拭って携帯を取り上げた。

開いた携帯を耳に当てた途端、その顔が曇った。

「あんた、どうしたの。泣いてるだけじゃ分からないよ」

こわばった声になっている。泣いてるだけじゃ分からないよ」

「一体何があったの。どうしたの。いまどこにいるの」

眉間に深い皺が寄っていた。よく見ると、化粧が浮いて細かくひび割れている。

「リリコ。泣いてるだけじゃ分からないよ。しっかりして。どこか怪我してるの」

相手はリリコだ。

「とにかくそのままじっとしてるんだよ。いまからすぐ行くから。十五分で着くからね。それま

134

では誰も部屋に入れちゃ駄目だよ」

唐突に電話は終わった。

布巾を持って美帆はカウンターに近づいた。かすみと目が合った。

「リリコちゃん、どうかしたの」

「また研一に殴られたのよ」

かすみが舌打ちするように言った。

駅前でタクシーを拾った。リリコのマンションまで十分程度だという。がらがらの国道をタクシーはスピードを出して走る。美帆もかすみも無言だった。

ニューオータニで丈二の両親と食事をしていたのが数時間前だった。それがいまはこうして片瀬の田舎道を元シャブ中の女と二人で若いホステスの部屋へと向かっている。丈二は自分が出馬する次期衆議院選挙の話をしていた。父親も母親もそれが当然のように息子の話を聞いていた。

一方、こちらではやくざ上がりの男に暴行を働かれた女が、泣き叫びながら助けを求めてきている。

研一は常習犯だとかシャブは駅までの道すがら、うんざりした口調で言っていた。

「シャブやってると、突然切れるのよ。もう何度目だか分からない。だから優ちゃんもケンとは早く手を切れっていつも言ってるのよ」

「そんな男とリリコちゃんはどうして別れないの」

美帆は素朴な疑問を口にした。かすみは遠くを見るような目つきになって、

「あの子が研一にぞっこんなのは、セックスのせいよ。きっといままでもシャブ使われて毎晩気違いみたいにイカされてるのよ。シャブマンやっちゃったらそれ以外のセックスできなくなるから。

135

と言った。

リリコもシャブ中とおんなじよ」

まるで同じ世界ではないみたいだ、と明かり一つ見えない国道沿いの風景を眺めながら美帆は思った。あれから何日も経ったような気がするだけではなく、まるきり違う世界に迷い込んでしまったような気がする。

鍵を開けてくれたリリコを見て美帆もかすみも玄関先で絶句した。

かすみは靴を脱ぎもせずにリリコを抱き締めた。リリコは腫れ上がった顔をかすみの首の付け根に押し当て、何も言わずにしゃくりあげた。

「もう大丈夫だからね。もう誰にもひどいことさせないからね」

彼女はリリコのくしゃくしゃの髪を撫でている。美帆は二人をその場に残して部屋に上がった。念のため、中の様子を確かめておきたかった。万が一、研一が潜んでいたら自分たちまで暴力の餌食になってしまう。

部屋は広めの1LDKだった。小さなダイニングテーブルが置かれたリビングも、隣の八畳ほどの寝室もめちゃくちゃになっていた。

リリコのあの有様からして予想はついたが、ここまで凄まじく荒らされた部屋というものを美帆は初めて見た。

これほどの暴力が吹き荒れた中で、リリコはよく生き延びられたものだ、という気がしたくらいだった。

五分ほどしてかすみが抱きかかえるようにしてリリコをリビングに連れて来た。割れた食器や

倒れた棚、砕け散ったサイドボードのガラス片などで足の踏み場もない。驚いたのは天井のシャンデリア型の電灯まで木っ端微塵になっていたことだ。棒かバットでも使って打ち壊さないかぎり、とてもこうはならない。

ガラス片を避けながら、かすみは壁際のソファまでリリコを運んで座らせた。彼女はそのまま服や衣装ケースが散乱する寝室へ入り、どこからか救急箱を見つけて戻って来た。コットンにマキロンをたっぷりしみこませ、優しく声を掛けながらリリコの顔の傷を消毒しはじめた。実に手馴れた感じだった。

左目は塞がるほどに腫れ上がっていた。右頬には深い裂傷があり、噴き出した血がすでに固まりだしている。唇は上下とも紫色に膨れ上がり、鼻からはぼたぼた鼻血がこぼれていた。口の中もぐちゃぐちゃだろうし、歯も何本か折れているに違いなかった。

顔の消毒が終わると、花柄の薄手のワンピースを着たリリコの全身をかすみはゆっくりとさすっていく。首、肩、腕、腰、お腹や胸、腿、膝、足首、爪先、そして尻や背中をまるで卑猥な手つきでくまなく撫でさする。部位ごとに少し指に力を込めて「ここ痛くない？」と訊いていた。リリコは幼児のようなしぐさで首を横に振っていた。

美帆が、床に散ったガラスの片づけから始めていると、

「大丈夫。骨は折れていないみたいね。でも顔がひどいし、内臓は分からないから」

と言ってかすみは立ち上がった。そばに置いていた自分のバッグから携帯を取り出した。

「美帆さん、優ちゃんを呼ぶけどいいよね」

と断ってくる。美帆は頷いた。

優司は十分ほどでやって来た。電話で美帆のことは伝わっていたので、顔を合わせても「お

う」と言っただけだった。ソファの上にへたりこんでいるリリコの顔を慎重に検分し、「この腫

れ方だと頬骨にひびくらい入ってるな」と呟いた。

「やっぱりいまから病院に行った方がいいと思う」

美帆が言うと、優司も頷いた。

「二人とも飲んでるのか」

と訊いてくる。

「私はもうすっかり醒めてる」

かすみが答えた。

「私も大丈夫」

美帆も言った。リリコの顔を見た瞬間にほろ酔い機嫌など吹き飛んでしまった。

優司がポケットから車のキーを出して、かすみに手渡した。

「二人ですぐに市民病院に連れて行ってやってくれ。医者には最初からDVだと伝えた方がよか。

そっちの方が変な勘繰りされんですむやろ」

「分かった」

かすみはリリコのそばに寄ると、中腰になって、

「リリちゃん、一緒に病院に行こう」

と言った。時刻は午前三時をとっくに過ぎていた。

「研一は何でこんなことをした。理由は何や」

138

かすみの身体につかまりながら立ち上がったリリコに優司は言った。この部屋に入ってリリコの無残な姿や室内の惨状を見ても、優司は眉一つ動かさなかった。リリコに対する態度にもさしたる同情は窺われない。問いかけにリリコが答えないでいると、

「だから、一体どうして研一がここまで暴れたんかと訊いとるやろうが。ちゃんと答えんか」

優司は苛ついた声でたたみかける。

「先週、お客さんに貰った時計のことが研ちゃんにバレちゃって……」

くぐもった声でリリコが言った。声まで別人のようだった。

「また、そげんくだらんことかい」

優司は吐き捨てるように言った。

「もうこれが限界やな。よかな、リリコ」

俯いたままのリリコがしばらくして小さく頭を縦に振った。

それだけ確かめると、優司は部屋の隅に移動して電話を掛け始めた。

「おう俺や、研一を見たらすぐに連絡頼むわ。何時でも構わん」

と言っている。あっという間に切った。また別の相手に同じことを言っていた。そうやって片っ端から電話をしている優司を残して、かすみと美帆はリリコを連れて部屋を出た。

四年前に足を洗ったというが、今夜の優司はどう見ても正真正銘のやくざにしか見えなかった。

139

十一月二十九日

以前に比べると永妻克子はやけに老け込んでいた。もともと年齢不詳の人物ではあるが、こうして面と向かってみれば、顔の皺は二倍に、白髪は三倍にでもなったかのようだった。永妻はいま一体幾つなのだろう。まだ四十前にも思えるし、もう五十間近であるようにも見える。化粧気のない浅黒い顔は、顎の骨が発達していて男のようだ。

ただ、目が美しい。澄み切っていながらも、相手の嘘やごまかしを一瞬で看破しそうな強い光を秘めている彼女の目。初めて会ったとき、即座に仕事を依頼しようと決めたのは、その目に魅せられたからだった。

「もし、ご結婚云々ということであれば、すこし慎重に考えられた方がいいお相手だと思いますが」

永妻は低い声で言った。この仕事を始める前は何をしていたのだろう。女性ではあるが、やはり警察官だったのか。どうしてこんな仕事をやっているのだろう。結婚はしているのだろうか。彼女でも好きな男の前では別の女に変身したりできるのか。

「そのようですね」

美帆は相槌を打った。

目の前のテーブルには分厚い調査報告書が置かれていた。「永妻克子調査事務所」はＪＲ新橋駅から虎ノ門方向へ歩いて十分ほどの場所にある。日比谷通りを渡って、西新橋の小さなビルが立て込んだ一角、四階建ての古い雑居ビルの三階だった。

ここ数日、雨や曇天の日がつづいたが、今日は朝からさっぱりした快晴だった。

すでに午後三時を回っているものの、初冬の日差しは、まだ十分に窓から降り注いでいた。窓を背負って座る永妻の顔が逆光のせいで余計に皺深く陰気に見える。

片瀬から戻って来てこの三週間、美帆はずっと体調がすぐれなかった。二度ほど病院にも行った。雨の日はとくに悪かった。久しぶりの晴天のおかげか、今日は比較的調子がよかった。

ニューオータニで別れてから、丈二とは一度も話していない。当日、翌日と何度か携帯に連絡が来たが、電源を切ったり、出なかったりでやり過ごした。翌々日の夜、東京に戻ってみると、部屋のドアの新聞受けに手紙が入っていた。

〈電話にも出ないし、ここにも帰っていないようなので一筆します。

一昨日は、一体どうしたのですか？ 急にあんなふうに怒り出して、僕も、父や母もただただ驚いてしまいました。何か、僕が美帆を傷つけるようなことをしたのではないか、と危惧しています。すくなくとも、こちらが気づかないうちに、美帆が僕に対して大きな不満を募らせていたのではないかと。

あのときのことは、もう何とも思っていません。

親たちもいずれは忘れてくれるでしょう。

美帆もいまはきっと冷静になっているのだと信じます。でも、しばらくはお互い気まずいかもしれない。

また、折を見て訪ねます。そのときは、とにかくこのドアを開けてください。

　　　美帆へ

　　　　　　　　　　　　　　　　　　　　　　　JOE2〉

この文面を読んで、美帆は、裏切りの匂いをうっすらと嗅ぎ取った。丈二という男には「時間を置く」などという発想はない。彼はあらゆる課題をその場で解決しようと欲する人間だった。

手紙を見つけてから二週間待って、美帆は永妻に丈二の素行調査を依頼した。ちょうど一週間前の二十二日月曜日のことだった。

予想通り、丈二は他の女性と付き合い始めていた。ニューオータニで四人で食事をしたのは七日の日曜日だったが、丈二はその週、十二日の金曜日に奈良に帰り、翌日には市内のホテルである女性と見合いをしていたのだった。その電光石火の早業ぶり、向こうの親たちの手回しのよさにはさすがに美帆も呆れるばかりだった。

見合いの相手は、桐山組の社長、桐山貞行の孫娘だった。名前は春奈。地元の女子大に通うまだ二十歳の学生だった。

永妻の報告書によれば、春奈は見合いの翌週も翌々週も上京し、丈二とデートを重ねていた。

添付の写真が撮影された先週木曜日には、丈二の高輪のマンションに彼女が泊まったことが確認

されていた。

写真で見る限り、どうということもない若い女の子だった。

日本テレビの女性記者と丈二が関係を持ったときのことを思い出した。

美帆に勘づかれた丈二は最初は白を切っていたが、そのうち平謝りに謝りだした。美帆には言葉は必要なかった。一刻も早く女と手を切り、これを潮時に記者の仕事を辞めて、もう一度弁護士を目指すと丈二が決めてくれれば許すつもりだった。だが、彼の口から出てきたのは「時間をくれ。きれいに別れるから」という無責任な一言だけだった。

美帆は、相手の女性に会いに行った。一目見て、

なんだ、この程度の人でもいいんだ。

と正直、拍子抜けした。

向こうは突然の美帆の出現にうろたえていた。

「あなたのしていることっておかしくないですか。だいいち彼の奥さんでも何でもないわけでしょう。あなたのような人がいるなんて、私、全然知らなかった。だから謝りようもないわ。でも、もう二度と彼と会わないことは約束します」

言葉は強気だったが、彼女は美帆と正対してしどろもどろだった。

その夜、丈二が美帆の部屋に怒鳴り込んできた。

「俺の仕事をめちゃくちゃにするつもりかよ。あの女とは同じ記者クラブにいるんだぞ。さっそく今日の夕方、うちのキャップのところへねじ込んできたそうだよ。一体どうするんだよ、俺の方が飛ばされたら。ただの遊びだって言っただろ。ほんとうなんだよ。あんな女、好きでもなん

143

でもなかったんだ。ちょっと生意気だから寝てみた、それだけなんだよ。なのに一体何てことをしてくれるんだ」

丈二はしたたかに酔っていた。

美帆の気持ちが一気に冷めたのは、この醜悪な一場を経験したあとだった。

手紙では「あのときのことは、もう何とも思っていません」だの「また、折を見て訪ねます」だの柔和な文句を書き連ねているが、両親、ことに母親の面前で美帆にあんな咬呵を切られて、プライドの高い丈二が憤激していないはずがなかった。彼がソフト路線を選択しているのは、美帆との別れで余計な傷を負いたくないからだろう。もっと露骨に言えば、いずれ選挙に出馬する人間として、長年付き合った恋人にあれこれ告発されるような禍根だけは残したくないのだ。まして、桐山社長の孫娘が相手となれば、それを知った美帆がどう出てくるのか一抹の不安もあるだろう。丈二としてはどうしても泥仕合は演じたくない。できるだけきれいに別れたいに違いない。

永妻の報告を聞き、案の定、そんなことかと美帆は思った。

桐山春奈との交際を知った以上、丈二と縒りを戻す可能性はほとんど無くなってしまった。だからといって丈二とあっさり別れるわけにはいかない。彼は相応の報いを受けるべきだし、美帆の側にも丈二といま一度、真正面から対峙せざるを得ない事情があった。

「これは直接、今回のご依頼とは関係ないのですが」

永妻がおずおずといった感じで一枚の紙切れを取り出し、美帆の前に置いた。

そのA4の文書を取り上げ、ざっと目を通した。

144

「今年の五月下旬に奈良県庁の課長級以上の職員宅に一斉に郵送された怪文書です。県の総務課の指示で直ちに回収されたそうですが、もちろんこうしてコピーが流出しました」

永妻が言う。

こんな怪文書のことなど丈二は一言も言っていなかった。しかし、知らなかったはずはない。

「出元がどのへんかは分かってるんですか」

美帆は訊いた。

「当然、一番疑わしいのは水上陣営でしょうね。ただ、黒川丈二さんに対してというより、黒川建設と黒川庸一氏にかねて恨みを持つ者の仕業だと言う人もいます」

「そうですか」

美帆は一つ息をついた。もう一度、文書に目を落とした。「愛人の子」、「朝鮮人」、「総連のスパイ」といった語句が太ゴチックで強調されていた。

「ひどいですね」

独りごちるように言う。この怪文書を初めて見せられたときの丈二の気持ちはいかばかりだったろうか。

「まあ、怪文書ですから」

永妻はあくまで淡々としていた。

「それに……」

彼女は言葉をつないだ。

「中味はまんざらデタラメというわけでもありません。丈二さんの実母であるみどりさんの亡く

145

なった父親は、昭和三十年代に活躍した朝鮮総連の幹部です。みどりさんは、その男が同じ朝鮮人の愛人に産ませた子供ですが、腹違いの兄はいまも総連で重要なポストに就いています。バブル崩壊直後には公安が黒川建設と総連との関係を調べたこともあったようです。不正取引などの直接の証拠は出なかったようですが、黒川建設の資金繰りが悪化していた一時期、総連系の金融機関から黒川が融資を仰いでいるのは事実です。現在でも、黒川庸一は要監視対象者のリストから外れていないという噂です」

永妻が説明した話の一部は怪文書にも記述されていた。公認が下りるかどうか瀬戸際の時期にこんなものをばら撒かれては、丈二にとっては相当のダメージだったろう。

こうした経緯を知ってみれば、次の選挙に向け、黒川家が地元の足場固めをしたくなる気持ちも分からなくはなかった。何の閨閥も背景も持たない孤児上がりの嫁など迎えるよりも、盟友とはいえこのままでは敵に回しかねない桐山貞行と縁戚関係を結ぶ方がはるかに得策に決まっている。

「今回もお世話になりました。料金は明日必ず振込んでおきます」

調査報告書の束をカバンにしまい、美帆は立ち上がった。

「お役に立てたなら光栄です」

永妻が一緒に立ち上がりながら、いつもの決まり文句を言った。

怪文書以外は何も置かれていないだだっ広いテーブルが二人を隔てていた。

そういえば、この事務所を訪れるのはもう四度目だったが、お茶の一杯も出たことがないな、

と美帆は思った。

146

十二月十二日

午後六時。

玄関のチャイムが鳴った瞬間に、丈二だと分かった。

二、三日前から、彼がもうすぐやって来るだろうという気がしていた。

あれから三十五日。丈二にとっての「ちょっとだけ」とはその程度の期間だったということか。

初めて知り合って別れるまでの六年間、離れ離れだった七年間、そして再会してからの二年。そのどれと比べてもたしかに三十五日なんて、ほんのちょっとだけに過ぎない。

彼は一体どういうつもりで訪ねてきたのだろうか。桐山春奈とのことを伏せたままで美帆との関係を解消させる妙手を編み出したのか。頭のいい彼のことだ、すくなくとも何らかの切り札は手にして、今回の訪問に臨んでいるに違いない。

そうやすやすといくはずがないとの予想もつけてはいるだろう。

だが、強い意志さえ貫き通すことができれば自ずと道は開ける、と安易に楽観していることも疑いない。

丈二は本質的にそういう人間だし、男というのは緻密な頭脳を持っているくせに、肝心なところで地に足のつかない希望的観測をしてしまう生き物なのだ。

そんな男の甘さを、今日は粉々に打ち砕いてやる、と美帆は決心していた。

一度裏切った人間は、また必ず裏切る。やはりその通りだった。

しかし、二人で蒔いた種は二人で刈り取るしかないのだ。この十五年にも及ぶ根深い関係を断ち切るには、互いに相当量の血を流す以外にない。理屈や計算などでは解決し得ない問題がこの世界には満ち溢れていることを、消し去ることのできない記憶として彼の脳裡に焼き付けてやらなくてはならない。

最終的には美帆がケリをつけるにしても、自分だけが泥をかぶるなんて真っ平御免だった。こうした事態に立ち至った責任の過半は丈二にあった。

彼の今回の裏切りがなければ、別の可能性もなくはなかったのだ。

すべてを台無しにしてしまったのは、間違いなく黒川丈二の方だった。

しばらく待たせてから美帆は玄関に行った。ドアを開ける。

「よっ」

丈二は満面に笑みを浮かべていた。手には紙袋をぶら提げている。ワインだ。彼は必ず赤と白の両方を買ってくる。そうした些細な癖にも性格が反映されている。もともと欲張りな男なのだ。

そして、こういう朗らかな笑みを浮かべているときの彼は、したたかな計算を腹中で働かせていた。

美帆は最初からワインを抜いた。部屋は十分にあたためてある。上着を脱がせようとすると丈二はやんわりと拒んだ。長居をするつもりはないのだろう。いつものようにリビングのダイニングテーブルを挟んで向かい合って座った。

148

シャンベルタンの赤を丈二のグラスに注ぐ。ナポレオンがこよなく愛したワインだと教えたら、彼はそれ以来すっかりシャンベルタン党になってしまった。一体、何回、一緒にこのワインを飲んだだろうか。

「元気そうね」

美帆は言って、先にワイングラスを口許へ運んだ。乾杯はもうできない。

「まあまあかな」

丈二もワインを口に含む。

「最初に言っておきたいことがあるんだけど、いい」

丈二の顔にかすかな期待が滲んだ。予想通りだった。

だが、これから告げる言葉でそんな期待は粉砕されることになる。

「私、あなたとは絶対に別れないわよ。来年の六月までには結婚してもらう。それが約束だったでしょう。それからもう一つ。私はあなたのご両親のことを自分の親だとは思わない。結婚しても一切のお付き合いは遠慮させてもらうわ。ただ、あなたがあの人たちと交流することは止めない。だってそれはあなたの自由だから」

丈二は意外な言葉、のっけからの想定外の展開に戸惑った表情を隠さなかった。

「ちょっと待ってくれないか。もうすこしちゃんと話そう。そのために一ヵ月以上もお互いに時間を置いたんだから」

グレーのジャケットの襟を一度ととのえて言う。初めて見る上着だった。グレーは彼の趣味ではなかった。

「これは、私が何度も考えて決めたことなの。私、初めて会ったときからあなたのお母様が嫌だったの。この人とはどんなことがあっても分かり合えないだろうって直感した。だから、結婚しても関わりたくないの。あの人のためにもそれが一番いいのよ」

丈二はテーブルにのせていた両手を持ち上げ、美帆を制止するように掌を広げた。

「だから、ちょっと待ってくれよ。何だか今日の美帆はおかしい。というより、この前からそうだ。うちのお袋とのあいだで何かあったんじゃないのか。九月に上京してきたとき二人で銀座に出かけただろう。たとえばそのとき、何か揉めたりしたんじゃないのか」

丈二は冷静な顔、落ち着き払った声で言う。まるでこちらを気遣っているようなその白々しい態度が気に障る。

「別に何もなかったわ。そんなんじゃないの。とにかくあの人とは合わないのよ。そういうことってあるでしょう」

ここでちょっと誘い水を向けてみた。

「だけど、もし結婚するとなれば、お袋とうまくやってもらえなくては困る。僕の親とは付き合わないなんて滅茶苦茶だよ。僕は来年には地元から選挙に出る身なんだ。身内がバラバラじゃあ、勝てる選挙だって勝てなくなる。それくらいは美帆にだって分かるだろう。きみがそういう姿勢だととても結婚なんて無理だ」

さっそく本音が滲み出てきた。

「だったら、政治家になるのなんて止めればいいじゃない。私と結婚することと選挙に出ることとどっちが大事なの」

150

「おいおい、あんまり無茶を言わないでくれよ」

丈二が苦笑する。

「だから訊いているじゃない。どっちが大事なの」

「そんなの答えられるわけないだろう。次元の違う話を混同するなんて美帆らしくもない」

美帆は残っていたワインを飲み干し、ボトルを摑んでなみなみと注ぎ足した。

「じゃあ訊くけど、あなたはどうして政治家になりたいの。政治家になって一体何がしたいと思っているの」

また丈二が笑みを浮かべた。

「そんなこといまここで話すようなことじゃないだろう。一言で言えるようなことでもないしね」

「もったいぶらないでよ。私は知っているわ。あなたは出世したいだけなのよ。大臣にでもなって皆を見返したり、威張ったりしたいだけでしょう。あなたの親たちが、あなたが代議士になるのを望むのも同じ理由よ」

「何だよ、それ」

丈二は大袈裟に手を広げてみせる。

「もう酔っ払ったのか」

と冷たい視線で美帆を見た。

「だから誤魔化さないでって言っているでしょう。正直に答えてよ。あなたは政治家になって何がしたいの。一つでもいいから言ってごらんなさいよ」

151

「一つと言わず幾らだってやらなくちゃならないことがある。だけど、一番は、この日本という国を真の独立国にすることだよ」

丈二は面倒くさそうな顔だったが、やがて表情を引き締めて言った。

今度は美帆が苦笑する番だった。

「何が独立よ。ばっかみたい。政治家なんてどうせ何もできないのよ。ただ、偉くなってでかい顔したいだけでしょ。しっかりそう自覚している人の方が、あなたみたいな中途半端な人よりよほど出世するんじゃない。すくなくとも自分に正直な分、許せるところがあるから。政治家なんてこの社会のクズよ。やくざとどっこいどっこいの最低な商売よ。結局、金と暴力を手に入れて、この世の中を自分のいいようにしたいだけなのよ。そのためならどんな人間だって利用するし、平気で身内や仲間だって裏切る。私たち女のことなんてどう思っちゃいないわ。政治家はみんな、女なんてどうせ子供を産む道具で、子供を育てる機械くらいにしか思っていないのよ。あなただって本音はそうでしょ」

「人を愚弄するのはいい加減にしてくれないか」

丈二の声に怒気が混じった。

「別に愚弄などしていない、と美帆は思った。ただありきたりの真実を指摘しているに過ぎない。当選のために自らの結婚さえ道具とする男に、誰が「国の独立」など語って欲しいと思うだろうか。

「この日本という国を真の独立国にする？　本物の日本人でもないくせに、よくもまあそんな偉そうな口がきけるわね。笑っちゃうわ」

152

丈二の顔色が一瞬で変わった。

「あなただってあいのこじゃない。みなしごの私と似たりよったりよ。それが国会議員になるだなんて、いい加減にした方がいいのはあなたでしょう。そんな馬鹿げた夢、早く捨てなさいよ。あなたはね、田舎の土建屋が朝鮮人の愛人に産ませたエセ日本人なのよ。それくらいの現実、もう大人なんだからそろそろ受け入れたら。まったく幾つになったら目が醒めるのよ」

「僕は日本人だ。正真正銘の日本人だし、誰よりもこの国を愛している」

丈二のこんな顔はかつて見たことがないと美帆は思った。歯を食いしばり、頬は真っ赤だったが目元や額は蒼白だった。その悲憤慷慨したような、自分自身に酔ってでもいるような表情が哀れで滑稽だった。正真正銘の日本人だの国を愛しているだの、男というのは他に信ずべきものを持てないのか。

「また嘘ばっかり。あなたは朝鮮人とのハーフで、愛人の子で、そのくせべらぼうな秀才で、子供時代から肩身の狭い理不尽な思いばかりしてきたのよ。だから、自分の味わってきた悔しさの代償が欲しいだけよ。誰よりも出世して、自分のことを虐げてきた日本人やこの日本社会に復讐したいのよ。そのくせ、そうした自分の本当の気持ちには気づかないふりばかりしてきた。あなたは要するにただの臆病者に過ぎないわ」

丈二の瞳が憎悪の光できらきらしている。

美帆はグラスのワインを一息に呷った。全身の肌がぴりぴりしてきていた。いままで感じたことのない興奮が身の内から湧き上がっていた。

この感じだ、と思う。リリコの腫れ上がった顔やめちゃめちゃに荒らされた彼女の部屋の情景

153

が脳裡に甦っていた。男と女が別れるには、本来あの程度のことは当たり前なのだ。二人を貼り合わせる接着剤を溶かすには、二人して燃え盛る火に飛び込むか、滾った湯を頭からかぶるかするくらいの荒療治が必要なのだ。

そうやって、私の心だけでなく、この私の身体の中からも完全に丈二を排泄しなくてはならない、と美帆は思った。

「自殺した女の娘にそんなこと言われたくもないね。きみこそ臆病者の子供だろ」

丈二が言った。その瞬間、ふっと彼の全身から力みのようなものが抜けるのが分かった。

「自殺した女の娘ってどういうことよ」

美帆は訊き返した。

「きみは自分の親がどんな人だったかも知らないじゃないか。うちの親はそういうこともひっくるめてきみを受け入れるつもりだったんだ」

ふたたび丈二の表情に余裕の色が浮かんできた。

「まさか、私の親のことを調べたの。この私に一言の断りもなく」

丈二がここでも嘘を語っているのは明らかだった。黒川家が美帆の出自を調べたのはごく最近のことだろう。ニューオータニで食事をしたときは、庸一もみどりも詳しい事情を知っている気配はまったくなかった。

「きみがこんなひどいことを言わなければ、僕だって黙っているつもりだった。だが、今夜ではっきりと分かったよ。僕はもうきみと金輪際一緒にはやっていけない。正直なところきみがこれほど卑劣な人間だとは思わなかった。やはり生まれ持った気質は変えようがないってことだな。

154

実感したよ」

　美帆は丈二がワインで喉を湿らすのを黙って見ていた。

「僕だって、きみの母親のことを聞かされたのは、きみがあんなことをして店を出ていったあとだ。それまでは知らなかった」

　それも嘘だ、と思った。丈二たちは、美帆と別れる理由が欲しくて、慌てて調査会社に彼女の過去を洗わせたのだ。

　これから丈二が口にすることが今夜の切り札に違いない。そのカードで美帆を切り捨てることができると彼は確信しているのだろう。

「きみの母親の名前は古川美和。彼女はきみが二歳のときに自殺している。きみを東京の養護施設に預けたのは古川美和の弟、古川隆志。つまりきみのたった一人の叔父さんだ。何しろきみは私生児だからね。この古川隆志は十五年前に亡くなっている。死んだのは八王子医療刑務所。彼は服役中だった。前科七犯。札付きの結婚詐欺師だったそうだよ。きみの叔父さんは女を食い物にして生きるしかなかった哀れで恥ずべき男だ。そして、お母さんは父親も分からないような娘を産んで、しかもその子を残して自殺してしまった。どんな事情があったにしろ、彼女の自殺は無責任の誹りを免れないだろうね。　要するにきみはそういう母親や叔父の血を受けた人間だということだ。ついでに言っておくと、お母さんや叔父さんもきみ同様に大層な美男美女だったらしいよ。　不倫や結婚詐欺にはうってつけだったってわけだ」

　美帆は丈二の話には直接反応しなかった。ただ頭の中におさめただけだった。

「それでも、あなたは私とは別れることはできないわ」

155

相手の皮膚になすりつけるように言った。

「馬鹿を言うなよ。僕のことをあいのこ呼ばわりする女とどうして一緒にならなくてはいけないんだ」

「もしも私を捨てたら、あなたはとんでもない代償を支払うことになるからよ」

「代償ってどういうことだよ」

「あなたが選挙に出ることになったら洗いざらいぶちまけてやるってこと。週刊誌にでも何にでも出て、あることないこと言ってあげるわ。私がそんなことすればどこだって飛びつくはずよ。この顔をカメラの前にさらさせばいいんだもの。孤児だという理由で私を捨てたこと、どうにもならない女好きだってこと、それにあなたの生まれ育ち。あなたが落選するために必要なことはどんなことでも、たとえでっち上げてでも喋ってあげる。そんな大恥を満天下にさらすのが嫌なら、このまま私とおとなしく結婚することね。もう他にあなたに残された選択肢はないわ」

丈二は愕然とした顔で美帆を凝視している。まさかこんな成り行きになるとは想像もしていなかったはずだ。美帆の日頃の性格からして、案外あっさり終止符を打てると思い込んでいたに違いなかった。

「一体どうしたんだ。まるで人が変わったみたいじゃないか」

眉間に皺を寄せて、丈二はいま作戦の練り直しを始めていた。

「変わったんじゃない。分かったのよ」

美帆は言った。

「何が」

156

徐々に暴力的な雰囲気が丈二の全身から生まれ始めていた。

どんどん凶暴になればいい、と美帆は思う。そうやって互いの感情をさらけ出して行き着くところまで行くのだ。

暴力は望むところだった。この身体の中に巣食った丈二を丈二自身の手で抹殺させてやりたいと願う。

「あなたのことが許せないということ。あのときのあなたの仕打ちがどうしても許せないってこと。あなたに復讐しない限り、私の心は絶対に満足しないってこと。そのためならどんなことでも自分にはできるってこと。だから、あなたが最も苦しむ方法であなたを苦しめることに決めたのよ」

「それが、そうやって僕を脅して、僕と結婚するってことか」

「そう。憎みあった者同士で結婚するの」

「狂ってるな」

「ええ。私は狂ってるわ。でも、私をこんなふうにしたのはあなたよ。あなただって言っていたでしょう。お前はずっと俺を恨んでいるんだって」

「同時に愛してくれていると思っていたよ。僕がそうであるように」

「私はずっと大きな錯覚をしていたの」

美帆は下ろしていた手をテーブルの上で組んだ。

「あなたと縒りが戻ってからの二年間、私はずっと思ってた。昔はあんなにあなたのことを愛していたのに、いまはもう愛せなくなった。どうしてなんだろうって。ほんとうに最近までそう思

っていたの。それがやっとそうじゃないって分かった」

そして、美帆は一つ息を整えた。

「私はこれまであなたを愛していると錯覚していたけど、本当は一度も愛したことなんてなかったんだって。私はあなたに、ただ傷つけられてきただけなんだって。私はあなたと一緒にいると、小さく心が死んでいくの。ああ、あなたと初めて出会った二十歳の誕生日からの十五年間、私はそうやってどんどんどんどん自分の誇りのようなものをあなたに奪われてきたんだなあって。そのことにやっと気づいたの」

「最低だな」

丈二が言った。

「自分だけが一方的な被害者ってわけか」

「そうよ、その通り。だから今度はあなたが重い罰を受ける番なのよ」

「冗談じゃない。きみは明らかに精神病だ。一刻も早く病院にいくべきだね」

「だからそれでもいいって言っているでしょう。私はあなたが一番大切にしているもののどちらかを奪うことに決めたの」

「どちらかってどういう意味だよ」

「そんなの分かりきっているじゃない。一つはあなたの政治家になりたいという夢。そしてもう一つはあなたの母親の幸福。あなたは今日この場でその二つのうちの一つを諦めなくちゃいけない。私を捨てればあなたの夢が、私と結婚すればあなたの母親の幸福が失われる。選ぶのはあな

158

「もううんざりだ」

丈二が立ち上がった。これでは埒が明かないと判断したのだろう。当然のことだった。だが一度幕が開いた舞台から立ち去ることなど彼には許されない。

「逃げる気」

美帆も立ち上がる。

「気違いと幾ら話したって無駄なだけだ」

吐き捨てるように丈二が言った。

「もう二度ときみの顔は見たくない」

陳腐な捨て台詞だと美帆は思う。

玄関へと向かおうとする丈二の前に彼女は立ちふさがった。

「ちゃんとした返事をくれるまで帰さないわ」

大袈裟に両手を広げ、通せん坊の恰好をした。

「どいてくれないか」

憤怒を抑えた口調で丈二が言う。

「あなたのお母さんは、あなたの思っているような女じゃない。あいつは性悪よ。あなたの父親も騙されてるだけ。早く目を醒ましなさいよ」

「もう……。そんなくだらない妄想に付き合っているひまはないんだ」

そこで美帆は突然のように声を荒らげた。「あかり」で飲んだ晩の優司の怒声を思い出しなが

159

ら精一杯に怒鳴りあげた。

「朝鮮人の子が偉そうな顔すんじゃないよ。日本人でもない女にどうしてこの私があれこれ言わ
れなくちゃいけないんだよ」

頬に激しい痛みが走った。

耳の奥にまで響く派手な音が聴こえた。

「これ以上、お袋の悪口を言うな」

美帆は張られた左の頬を押さえ、怒りに歪む丈二の顔を見据えた。

丈二が大声を出した。やはり男の声は桁違いだ。

「あんた、女を殴ってただで済むと思ってんの」

腹の底からいま一度声を絞り出した。

「甘えるんじゃないよ！」

美帆は頭から丈二に突っ込んでいった。丈二の胸の骨に自分の頭頂部が激しくぶつかるのが分
かる。相手が一歩あとずさった。

直後、ものすごい力が襲ってきた。

一瞬で、美帆は後方に弾き飛ばされていた。後ろにたたらを踏むまでもなかった。全身が宙に
浮いてそのまま尻から床に落ちていた。激しい衝撃と痺れるような痛みが腰から背中へと突き抜
けた。

すぐさま美帆は立ち上がった。ここで怯むわけにはいかない。怒りを喚起し、黒川丈二という
男のすべてを身をもって否定するのだ。

160

「殺してやる。お前なんか殺してやる」

壁の書棚の中段にあった陶製の置時計を摑んだ。ひらべったいミントンの時計だった。それを右手に振りかざして、仁王立ちになっている丈二へと突進していった。目をつぶり、彼の頭めがけて全力で右腕を振り下ろす。ゴツンという鈍い音としたたかな手ごたえがあった。

「何するんだ、この野郎」

獣のような叫びが上がる。美帆は時計を床に捨て、そのまま肩の辺りをおさえている丈二に食らいついていった。彼の顔や首を手当たり次第に引っ掻き、腹や胸を渾身の力を込めて殴りつける。

人間をこんなに本気で殴ったのは初めてだった。

だが、それももののの数秒のことだった。最初とは比べものにならないほどの力で、美帆は吹き飛ばされた。

壁に並んだ書棚の一つに身体ごと打ちつけられた。書棚が揺れ、うずくまった美帆の上に本や雑誌が降ってきた。

必死で立ち上がろうとした。この程度ではきっとまだ足りない。リリコのようにもっともっと殴られるのだ。

だが、立てなかった。どこかの関節を痛めたのかもしれない。足に力がどうしても入らなかった。

丈二が歩み寄ってくる。美帆はかろうじてよつんばいになった。首を起こして近づく丈二を犬のような恰好で見上げた。

161

「来るな」

一喝した。

丈二は蔑んだ瞳で一瞥をくれたあと踵を返した。出て行くまでの後ろ姿を目で追うことはできなかった。ドアが荒々しく閉じられた音を聞いて、美帆はふたたび床にくずおれてしまった。身体の節々がじんじんしていた。しばらく背を丸めていた。身体の節々がじんじんしていた。首も腕も足も十本の指も決定的なダメージは受けていないようだった。呼吸を整えて各所を動かしていく。美帆はゆるゆると立ち上がり、窓のそばのソファまで歩いて、静かに身を投げた。ソファに仰向けに寝そべり両手を下腹に置いた。

レースのカーテン越しにほのかな明かりが射し込んでいた。今日は日曜日だった。壁の掛け時計を見るとまだ七時を過ぎたばかりだ。表参道は人で一杯だろう。通りの店々のショーウィンドーには、早くもクリスマスの飾り付けが施されていた。

丈二が今日という日を選んだのは、何となく分かる気がした。あと二週間もすればクリスマスイブだ。そのイブを心おきなく桐山春奈と祝うためには、今日が別れ話を持ち込むぎりぎりのタイミングだと判断したのだ。もう彼の中には、そのイブが美帆の三十五回目の誕生日であり、二人が付き合い始めて十五年目の記念日だという思いは一片すらなかった。そのことが今夜、丈二と会ってみてはっきりと分かった。

十五分ほど寝そべっていたが下腹部に期待していた違和感は生まれなかった。

美帆は目を閉じる。

ちくしょう、ちくしょう、ちくしょう……。

162

目を瞑った途端にみるみる涙があふれてきた。美帆は両手で自分の腹を殴りつける。

泣きながら何度も何度も殴りつづけた。

美帆は、この世に生まれてきたことをずっと呪いつづけてきた。

そしていま、女として生まれてきた自分が無性に許せなかった。

昭和六十一年九月二十日

スプーンは真っ白な猫だった。

弟の正也が一歳になった年に父が知り合いから貰ってきた。まだ生後二ヵ月ほどの仔猫だった。キャットフードをなかなか食べなくて、美帆がスプーンにフードをすくって口許まで近づけたところ、やっと食べてくれた。それでスプーンという名前になった。雑種のメスだったが、穏やかで優しかった。美帆が沈んでいたりすれば、そばに寄り添ってっと見つめられているような心地になった。大きな瞳は青みがかっていて、じそっと見守ってくれるような猫だった。美帆も正也もスプーンのことが大好きだった。

小学校五年の春、植皮手術を受けた美帆が無事退院し、自宅で一週間ほどの休みを取っているとき、早苗がスプーンをベランダから投げた。美帆はちょうど庭に出て日向ぼっこをしていた。スプーンの悲鳴が頭上から聞こえて、顔を上向けた。ふだんはそんな大声を出す猫ではなかった。

163

スプーンを両手に抱えた母がちょうど手すりから身を乗り出すところだった。

早苗はまるでサッカー選手のスローインのようにスプーンを放った。スプーンは声も出せずに、見上げる美帆の頭をはるかに越えて、当時庭の中央に掘られていた池のすぐ近くまで飛んでいった。

そして、池の縁石に半身の体勢で打ちつけられ、左後ろ足に大怪我を負ったのだった。

それからは、その瞬間の光景が頻繁に夢に出てくるようになった。しかも現実とは違って、夢の中のスプーンは、庭の芝生に座り込んでいる美帆の頭上めがけて全身をばたつかせ、金切り声を上げながら真っ逆さまに落ちてきて、目の前の地面にしたたかに叩きつけられた。

そのたびに美帆ははっとしてベッドから跳ね起きねばならなかった。

それでもスプーンは力強く生きた。彼女が亡くなったのは正也が東京の大学に進学する直前だった。

もう二度と母に心を許すことなく、スプーンはその後、実に十一年の長い歳月を見事に生き抜いたのだった。

高校二年の夏休み。

美帆は吹奏楽部に所属していた。連日登校して、他の部員と共に練習に励んでいた。文化祭での演奏会が九月に迫っていた。美帆の扱っていた楽器はクラリネット。本当はサックスかコルネットを吹きたかったのだが、入部のときの抽選で負けてしまった。

八月末のことだった。

音楽室で練習していると、何やら外が騒がしくなった。演奏を止め、部員の一人が偵察に行った。「誰かが屋上のフェンスを越えて、飛び降りようとしている」という報告で、全員が楽器を

164

放り出して校庭に飛び出した。

朝礼台の周辺に大勢の人間が群がっていた。登校していた生徒たち数十人のほかに教師も幾人か混ざっていた。みんなが真上に顔を向けていた。まだ警察は来ていなかった。

制服姿の女子生徒が一人、屋上のへりに立っていた。

美帆は野次馬たちとはすこし離れた場所から彼女の姿を見た。

校舎寄りに陣取っていた。そちらからの方が女子生徒の様子がよく見えたのだ。

美帆が到着して、山口さんが身を投げるまでには三十秒もなかった。

「あれ、三年の山口やろう」

という誰かの声が耳に届いた。山口と聞いても美帆にはピンとこなかった。

彼女はあっさりと虚空に舞った。

大きくてがっちりした木製の朝礼台の手前にいるのは美帆一人で、他の人々は台の向こう側、

風に乗ったわけでもないだろうが、ダイブした身体は想像以上に遠くまで飛んだ。真っ青な空を背景に、すーっと大きな弧を描いて群集の頭を越え、山口さんの目の前に落下してきた。

物凄い音と地響きとが立った。

美帆は墜落するまでのわずかな時間に、数歩後ずさっていた。が、それでも大音響と風圧のようなもので地面に尻餅をついた。

山口さんの身体が朝礼台の天板に衝突し、一度小さくバウンドするのが見えた。周囲では何十人もの甲高い悲鳴が一斉に湧き上がった。

美帆は声も出せなかった。

山口さんは病院に搬送された。救急車が到着したときはまだ息があったという。

165

彼女が亡くなったのは翌日の昼だった。

美帆は意識が朦朧としてしまい、友人に保健室へ運ばれたので、あとのことは一切見ていなかった。

仲間優司が川土手から濁流へと落ちていく光景。

スプーンが美帆めがけて落下してくる光景。

身を投げた女生徒が目の前の朝礼台に叩きつけられる光景。

保健室のベッドに横たわっている時間、この三つの光景がきれいに重なり合った。それは、三つの錠のついたドアが、ようやく手に入れた三本の鍵で、いま初めて開かれたような感じだった。

ずっとずっと封印してきた記憶が、ドアの向こうからねっとりとせり出してきた。

死にたいと思った。

保健室を出て、吹奏楽部の仲間たち二人に付き添われて帰宅したときは、絶対に死のうと決めていた。自分はとても冷静だと思った。必要なのは、今日の午後に取り戻した記憶の細部をより正確に思い出すことだけだった。誤解ないしは錯覚に基づいて自殺するのは余りに馬鹿げている。数日を費やして思い出せるだけ思い出し、それから幾つかの身辺整理を行なって死ぬつもりだった。方法は決まっていた。どこか高いところから飛び降りるのだ。

あの母のように……。

その日は、自殺決行日の前日だった。

学校が終わると、美帆は片瀬駅前の福岡銀行で預金を全額引き出し、福岡行きの西鉄電車に乗

166

った。天神のデパートで買いたいものがあったし、一度行ってみたかった大名の人気の美容室で髪を整えたかった。イギリスの皇太子夫妻が五月に来日してからというもの日本中にダイアナフィーバーが巻き起こっていた。美帆も一度ダイアナカットを試してみたいと思っていたのだった。

下着や洋服を買い、髪を切って西鉄福岡駅に戻った。時刻は六時を回り、土曜日夕方の天神界隈はたくさんの人々で混雑していた。

明日の計画はすでに立ててあった。今日買った下着と服を身に着けて、午前中に家を出る。母には部活の友だちと新町の楽器店に行くとでも言えばいい。

昼過ぎには、石川町の県営団地に着く。何度かの下見で目星をつけた場所だ。団地の中央にある十二階建ての十号棟に入る。屋上に通ずるドアは締切りだったが、最上階までのぼれる外階段がついている。この外階段の柵は美帆の胸の高さ程度だった。十二階の踊り場で靴を脱ぎ、服と一緒に買ったピンクの帯締めで足を縛って、そのまま腕力で上半身を柵の外へ乗り出す。弾みをつけて頭からまっ逆さまに落下していく。そうすればアスファルトの地面に激突した瞬間に即死するだろう。

帰りの電車は意外に空いていた。ベンチシート型の座席に座り、デパートの紙袋を膝に置いて、暮れなずむ景色を車窓越しに眺める。もう自分の心はこの世界にないような気がした。目に映るものすべてが現実味を薄くしていた。それはとても軽やかで心地よい感覚だった。

死ぬことなんて簡単だ、と美帆は思った。

自分は明日、何のためらいもなく飛ぶことができるだろう。

そう確信した。

167

三つ目の駅に停まったとき、一人の少年が電車に乗ってきて、美帆の正面に座った。

一目見て、仲間優司だと分かった。

優司もすぐに美帆に気づいた。席を立ち、網棚に載せていた柔道着を取ると、美帆の目の前に来てつり革に片手を掛けた。

「何やその髪型は」

二年ぶりの再会にもかかわらず、ぶっきらぼうに言う。

「ダイアナカット」

「ダイナシカットか」

優司が言った。美帆が何も返事をしないと、さらに追い討ちをかけてきた。

「小柳には全然似合わんな」

「座ったら」

美帆は言った。右隣が空いていた。

「よか」

それからしばらく口をきかなかった。美帆は優司を見上げた。中学時代は背が高い印象があったが、いまはさほどでもなかった。高校に入ってそんなに伸びなかったのかもしれない。身体つきは見違えるようだった。肩や胸の辺り、腰部などががっしりとしていた。もうほとんど大人の身体に近かった。髪型は余り変わっていない。大きな瞳と高い鼻が印象的な顔にも変化はない。

ただ、こうして見ていると優司はなかなかの美男子だった。そんなふうに感じたのは今日が初め

168

てだった。

五つ目の駅で、

「小柳、降りるぞ」

と優司が急に言った。

「え」

美帆はきょとんとしてしまった。

「早よせい」

優司の腕が伸びてきて二の腕を摑まれた。あれよという間に立たされていた。膝から落ちそうになった紙袋を慌てて持った。

そのまま電車を降りた。「川尻」駅だった。「片瀬」まではまだだいぶある。

優司は手を離すと、黙って駅の階段に向かって歩き出す。美帆がついてくるのが当然という様子だった。

「ラーメンでも食うか」

駅を出ると、優司が言った。柔道着を縛った帯と薄い学生カバンの取っ手を一緒に握り込んで肩に担いでいた。帯は黒帯だった。

南口を出て十分ほど歩いたところにあるラーメン屋に入った。優司はちょくちょく通っているらしく、店の大将とも顔馴染みのようだった。優司に勧められてチャーシューメンを注文した。

優司はカウンターの下の棚に置いた柔道着がはみ出しているのが気になるらしく、何度も両腕で奥に押し込んでいた。半袖のシャツから剝き出しの上腕は以前よりさらに太く逞しくなってい

169

た。

「仲間君、柔道うまいの」

五分ほどで届いたチャーシューメンを並んで食べながら訊ねた。

「もしかしたら柔道で大学行けるかもしれん」

優司はそう言って少し照れた顔になった。

「じゃあ、うまいんだ」

「あのなあ、柔道は上手い下手やないとばい」

「じゃあ、何て言えばいいの」

「強いか、弱いかたい」

「じゃあ、仲間君、強いんだ」

「俺は強か。試合で負けたことがなか」

これは別に照れるでもなくあっさり言った。

優司は瞬く間に食べ終わり、替え玉を頼んだ。

「隣のえらい別嬪さんも替え玉いらんね。サービスしとくばい」

優司のどんぶりに替え玉を放り込んでいた大将が話しかけてきた。

「じゃあ、もうちょっとしたら硬麺でお願いします」

美帆は笑顔を浮かべてみせた。

「了解」

大将は言って、美帆たちの前から離れていった。

170

「仲間君はいいね。自分に自信が持てるものがあって」

美帆は言った。

「小柳にもあるやろ」

「私なんて何もないよ」

「小柳は頭がよかやないか」

「それはね、塾とか行って一生懸命勉強してるから。それだけ」

「そいでも勉強ができることに変わりはなか」

優司は豪快な音を立てて麺をすすっていく。

美帆のどんぶりに入った替え玉も半分は優司の方に回した。

「仲間君、私、ほんとうは貰いっ子なんだよ」

箸を置いて美帆は言った。スープもきれいに飲み干した優司は、水差しから何度も氷水を注い

でがぶ飲みしていた。

「知っとるよ」

意外な言葉が返ってきた。

「何で？」

訊き返す。

「だいぶ前、小柳先生に聞いた」

「いつ？」

「忘れた」

171

面倒くさそうに言う。

店を出て駅の方角へ歩いた。時刻は七時になるところだった。どうして優司がわざわざ途中下車させてまで強引に自分を誘ったのかが美帆にはよく分からなかった。

「仲間君、この近所に住んでるの」

「北口からちょっと行ったとこの団地」

優司の通っている高校が博多南工業であることは鞄の校章で分かっていた。駅ビルが見えてきたあたりで、美帆は、

「仲間君、どうしてあんなこと言ったの」

迷った末に訊いた。どうせ明日には死んでしまうのだ、と思うと迷いが消えた。

「あんなことて何ね」

優司はすぐには思い出せないふうだった。

「だから、三年前の夏、市民病院で私に言ったこと」

尚も優司は無反応だった。

「仲間君、憶えてないの」

やはりあれはうわごとだったということか。美帆は拍子抜けした気分だった。

「憶えとる」

ぼそりと優司は言った。

「やけど、なしてそげん理由なんか知りたいとか」

その一言に、美帆は何だか自分が小馬鹿にされたような気がした。人が、死の前日に口にする

172

問いかけに理由なんているものか、と思った。小柳のためならいつでも死んでやると言ったのは優司の方だ。だったら、明日死んでしまう自分に対して、あの約束をどうやって果たすつもりなんだ、と詰め寄ってみたくなった。

美帆は先月亡くなった女子生徒のことを話し、さらに、

「私は芝生の上に寝そべっているの。薄曇りの空が広がっていて、自分がどうしてこんなところに寝そべっているのか不思議な気持ちでいるの。身体中がじんじんして、でも全然痛みはないの。そしたら、空から大きな黒い固まりのようなものが降ってくるの。まるで私に向かってくるみたいに。その固まりがだんだん人の形になって、気づいたら物凄い地響きがして、ほんのすぐそば、私から一メートルも離れていない場所に落ちたの。気味の悪い何かお茶碗が割れるみたいな音が聞こえて、真っ赤なものや白いゼリーみたいなものがさーっと私の顔に降りかかってきた」

この三週間くらいで少しずつ思い出した記憶についても優司に語った。

「あの山口さんという三年生が、朝礼台に墜落したとき、私はその小さいときの記憶を取り戻したの。ああ、おかあさんは、私の目の前で飛び降りて死んだんだって。おかあさんのことなんて何一つ憶えてなかった。顔も声も姿も何にも憶えてなかった。毎日鏡を見るたびに、自分の顔を眺めながら、どんな人だったんだろうって考えてた。それが、あのとき、はっきりと思い出したの。おかあさんは私にとても似ていて、いつも哀しそうな顔ばかりしていて、そして、幼なかった私を置き去りにして飛び降り自殺してしまったんだって」

優司は黙って聞いていた。駅前に着いたが構内には入らず、ロータリーの隅に置かれたベンチに美帆を誘った。美帆は座ってからも喋り続けていた。改札口から吐き出された大勢の人たちが

173

二人のそばを通り過ぎていく。

「そうやって本当のおかあさんのことを思い出した瞬間、思ったの。もうこれ以上、絶対生きてなんてやるもんかって」

美帆はある一つのことを除いて、洗いざらい優司に話していた。自分の生い立ちや家族に関して——俊彦が浮気を繰り返していること、早苗がスプーンをベランダから投げたこと、あの片瀬川での事故以来、正也が父親を決して許さないことなどなど。自分でもどうしてそんなことまで明かしているのかよく分からなかった。

「小柳、死ぬんはそげん大したことやなかぞ」

改札の方を眺めやりながら、優司はさらりと言った。

「俺は、あんとき死にかけたけん、ちょこっとだけ分かっとる」

彼は顔を美帆に向けた。

「死ぬのはいっちょん苦しくなか。寝るのと大して変わらんばい」

優司の目が真剣な色を帯びているのに美帆は気づいた。

「それに、きっとまた目が覚めてしまうと」

「目が覚めてしまうって？」

美帆には優司の言っていることがよく理解できなかった。

「俺は死んだと思ったら、目が覚めとった」

「そんなの当たり前だろう、と美帆は思う。優司は死ななかった。

「目が覚めたって？」

174

もう一度同じ質問を繰り返した。

「はっきりとは憶えとらんけど、俺は龍になっとった」

「龍？」

優司が頷く。

「龍って、あの蛇みたいな龍？」

「龍は蛇やない」

優司の声がきつくなった。

美帆は奇妙なことを突然言い出した優司をじっと見た。

「どうして龍になったたって思ったの。自分の身体がじっと見えたの」

余りに突飛な話だったが、なぜか嘘や妄想のたぐいだとは思わなかった。

「目ば覚ました瞬間に俺の心が教えてくれたと。うまく言えんけど、俺は龍の心になっとった」

「龍の心？」

「うん」

優司は大きな瞳を見開いて、こくりと頷いてみせた。その素直な反応になぜだか美帆の胸は熱くなった。

「小柳」

優司は言った。

「俺はあんとき、魂っていうんは固まりやないんやって分かった気がすると。何か知らんけど、魂は心の真ん中にドカンとあるんやなくて、心の一粒一粒に入っとると。俺の心にも小さか魂が

いっぱい詰まっとった。そいが、龍のごとあった。溺れて意識がなくなった途端、その小さか龍が一個一個の心の粒から飛び出して、でかい一匹の龍になった。俺らがふだん魂に気づけんとは、心にそげんして魂が小さくなって心の中に散らばっとるけんたい。俺にとって死ぬていうのは、心にちりばめられとった龍が、大きな一匹の龍になることやった気がする」

優司はいかにも懐かしそうな表情になっていた。美帆にはやっぱり彼の言っていることはよく分からなかった。龍の心。心の龍。ずいぶんカッコいい話だと思った。ただ、龍というのは仲間優司にはいかにもふさわしいもののように感じられた。

しかし、どうして龍なのだろうか？

「小柳」

ふたたび優司が名前を呼んだ。

「ちゃんと生きれんやつは、ちゃんとも死ねん。生き死には一つやろ。いまのお前は、龍にはなれんばい。死にたいなんて言うやつは絶対大したもんにはなれん」

美帆は優司の目を見返した。私だって全部を打ち明けたわけじゃないと思った。

「だったら、いまの私は何にだったらなれるっていうの」

口をわざと尖らせて言い返した。

優司はしばし考える表情になった。

「まあ、せいぜいネズミかウサギくらいやろ」

やがて彼は言って、にやりと笑ってみせたのだった。

176

平成十七年一月四日

　片瀬駅はJRと西鉄が乗り入れている大きな駅だった。新町はこの片瀬駅を取り囲むように広がっていて、南口側が一、二丁目、北口側が三〜五丁目となっていた。どちらにも大きな商店街があるが、より繁華なのは「あかり」がある南口方面だった。

　「片瀬駅北口」でバスを降りると、美帆は正面に見える新町北商店街へと入っていった。三が日が明けたといってもシャッターを閉めた店も多かった。人通りもまばらだった。都会では初売りがおおかた二日、元日から営業している店もたくさんある。

　閑散とした商店街を歩きながら、東京とこの田舎町とでは時間の流れそのものが異なるのだと実感していた。

　「焼鳥の富士本」は商店街のアーケードを五十メートルほど進んだ左手にあった。間口二間ほどの小さな店だった。二階建てのしもた屋ふうの作りだが、一階が店舗、二階が優司の住まいだとかすみに聞いていた。店の扉には「六日から営業します」と書かれた貼り紙があった。

　美帆は時間を確認した。午後一時半。優司が在宅しているといいのだが。

　チャイムを探したが見つからなかった。といって店の入口以外には出入り口はなさそうだった。美帆は仕方なく、店の引き戸を叩いた。叩きながら「仲間くーん」と優司を呼んだ。最初は遠慮がちに叩いていたが、一向に返事人気がないといっても時折は誰かが通りすぎる。

がなかった。途中からかなり力を込めて叩いた。声も高くした。

五分ほどして店の明かりが灯った。黒い影が近づき、すぐに戸が内側から開かれた。

「あけましておめでとう」

美帆が言う。優司の方はもそっとした風情で美帆を見ていた。およそ正月気分とはかけはなれ

たたずまいだった。

「寝てたの」

「どうしたと？」

優司は不思議そうな声を出す。

「今年は帰ってきたから、東京に戻る前に仲間君にも会っていこうと思ったの」

昨年の正月はイタリアに行っていた。その埋め合わせにと春のお彼岸に帰省して、十八年ぶり

に優司と再会した。

「入れてくれる。寒いんだけど」

美帆が言うと、

「汚れとるばってん」

と言いながら優司は慌てて戸を大きく開けた。

美帆は老松町のスーパーで揃えてきた食材を右手に提げて、店内に足を踏み入れた。

ふくらんだレジ袋に気づいて、優司が荷物を引き取る。

「どうせお雑煮も食べてないんでしょ」

美帆が言うと、

「雑煮かあ」

と呟く。やっぱり寝起きのようだった。こんな優司を見るのは初めてだった。

「食べさせてあげようと思って材料買ってきたの。キッチンは上にもあるの？」

優司は無言で首を振る。

「冷蔵庫も」

今度は頷いた。

美帆はため息をついて、レジ袋を取り戻すと、カウンターの中へ入っていった。焼き台の横の調理スペースに買ってきたものを並べて、肉や魚、野菜などを大きな業務用の冷蔵庫にしまっていった。

十坪足らずの小さな店だった。

入ってすぐ右側にカウンター。席数は八。カウンターの向こうが変形のテーブル席。テーブルを囲む席数が十三。合計二十人ほどが入れば満員の店だった。席数は絞って、客の回転率を上げることで儲けを出す。焼き鳥屋の鉄則だった。

繁盛店だとかすみは言っていたが、中に入った途端に、美帆もそう感じた。長年の取材経験で流行店の持つ雰囲気は知悉していた。その雰囲気が「焼鳥の富士本」にもはっきりとあった。

「仲間君、カツ丼は好き？」

入口に突っ立っている優司に訊く。

「うん」

「じゃあ、お雑煮とカツ丼作ってあげる」

「ちょっと二階に上がってお茶でも飲まんね」

優司は困惑した顔つきで言った。

二階には三つ部屋があった。入口の左にある階段をのぼると、前後に二間つづきの和室。つきあたりが風呂と洗面所、トイレ。その右にもう一つドアがあるので、おそらくそこが三つ目の部屋だと美帆は思った。とにかく全体が古びていた。築二十年は優に越えていよう。一階を店舗スペースにしたため慌てて二階に水回りを持ってきたのだ。もともとは普通の家屋だったに違いなかった。

手前の八畳ほどの和室に通された。畳を覆うように灰色のカーペットが敷かれ、中央に炬燵が据えてあった。窓はアーケードに面した壁と右の壁とにあった。どちらも磨ガラスが嵌っているので外の景色はまったく分からない。炬燵の他には旧式のテレビと茶箪笥しかなかった。茶箪笥の上には電気ポットが置かれていた。目につくものと言えば、あとは巨大なトラバサミのようなものが壁に掛けられているくらいだった。

優司が茶箪笥からお茶の道具を出して、日本茶を淹れてくれた。

湯飲みを二つ持って美帆の座る炬燵までやって来る。彼は窓の一枚を背負って斜向かいに腰を下ろした。そこが定位置なのだろう。

「侘住まいとはこのことね」

美帆はそう言ってからお茶をすすった。

「おいしいわね」

180

思わず呟いた。茶箪笥の上で何気なく淹れていたのだが、一服すると香りが口の中に広がった。こんなにおいしいお茶は久しぶりだと思った。

「どこのお茶」

優司は茶箪笥の茶筒を見て、

「これは八女やな」

と言った。

お茶一杯で彩りのない殺風景な部屋がすこし温かくなった気がした。優司は黙ってお茶を飲んでいる。上は厚手のトレーナー、下はくたびれたジーンズ。いまの彼はどこから見ても、焼き鳥屋のおやじといった風情だった。

お茶をすする音だけがしばらくつづいた。そうやって黙り込んでいても気詰まりではなかった。

「あれは何」

美帆が壁に掛けてある白い物体を指差した。優司が首を回した。

「あれはホオジロザメの顎や」

たしかにトラバサミのようなそれは、巨大な魚の顎のようだった。大きく開いた口は上下とも鋭い歯でびっしり埋まっていた。

「どうしたの、あれ」

「マグロ船に乗っとるとき、あいつに嚙みつかれた」

優司は事も無げに言った。

「揚げ縄んときようサメがかかってくると。あいつもいつも甲板でずたずたに殺したつもりやったんや

181

けど、神経が生きとったんやろな、ぐちゃぐちゃ血まみれの身体で突然、俺に食いついてきたとさ。長靴の上からやったけん大したことなかったけど、下手すりゃ足は食いちぎられとこやった」

優司は言うと、炬燵から右足を出して、ジーンズの裾をたくし上げた。

「見てみい」

筋肉が盛り上がったふくらはぎには、何かに噛まれたような歯型がくっきりと残っていた。

「こんときは食いつかれただけやなくて、ちょうど横たくりの波ば食らって、俺一人海に放り出されたと。延縄のブイに何とか摑まって、仲間の投げてくれた命綱で引き揚げてもろうた。あいつのせいで危うく死ぬところやった」

優司は顔を上げて、もう一度壁のホオジロザメを見た。

「そいで、顎ば切り取って持って帰ったと。船の中で毎日やすりで磨いて、あげんぴかぴかにしてやった」

「だけど……」

大したことなかったといっても、この傷からして大怪我だったはずだ。

「こんな怪我して、そのあとも働いたの」

「マグロ船で身体動かせんようになったら、人間扱いしてもらえんごとなる。その場で漁労長に傷口は縫うてもらって、ペニシリン打って、次の日にはもう甲板に出とった。二年近くも航海しとったら、誰やって一度はそれくらいの怪我はしよる。そいでも死なんだけましゃった」

浅草で一緒に食事をしたとき「航海中に二人死んだ」と優司が言っていたのを美帆はまざまざ

182

と思い出していた。

「すごい体験ね」

それくらいしか言いようがなかった。

優司は立ち上がって、お湯を入れた急須を持ってきた。双方の湯飲みにお茶を注ぎ、

「どうやろうな」

と遠くを見るような表情になった。

「ときどき思い出して、懐かしくなったりする？」

美帆が訊く。

「懐かしいことはなかけど、あんときの俺はちゃんと生きとった気がする」

優司は言った。

お雑煮とカツ丼を作って食べさせた。家で時間をかけて取った出汁をポットに詰めてきたので、どちらもあっという間にできあがった。

「うまか」

と言って優司は食べた。男が自分の作った物をがつがつ食べるのを見るのは楽しい。

「リリコちゃんは元気にしてる？」

カツを頬張っている優司に訊く。

「高知市内のスナックでバイトしよる。早く帰りたいて毎晩かすみ相手に愚痴こぼしよるみたいや」

リリコが高知に行ったのは十一月半ばのことだった。あの一件のあと、リリコはかすみの店の

183

二階に匿われていたが、一度は優司の説得に応じたかに見えた研一が、一週間もすると「あかり」に押しかけてきた。かすみはすぐに優司を呼んだ。結局、店の中で大喧嘩となり、研一が優司の頭をビール瓶で殴って、警察が来る騒ぎになったのだった。

かすみによれば、優司はふだんのような獰猛さを発揮しなかったという。「やっぱり研ちゃんのことが可愛いのかなあ」と彼女は不思議そうにしていたが、美帆は、あの隅田公園での一件が影響している気がした。

結局、優司の言うとおり美帆たちに捜査の手が及んでくることはなかった。が、一度は一命を取り留めたと伝えられた少年も亡くなり、死者の数は三名となった。逮捕された海江田容疑者への同情論もその犠牲者たちの前に次第にかすんでいった。とくに海江田が元暴力団員だという事実が報じられたことで、世論の流れは一気に変わってしまったのだ。

「あかり」での乱闘騒動のあと、優司はリリコを高知に住む知り合いの元へ送った。優司が被害届を出さなかったので研一はすぐに釈放された。いつまたリリコを探しに来るか分からなかった。

その研一に逮捕状が出たのは、年の暮れのことだった。

「研一さんはまだ捕まってないんでしょ」

優司が頷く。

「まさか高飛びしたわけもないやろうが」

箸を止めて浮かない顔つきになった。

「あいつは俺がサツにタレこんだと思い込んどるやろ」

美帆は一連の経緯をかすみから聞いていた。研一が釈放されたあと、かすみが電話してきて、

184

しばらくリリコを東京で預かってくれないかと言ってきたのだが、あとになって優司が割って入り、リリコは高知行きと決まった。以来、たまにかすみとは連絡を取り合っていた。

「手っ取り早く金が欲しかったんやろが、馬鹿なやつや」

研一は昔の仲間とつるんで博多の大手建材会社の社長を恐喝したのだった。社長が脅しに屈せず警察に届けたため悪事が露見してしまった。仲間二人は逮捕されたが、研一は捜査員が家に踏み込む寸前に逃走した。

恐喝のネタはあったようだ。社長には二人の息子がいて、次男は跡取りとして本社で働いていたが、できの悪い長男はマニラ支店の支店長として出されていた。その長男がマニラの邸宅に十三歳の少女を監禁してさんざん玩具にしていた。日本人社会でも問題化し、マニラ市警も動いたが、長男は少女の両親にたっぷり金を握らせて事実を揉み消そうとした。この話が研一のかつての組仲間のところへ回ってきた。さっそく組仲間の二人はマニラに飛び、少女の両親を丸め込んで証言ビデオを撮影し、またメイドを使って長男の屋敷に隠しカメラを仕掛け、彼が少女に行なっていた変態行為の一部始終を録画した。

そのビデオをネタに研一も含む三人で社長をゆすったのだった。

「被害者が警察に届け出たんでしょ」

美帆が言う。

「そうらしいな」

優司は何となくぼやけた物言いをした。

185

食器を片づけ、美帆は暇乞いをした。案の定、優司が車で老松まで送ってくれると言う。いつの間にか時刻は五時を回っている。外に出ると正月の空は冷たい闇に染まり始めていた。車は店の裏手にとめてあった。助手席に座ると胴震いが出る。黒のレザーシートが冷え切っていた。優司がシートヒーターを入れた。

「どうしていつもサングラスしてるの。仲間君、もうやくざじゃないんでしょ」

美帆が言う。この真冬の夕暮れ時にサングラスは理解できなかった。

「腎臓ば刺されたあとから、どうかした拍子に視界が一瞬真っ白になって何も見えんようになると。特に昼間の太陽とか、夜の車のライトとかがいかん。こればっかりは手術しても治らんかった。慶応の医者にも聞いたけど、原因はよう分からんって言われた」

「そうだったんだ」

「かすみが知り合いの漢方の先生に聞いてくれたら、腎臓と目はつながっとるらしか。たまにそげん症状の出ることがあるって言われた」

話しながら優司はゆっくりと車を出した。

老松まで三十分ほどかかった。

美帆の家のそばで車は止まった。

「今日はごちそうさん」

優司が言う。すぐ目の前に広い芝庭の大きな家がある。正也は昨日の夕方の便で帰っていった。美帆もあと三、四日で東京に戻るつもりだった。この広壮な家に母一人きりの暮らしはいかにも寂しかろう、とあらためて感じた。

エアコンが効いた車内はすっかり温もっていた。

「仲間君、私、仲間君にどうしても頼みたいことがあるんだけど」

美帆は膝に置いたハンドバッグの取っ手をいじりながら言った。このためにわざわざ新町まで優司を訪ねたのだった。

「何ね」

優司がサングラスを外して美帆を見た。

「一度でいいの。私にシャブマンっていうのを教えてくれないかな」

優司の眉がわずかに動いた。

「小柳、お前、シャブマンっていうのが何のことか知っとるんか」

「知ってる。だから、こんなこと仲間君にしか頼めないでしょう」

さすがの優司も呆気に取られているようだった。

「本当に知っとるんか。シャブマンいうのは、覚醒剤は使って男とセックスすることなんぞ」

「うん」

美帆はできるだけ感情を表に出さずに頷く。自分でも意外なほどに落ち着いていた。

「何でそげんことがしたいとか」

当然の質問だった。

「かすみさんもリリちゃんも、すごいって言ってた。女に生まれたからには私だって一生に一度くらい経験してみたいの」

優司の怪訝な顔つきに変化は見られなかった。

187

「俺が訊いとるのは本当の理由たい」

美帆はすこし口を噤む。ため息をついて、視線をフロントガラスの先に向けた。寒々とした丸裸の木々が見えた。

「私ね、不感症なのよ。いままで一度もイッたことがないの」

ここで一気に喋るしかないと美帆は感じた。

「男の人はお金を出せば幾らでも気持ちいいことできるでしょう。でも、女はそうはいかない。それに女はたくさんの男と寝ても、それだけで気持ち良くなれるわけじゃない。同じ女でも、気が狂うほどの快感を得られる人もいれば、私みたいに全然感じられない女もいる。シャブマンをしてみて、もしも感じることができたら、私は自分の身体を見直してあげられる。それだけでも救いなのよ。だから一度、どうしても試してみたいの」

優司は腕を組んで美帆の話を聞いていた。いつの間にかサングラスをかけていた。

「シャブマンていうたって、上がる花火が六尺玉になるだけたい。花火はたかが花火よ」

ぽそりと言った。

「恥を忍んでこうして頼んでるの。お願い、一度だけ私として。明日のこの時間、ホテルに部屋を取ってから仲間君に電話する。そしたら来て。クスリはそれまでに用意しておいてね」

優司は長いこと黙っていた。

「お雑煮もカツ丼も食べたじゃない。仲間君、食い逃げするつもり?」

美帆が冗談めかして返事を催促した。そこでようやく、優司の頬がゆるんだ。

「そいで今日、俺のところにやって来たんか」

188

優司はサングラスのまま美帆をじっと見た。

「小柳、お前、何ば企んどるんか。こげな法外な頼みでも、俺がハイハイ言うて聞いてくれると思うとったんか」

もとより優司がすんなり乗ってくるとは美帆も思ってはいなかった。

「別に何も企んでなんていないわ。仲間君がすぐにOKするとも思ってなかった」

「じゃあ、何でそげなことは言い出した」

「理由なんてない。このところいろんなことがあって、私ちょっとおかしいのよ。仲間君がノーだったら、誰か他の人を見つけて頼むことにする。自分をめちゃめちゃにできればそれでいいんだから」

「ふーん」

サングラスのせいで優司の表情はつかめない。

美帆は息を詰めて、その反応を窺う。彼も所詮は一人の男だ。釣る気にならない魚でも他人の網に飛び込むと言われれば竿を引く程度のことはするかもしれない。まして誘っているのはこの私なのだ、と美帆は思っていた。

「よう分からん話やな」

優司は呟き、

「好きな男に捨てられて、捨て鉢ってか」

と言う。

「何とでも言ってもらっていいわ。どうせ仲間君には関係ないことだから」

美帆はそう言って、助手席のドアレバーに手をかけた。今日が無理ならば、まだ明日、明後日
と時間はあった。できれば優司にはこんな誘惑に乗って欲しくはなかった。もしも、彼がその気
になってしまえば、そのときは丈二の肩代わりを優司がしなくてはならない羽目になる。

「やったら一回だけやぞ」

ドアを開けて車から降りようとする美帆の背中に声がかかった。美帆はドアを閉めなおして優
司の方を見た。

「そんかわり、いまからや」

「いまから？」

優司が頷く。

「肉の仕入れで、俺は明日からしばらく宮崎や。今日しか空いとらん。博多は無理やが久留米な
らダチもおる。シャブはそいつに用意させる。今夜が駄目なら、こん話はなかったことにする」

優司は淡々と言う。

「分かったわ」

美帆は内心の落胆を隠して、承諾した。

西鉄久留米駅前に着いたのは午後七時。帰省ラッシュにぶつかることもなく、優司のベンツは
九州自動車道を時速二百キロ近くで走りつづけた。猛スピードに美帆は助手席でずっと身を固く
していた。

駅前の駐車場に車をとめ、優司は駅ビルの近くにある古びた喫茶店に入っていった。美帆は地

190

面に足を降ろすことができてほっとしていた。席に座り、コーヒーを頼む。ウェートレスに注文を訊かれた優司は手を振って断った。すぐに席から立ち上がる。

「二十分くらい待っといてくれ」

そう言うと、店を出て行ってしまった。去り際に美帆の耳元で、

「引き返すんならいまのうちやぞ」

と言った。

三十分を過ぎても優司は帰って来なかった。次第に美帆は不審に思い始めた。どう考えてもさきほどの自分の依頼は突拍子もない話だ。いままでの優司からすれば、こんなふうに気安く応ずるなどあり得ないことだった。

もしかしたら優司は自分を置いてけぼりにしたのではないか。そうやって頭を冷やさせる魂胆ではないかと美帆は気づいた。

七時四十五分を回り、駐車場に行ってみようと美帆が席を立ちかけたとき、ようやく優司は戻ってきた。

手には茶色い紙袋を持っていた。

「じゃあ、行くか」

詫びの一つもなく、テーブルの伝票を摑んだ。

サングラスをかけたその顔は、次第に凶暴さを増しているような気がした。口調もどことなく荒々しくなってきていた。

車は夜道を大牟田方面に走った。美帆にはここがどこだか皆目見当もつかなかった。細い道の

191

両側は明かりの乏しい田んぼや畑ばかりだった。「リバーサイド2」と看板にあるから、きっと川のそばなのだろうが、水の気配はまったく感じられなかった。

優司は迷うことなく電飾の矢印が光る入口へと車を寄せた。巨大なビニールのすだれをくぐると左に建物があり、建物に沿ってそれぞれブロック塀で仕切られた駐車スペースが並んでいた。車はさらに奥へと進んでいく。グレーの壁に突き当たり、左折するとまた駐車スペースが広がっていた。優司はちょうど真ん中のスペースにバックでベンツを入れた。

「着いたぞ」

野太い声で言う。物慣れた感じに、

「仲間君、ここ来たことあるの」

と美帆は訊いた。

「ずいぶん昔な」

返事はそっけない。

美帆は生まれて初めてラブホテルというものに入った。

先に車を降りた優司が入口横の壁に嵌ったライトパネルに近づいた。美帆もその背後に立つ。優司は、パネルの下についたボタンを押した。「どうぞ中にお入りください」というアナウンスが流れた。

美帆は、パネルの写真に目を奪われていた。鉄格子があって、壁や天井からはチェーンや拘束具らしきものがぶら下がっていた。奥にベッドが見え、手前には奇妙な形をした赤い椅子が据え

192

つけられていた。

優司はさっさと鉄製のドアを開けた。美帆も後につづいた。暗い階段だった。周囲の壁も階段も真っ赤に塗られていた。上がると右手にもう一枚ドアがあった。施錠されておらず、ノブを回すと簡単に開いた。狭い玄関があって、その向こうはパネルの写真で見たままの鉄格子の部屋だった。

「早よ上がらんか」

せかすように優司が言った。さらに尻を手で強く押された。急いでブーツを脱ごうとすると「そのまま上がればよか」と言われた。仕方なくブーツのまま鉄格子の扉を通って部屋に入った。

今日の美帆は膝丈のスカートとカシミアのセーター、上にロングコートという地味ないでたちだった。

優司も靴のまま入ってきた。背後から美帆のコートを脱がせると、手荒く丸めて遠くのベッドに放った。最近買ったばかりのプラダのコートだった。

優司は黒のトレーナーを脱ぎ、その下のシャツも脱いで、上半身裸になった。美帆は素早い優司の行動に内心驚いていた。彼の裸体は素晴らしかった。発達した大胸筋が、腕を動かすたびに盛り上がった。腹筋は見事に六つに割れている。そして、背中にはあの一匹龍がとぐろを巻いていた。天井の蠟燭型のランプの光が赤みを帯びているからだろうか、龍は血の色を濃くしていた。

病室で見たときとはちがって不気味だった。

優司は紙袋から素焼きの皿と精製水のボトル、それに大きなハサミを取り出した。ジーンズのポケットからは慎重な手つきでビニールの小袋を出した。

193

カラオケの曲集や食事のメニューなどが置いてあるチェストに皿を載せ、小袋の端をハサミで丁寧に切って、白い粉を皿にあけた。そこへ精製水を、これも注意深い手つきで少しずつ注いでいく。美帆は手持ちぶさたで、優司のやることを黙って見ていた。水を注ぐと薬指で粉と水とを混ぜ合わせ、二度ほど指をしゃぶって味見をしていた。

「よし」

終始無言だった優司が声を出した。背後の美帆の方へ振り返った。

「小柳、その椅子に座れ」

と言う。サングラスは部屋に入ってすぐに外していた。優司の大きな瞳が険しさを加えていた。

椅子は奇妙な構造をしていた。黒い支柱からブランコのようにチェーンで吊り下げられていた。背板部分と座板部分とに分かれ、背板に二箇所、座板に二箇所チェーンで繋がれていた。背板はリクライニングチェアのような普通の形だったが、座板の方は正方形の板が凹型にくり抜かれていた。共にウレタン素材に真っ赤なビニールを張ったものだった。

黒い台座からのびた支柱には他にも四本のチェーンが吊られていた。四本とも大小二種類の黒い革製のバンドが取り付けられていた。二つは手首を拘束するもので、あとの二つは足を拘束するもののようだった。

美帆が訝しげに優司を見返すと、

「いいから早く座れや」

と言う。

194

美帆は支柱に両手を添えて、ゆっくりとその椅子に腰掛けた。ぐらぐらと揺れてまるでブランコだった。

優司が近づき、美帆の両手首をベルトで拘束した。さらにスカートを捲り上げてふとももを露出させると、ロングブーツの途切れたあたりに脚用のベルトを巻きつけ、かなりきつく絞って尾錠を留めた。

優司の意図が摑めず、勝手にさせていたら、あっという間に身動きが取れなくなってしまった。が、まさかこのまま行為を始めるわけではないだろうと思った。服を着ているし、シャワーだって浴びていなかった。

だから、足元に移動した優司が美帆のストッキングをハサミで切り裂き始めたときは心底驚いた。

「ちょっとやめて。服くらい自分で脱ぐわ」

自分でも声がひどく慄えているのが分かった。

優司の手が止まった。怒ったような顔が両膝のあいだから美帆を凝視していた。

「シャブマンやるとに裸になってどうすっとか。シャブが効いてきたら、暑さと興奮でお前の方からこのハサミば下さいて哀願するようになる」

優司は右手のハサミをゆらゆらさせ、蔑むような笑みを浮かべていた。

「それ、どういうこと」

美帆は首だけ起こして優司を睨みつけた。

「この高そうな服ば、自分でずたずたに切り裂くったい。そいでなおさらお前は興奮すると」

195

優司はあっさり言うと作業を再開した。ブーツから上の部分のストッキングを完全に剥ぎ取り、今度は美帆の下着に手をかけた。

「やめて、恥ずかしい」

美帆は余りの成り行きに甲高い声を上げた。

手足をばたつかせて懸命に抵抗する。

「お前が、シャブマンやってくれて言うたんやろうが」

優司は一喝すると、美帆の腰をすごい力で押さえつけてきた。

「何すんのよ。ふざけないで！」

美帆は怒声で言い返す。だが優司は取り合いもせず、下着をつまむとそれをハサミで切断した。

その瞬間、美帆はショックで全身が硬直した。

「何や、小柳もう濡れとるやないか」

嘲笑まじりの呆れた声が響く。

優司の指が躊躇なく膣の中に侵入してきた。

「ほら、ぬるぬるやぞ。不感症やなんて大嘘かい」

「やめてー！」

美帆の口から大声が上がった。羞恥心で今度は全身が震え出していた。頬が火のように熱かった。

優司が太い指を出し入れするたびに、尾骶骨のあたりから痺れるような快感が湧き上がってきた。

美帆はそれを気取られぬようにと必死で歯をくいしばった。

196

額と脇の下から汗がどっと噴き出してきた。

ふと気づくと優司が美帆の肩越しに顔を覗き込んでいた。いつの間に足元からこちらへ来たのか分からなかった。手に素焼きの皿を持っている。

「じゃあ、さっそくこれをたっぷり塗り込んでやるけんな。この分やったらお前、気い狂ったみたいに吼えまくるわ。シャブマン天国や。楽しみにしとけ」

優司は言って、皿の中をぐるぐるかき回す。薬指につけた覚醒剤の溶液を音立ててしゃぶった。

「混ぜ物なしの上物や。しょんべん百回漏らすぞ」

美帆はもう何が何だか分からなくなってきていた。ただ無性に涙が溢れてきた。自分がどうしてこんな場所でこんな目に遭わされているのか、それが理解できない。

「小柳、いいんやな。どうなっても俺は知らんぞ。万が一、腹にガキでもおったら、ガキはただではすまん。それは心配ないやろな」

優司はふたたび美帆の足元へと戻った。局部に掌をあてがいゆっくりと揉みしだく。恐ろしいほどの快感に美帆はたまりかねて喘ぎ声を漏らした。

「シャブ汁ば塗るぞ」

優司が言った。

「待って」

美帆は叫ぶ。

「お願いやめて」

美帆は頭を振り立て、「やめて、もうやめて」と絶叫を繰り返した。

「お願い、もうイヤ。やっぱりできない」

両手両脚を縛りつけたチェーンがガチャガチャと盛大な音を立てる。

「なんばいまさら言いよっとか。ここで止めてもまたどうせ別の男に頼むんやろうが」

剥き出しの局部にあてがわれた優司の手にさらに力が込められる。

「自分ばめちゃめちゃにしたいんやろうが。ほらシャブ汁いくぞ」

優司の手が一旦離れ、腿のあたりに液体の冷たい感触が広がった。

「ダメー」

美帆は声を振り絞る。

「何が駄目か!」

優司が怒声を張り上げた。

「何ば企んでこげんことしようとした。シャブばやるなんてクソみたいなこと、どうして言い出した」

優司の指がふたたび股間に突き刺さる。

「ダメ、ダメ、ダメー」

美帆は必死で腰を振って、その手から逃れようとした。チェーン同士がぶつかり、椅子を吊り下げているフレームが軋んで不気味な音を立てた。

「お願い、やめて。赤ちゃんがいるの。私、お腹に赤ちゃんがいるのよ」

美帆は悲鳴を上げてついに泣き崩れた。

198

椅子から下ろされベッドに連れて行かれると、彼女はマットに突っ伏して一時間以上泣きつづけた。

どうしよう、どうしよう。怖いよ、怖いよ。母親になんてなりたくない。母親なんて絶対イヤだ。

ぶつぶつ呟いているのは分かるが、自分が何を喋っているのか、何をしているのかは混乱した頭ではうまく掴み取れなかった。美帆はただ、全身で泣いた。

優司は「どうせ、そげんことやろうと思うとった」と言ったきり、黙ってそばに座っていた。ラブホテルを出たのは十時過ぎだった。泣き疲れた美帆は車の中で眠ってしまった。優司に肩を揺すられて目を覚ました。老松の自宅が目の前に見えた。あたりはもう真っ暗闇だった。久しぶりによく眠れたと思った。さきほどまでの数時間が夢だったような気がした。運転席の優司はサングラスをかけて普段と変わらぬ様子だった。

優司が紙コップを差し出してきた。そういえばコーヒーの香りが車の中に立ち込めていた。美帆はあたたかいコーヒーをすすった。三分の一ほど飲んだところでだいぶ意識がはっきりしてきた。

「何で女だけが子供産まなきゃいけないの。よりによってどうして私に決めさせようとするのよ」

ぽつりと言う。

「やったら産まんかったらいい。いまどき中絶やってわけないやろ」

すぐに言葉が返ってきた。

199

「そんな単純な話じゃない」

「半分女やるけんそげんことになる。やるなら全部女か女捨てるかどっちかにしろ」

こんなやり取りをしていても、優司といることでどこか安心している自分がいた。

「父親のいない子を産むのがイヤなんじゃない。自分が母親になるのがイヤなの」

優司がゆっくり息を吐き出した。

「だったら、さっさと堕胎すればよかやないか。お前自身が産みたい気持ちばどうしても消しきらんけん、さっきみたいなことするんやないとか」

美帆は黙ってコーヒーをすすった。

「小柳」

優司が名前を呼んだ。

「お前が産むんやない。その腹の子がお前を選んで生まれてくるんや。やから、そいつが本気で生まれたいと思うとったら、お前がどげんことばしてみても無駄なだけやと俺は思うぞ」

「じゃあ、私も仲間君も自分の親を選んで生まれてきたっていうの」

「おそらくな」

「私は絶対に違う。自分を捨てるような母親なんて選ぶわけがない」

「やけど、お前は現に生まれてきとる。それはやっぱりお前自身の力やろ。俺たちみたいな人間は、そうでも思わんと生きていけんやないか。俺は、やくざから足を洗ったとき、俺は自分の意志で自分の力だけで生まれた人間なんやと思うことに決めた。顔もよう知らん親のことなんかどうでもよか。俺の親は、俺を産んだ途端に、俺の方からクビにしたんやと思うとる」

200

「クビ?」

「そうや。小柳も、お前が自分の母親ばクビにしたと思えばよか。お前の母親が自殺したんは母親自身の問題で、お前とは何の関係もなか」

自分の意志で自分の力だけでこの世界に生まれてきた——美帆はいままでそんなふうに考えたことは一度もなかった。

そっと下腹に手を当てた。気づいてみると一日に何度も何度もそうやっている。

この子も自分の意志で自分の力だけで生まれてくるのだろうか。それならば、私が思い悩む必要などどこにもないのではないか。通りすがりの人間のように、ただこの世界への道案内さえすれば、それでいいのだから——美帆はふとそんな気がした。

三月二十七日

〈大豆、にがり、水——豆腐の原材料はたったそれだけ。だからこそ、その味は素材の質と作り方で決まってしまう。いまでこそ、国産大豆と天然にがりはこだわり豆腐のシンボルのようになっているが、戦前はそれらがごくふつうに使われていた。

当時は、絹ごし豆腐を美味しく作るのはとてもむずかしかった。豆乳ににがりをまぜるとすぐに凝固しはじめるため、味や舌触りを一定に保った絹ごしを大量に製産するのは容易ではなかっ

たのだ。豆乳の濃度と温度、にがりの濃さを巧みに調整するのは腕の良い職人だけにできる仕事だった。

しかし、戦争が始まるとにがりは軍需統制品となり、代わりに「すまし粉」と呼ばれる硫酸カルシウムが使用されるようになった。

この「すまし粉」の登場が、それまでの職人技に頼っていた豆腐作りを劇的に変えてしまう。

「すまし粉」は豆乳とまぜてもゆっくり固まってくれるため、職人たちの出番はなくなったのだ。絹ごし豆腐は手軽に量産できるようになり、しかし、にがりに含まれる豊富なミネラル分は、豆腐の中からまたたくまに消えてしまった。

そして戦後を迎えると、原料の大豆も価格の安い輸入大豆がもてはやされるようになる。豆腐作りは味や質よりも価格が優先される時代となった。〉

ここまで書いて、美帆は手を止めた。パソコンの画面から目を離し、両腕を持ち上げて大きく伸びをした。

デスクの上の時計を見た。いつの間にか午前二時を過ぎていた。深呼吸をしながら腕を下ろすと、空腹であることに気づいた。昨夜はかすみとリリコと三人で表参道の行きつけのイタリアンレストランに繰り出し、さんざん食べてきた。部屋に戻ったのが十一時頃だったから、まだ三時間しか経っていない。どうしてこんなにお腹が空くのだろうと我ながら不思議になる。

つわりにも二種類あると知ったのは妊娠してからだった。つわりと言えば、炊き立てのご飯の匂いにさえ吐き気を催すという、あれだとばかり美帆は思っていた。よもや、その「吐きつわ

202

り」とは正反対に、始終何か口に入れていないと気持ちが悪くなってしまう「食べつわり」なる

ものがあるとは思ってもみなかった。

それにしても、もう二十三週目に入っている。そろそろ「食べつわり」からも解放されたいの

だが、なかなか思うようにはいかなかった。

いま美帆が書いているのは、大手食品メーカーの広報誌用の原稿だった。彼女は、この広報誌

の中の特集ページ、十ページ分の制作を毎月引き受けていた。企画、取材、執筆、撮影、デザイ

ン出し、入稿、校正とすべてこなしてページあたり五万というのは決して割のいい仕事ではない。

企画によっては地方出張もするし、取材の回数も多い。カメラマンへの支払いはむろん別会計だ

が、それでも取材経費やデザイナーへのギャラを差し引くと残るのは三十万弱に過ぎなかった。

ただ、その分、勉強にはなった。三年もつづけているのはそれゆえだった。

テーマには毎回、食の素材を選んできた。水から始めて、味噌、醤油、みりん、唐辛子といっ

た調味料・香辛料類、茄子、蕪、大根、人参、ゴボウ、ねぎ、玉ねぎ、葉物にキノコといった野

菜類、とり、豚、牛、羊などの肉類、魚介、昆布、鰹節、乾物類、それにお米や餅などなど。調

べだしたら素材の種類にはかぎりがなかった。

今回「豆腐」を取り上げたのは、現在の美帆の体調とも関わりがある。食べつわりがひどかっ

た時期、特に脂っこいものが無性に欲しくて、一週間で三キロも太ったことがあった。他のもの

で何とか誤魔化そうと、出産経験のある友人の話やネットの情報などを参考に、ブドウ糖キャン

ディー、ウイダーinゼリー、ドライフルーツ、ナッツ類とさまざまに試した。その末に行き着

いたのがなんと豆腐だった。脂っこい物をやめても、豆腐を口にするとなぜだか胸のむかむかが

203

おさまった。

さっそく「豆腐」を取材してみることに決めた。

この広報誌の他にも定期の仕事が幾つかあった。一番大きいのは、ある流通系出版社の月刊料理雑誌を丸ごと請け負っている仕事だった。九十ページほどの雑誌だが、編集料とライティング料で九十万円ほどになった。料理本やムックなどの企画、編集も月に最低一本はやっていた。この種の仕事のギャラは内容にもよるし、印税計算で支払われる場合もあったが、平均して五十万くらいにはなる。そうやってあれこれ合算していくと、ここ数年の美帆の年収は大体、二千万円ほどに達していた。

この年収からすれば、彼女はフードライターとしては売れっ子の部類に入る。その代わり、日々の仕事はハードだった。徹夜もしばしばだし、今日のように泊り客を二人も招き、遅くまで外食をしてきた晩でも、こうやって締め切りの迫った原稿を夜っぴて書かなくてはならない。土日に取材が入ることも再々だし、フリーとは名ばかりでまとまった休みを取ることもなかなかできなかった。

かすみは今晩一泊だが、リリコの方は三日前から泊まっている。リビングの隣の寝室を明け渡して、美帆は仕事部屋のソファベッドで寝ていた。リリコはしきりに気の毒がったが、抱えている原稿もあるので、そうするしか手がなかった。今夜は美帆のベッドに二人並んで眠っているはずだ。

玄関右手の仕事部屋を出て、リビングに通ずるガラスのドアを開けた。明かりを灯し、キッチンに入って冷蔵庫の中身をあらためていると、寝室のドアが開いてかす

204

みが出てきた。モスグリーンのかわいらしいパジャマを着ていた。こうして見るとかすみはまだ十分に若々しかった。

「うるさかった?」

キッチンカウンター越しに話しかけた。

「やっぱり眠れなくて」

この数日ですっかりやつれたようだ。母親を亡くしたのだから仕方がない。

「そう……」

「美帆さんの方はお仕事大丈夫ですか。忙しいときに押しかけてしまって、ほんとにごめんなさい」

かすみが頭を下げた。

「全然構わないわよ。締め切りは今日の夕方だから、まだ時間たっぷりあるし」

「たいへんですよね。 物を書く仕事って」

「そんなことないよ」

千葉に住むかすみの母が急逝したのは、二十一日、彼岸のさなかのことだった。かすみはリコと二人で二十二日に上京してきた。当日の通夜、翌日の葬儀が済んで、リコだけ二十四日に美帆の家にやって来た。そして昨日、かすみがリリコを迎えに来た。二人は、今日の昼間の便で福岡に帰ることになっていた。

「かすみさん、一杯やる?」

美帆が訊いた。

「いいんですか」

「私もそろそろ休むから。昔みたいに完徹はできないし」

昔と言ってもわずか数ヵ月前だった。だが、いまの美帆にはその言葉がしっくりくる。妊娠が女性にとってどれほど大きなことかを否応なく思い知らされる日々がつづいていた。

「ワインでいい？」

「もちろん」

美帆は冷蔵庫からシャブリを一本出した。妊娠中の飲酒は医師から固く禁じられているので美帆は飲めないが、来客用のワインは欠かしていなかった。銘柄は、ドメーヌ・アムラン。値段は手頃だがすっきりした口当たりの美味しいワインだった。

つまみは豆腐だ。熊本の豆腐のみそ漬け、鳥取の豆腐ちくわ、それに岐阜のこも豆腐などを大皿に盛りつけてリビングのテーブルに置いた。今回の取材のために日本全国からさまざまな変わり豆腐を取り寄せていた。

差し向かいで座って、かすみのグラスにワインを、美帆のグラスにはペリエを注いだ。

「かすみさん、ほんとに大変だったわね」

と言って美帆は自分のグラスを持ち上げた。

「こちらこそお世話になりました」

二十三日に千葉市内で執り行なわれた葬儀には美帆も参列した。

「でも、お父さまがやっぱり心配ね」

夕食のときにかすみの実家の事情をつぶさに聞いた。七十一歳になる父親は膝の具合が悪く、

206

一人での遠出は無理だという。いままでは八つ年下の母親が家事全般はもとより車の運転もこなして夫の面倒を甲斐甲斐しく見ていたが、今回、心臓発作で急逝してしまい、残された父親は途方に暮れているとのことだった。

「妹もすぐに戻ってくるわけにもいかないみたいだし」

かすみが嘆息するように言った。たった一人の妹は、いまは夫の転勤で旭川に住んでいるのだそうだ。

「あの父が一人で暮らすなんてとても無理だろうし」

離婚してからの八年間、かすみは両親とは一度も連絡を取ったことがなかったという。

妹とは「あかり」を開店した三年前からやっと電話しあう仲に復していた。

「思い切って、かすみさんが千葉に戻ったら」

この数日考えていたことを美帆は口にした。さきほどはリリコと三人だったので言いそびれてしまった。リリコは二月に高知から戻って、いまは「あかり」で働いていた。部屋も新たに借りて引っ越していた。研一の行方は杳として知れないが、逮捕状が出てからは一切の接触がないようだった。

「妹ともその話はしてるんです」

かすみが言う。

「私はそうしたらいいと思うよ。お店を手放すのは残念だけど、まだかすみさんは若いし、こっちで一からやり直す手だってあるもの」

「五日間、久しぶりに父と一緒にいて、母の分まで償いをしなきゃなとは思いました」

207

しみじみと彼女は言う。この女性が一度は覚醒剤中毒で家庭を壊し、あげくやくざの情婦にまで身を落としたとはとても信じられなかった。

美帆は豆腐ちくわを手でつまんで食べていた。まろやかな味がおいしい。

「娘さんと遠く離れるのがつらいんでしょ」

ちくわを一本食べ終えて、美帆は言った。「それに、仲間君とも」という言葉はつけ加えなかった。

「それもあります。どうせ二度と親子には戻れない関係ですけど」

「そんなことないわよ。あかりちゃんも大人になれば、お母さんの気持ちがきっと分かるときがくると思う」

そう言いながら、美帆は自身のことを考えていた。すくなくとも自分にはあの母の気持ちは分からないし、分かりたくもない。

かすみはワインを飲み干し、手酌でふたたびグラスを満たした。

「私ね、もう一人子供が欲しかったんです」

グラスの中を見つめながら言った。

「男の子が欲しくって。小さい頃からそうだったんです。子供を持てたら男の子と女の子の両方を絶対に産みたいって。それで主人に頼んだんです。セックスは無理だけど、体外受精だったらできるんじゃないかって。実は、病院に行って相談も済ませていたんです。そしたら、主人がものすごい剣幕で怒り出して。普段は身体のこともあるからそんなふうに怒るなんてあり得なかったんです。俺は、お前が子供を産むための道具なのかって。主人にしたら不安だったんだと思い

208

ます。いつ死ぬか分からない身で二人目の子供を持つことが。でも、それでも私はどうしても産みたかった。主人がいつ逝くか分からないからこそ、男の子が欲しかったんです」

「そうだったの」

美帆はかすみの話を聞き、そのときの彼女の気持ちがよく分かるような気がした。

「それで自棄になって、私、出会い系なんかに手を出してしまったんです。だから、本当は後腐れのないセックスがしたいだなんて嘘だったのかもしれません。実は、私は誰の子でもいいから子供が欲しかったのかもしれない。女にはセックスだけなんて、実際はあり得ないんじゃないかって、いまになって時々思ったりします」

美帆は、かすみの言うことにも一理あるような気がした。男性の場合はセックスのためのセックスが十分に可能だと思う。男性のセックスというのはそちらが主流なのかもしれない。女性の場合は、どうしても妊娠という前提がつきまとう。これは男女のあいだの根本的差異の一つだろう。

「かすみさんは、あかりちゃんを身ごもったとき、ご主人の子供でよかったって心から思えた？」

男性にセックスのためのセックスがあるように、女性には妊娠のためのセックスがあるような気がした。

かすみが怪訝な顔で美帆を見返した。

「だから、誰か別の人の子供だったらよかったのにって思ったことなかった」

美帆は言った。

209

「美帆さんはそんなふうに思ってるんですか」

かすみは美帆の妊娠にまつわる事情はおおかた心得ていた。

「私の場合は、父親のいない子を産むわけだしね」

問い返されて、美帆は言葉を濁した。

「たとえば優ちゃんが父親だったらよかったとか」

しかし、彼女は核心をついてくる。

「そういえばそうかな」

美帆は正直に答えた。

「ただし、それは別に私が仲間君のことを好きだってことじゃないのよ。本当の父親と比べてみたら仲間君みたいな人の方がよかったのになって思うだけ。かすみさんなら分かるでしょ」

実際、正月に会って以来、優司とは電話で話すこともしていなかった。

「でも、それって好きよりもっとすごいことかも」

かすみが言った。

「そんなことないよ」

ふと口走った言葉に、美帆自身が戸惑っていた。

だが、かすみはにわかに真剣な面持ちになって美帆を見つめた。何か思い悩むように眉根を寄せて、口許に右の人差し指を当てていた。

「美帆さんなら、あの人に勝てるかもしれませんね」

不意に言った。

210

「あの人って」

美帆は訊き返す。

「いつか少しだけお話ししたことがありますよね。富士本美由紀さんって人のことです」

かすみはふっと一つ息をこぼすと、宙を見つめるようにして言った。

四月五日

「とうさんが亡くなって八ヵ月だよ。幾らなんでもみっともないよ」

まだ二杯目のギネスだったが、正也の顔はすっかり赤くなっていた。彼はあまり酒が強い方ではない。父にではなく母の早苗に似たのだろう。母は一滴も飲まない人だった。

以前、優司と行った表参道のアイリッシュパブだった。あれ以来、美帆はたまにこの店に顔を出していた。一人のときもあるし、仕事仲間を連れてくることもあった。

アイリッシュビールの生を飲むと、他のビールはちょっと飲めなくなる。

「雅光兄さんが相手だなんて、かなり意外ね」

美帆は最近はもっぱらジンジャーエールだった。

「どうもだいぶ前からの関係らしいよ。とうさんが桜花園に勤めていたときにも、そういう噂があったらしいし。新庄も、今回初めて古株の職員からそのことを聞かされたそうだけど」

父が「かたせ桜花園」で働いていた時期といえば、母はまだ四十手前、本多園長は三十前といういうことになる。その頃の母であれば、若い雅光兄さんを籠絡するくらい造作もないことだったろう。

「まあ、仕方がないじゃない。一人で生きていくのは、あの人には無理なんだから」

「それはそうだけど。一応、僕にとっては本当の母親だからね」

「正也はショックなわけ」

「ショックっていうのとも少し違う気はするけど」

相手が雅光兄さんと聞いて、美帆は思い当たるふしがあった。なるほど母と雅光兄さんは、父が桜花園にいる頃から関係を結んでいたに違いない。正也が片瀬川で流された折、後から駆けつけた雅光兄さんが美帆のためにあれほどのことをしてくれたのも、彼と母とがそういう間柄だったとすれば十分に納得できた。

新庄というのは、あのとき「あれは誰やー」と指導員に聞かれて「小柳君です」と真っ青な顔で叫んだ子のことだった。桜花園で高校まで過ごし、大学を出ると児童指導員としてふたたび園に戻ってきた。正也と彼とは二十年来の親友でもあった。

その新庄君が園長と母との関係が噂になっていると、最近、正也に電話で報告してきたというのだ。

「まさか」

「結婚する気なのかしら」

美帆が言った。

212

「でも、雅光兄さんって結婚したことないんでしょう。もしかしたら、おかあさんのことをずっと好きで、この日を待ちつづけていたのかもしれないじゃない」

どうしても本多園長と呼ぶより雅光兄さんの方がしっくりきた。

「アホくさ」

正也が苦笑した。

「どっちにしても、おかあさんが寂しくないなら、それでいいじゃない。雅光兄さんも悪い人じゃないだろうし」

正也は納得できない顔つきをしている。

「うちの財産目当てだったらどうする」

「アホくさ」

今度は美帆が笑った。

美帆も正也も子供のときから両親を突き放して見る習慣がついていた。貰いっ子の美帆がそうなるのはやむを得ない面もあるが、俊彦と早苗の実子である正也も、両親との関係はかなり淡白だった。長女の美帆の目線が自然に正也に乗り移った部分もある。その点は弟に悪いことをしたかな、と思わないでもないが、一方で、年中浮気を繰り返している父とわがままで何事も気分次第の母とのあいだに育てば、賢ければ賢いだけ、子供が冷静な目で親たちを見るようになるのは当然だと美帆は思っていた。

正也は幼い頃から美帆によく懐いた。小さい子供もやはりきれいな女性が好きなのだ。中学時代も美帆が桜花園に顔を出すたびに園児たちが群がってきたし、いまでも子供のいる家に行くと、

213

必ずと言っていいほど擦り寄ってきた。

母の早苗も美しい人だったが、弟の正也は、幼心にも姉の美貌の方に軍配を上げたのだった。

早苗はごくたまにだが、ヒステリーを起こした。そういうときは、子供たちの失敗を見つけては家の外に締め出した。一度大雨の真夜中に正也が出されてしまい、美帆が幾ら抗議しても哀願しても、早苗はずぶ濡れの正也を家に入れなかった。美帆は傘と毛布を持って自分も外に出て、一晩中、雨の中で正也を抱き締めていた。正也がまだ四つくらいの頃のことだった。

早苗に似た正也は美しい顔立ちをしていた。仕事は忙しいだろうが、その気になれば幾らでも相手はいるはずだ。が、この弟から女っ気を感じたことはほとんどなかった。いままで正式に彼女を紹介されたこともない。「姉ちゃんと会わせると、向こうは絶対引いちゃうから」と言い訳しているが、決まった女性と付き合ったことがないのではないか、と美帆は睨んでいた。

正也には、自分たちが母親の違う実の姉弟であることは伝えてあった。

五年前、永妻克子の報告書を見せながら、正也に説明したとき、

「どうりで、姉ちゃんはとうさんに似てると思ったよ」

とさほどの驚きを見せなかった。

美帆自身は、母や叔父の素性を初めて知ったこと以上に、自分が俊彦の実子だったという事実に驚愕していたので、この正也の淡々とした反応は意外だった。

「おとうさんにもおかあさんにも何も言わないつもりなの。その方があの二人のためにもいいでしょ」

美帆が言うと、

214

「とうさんに真実を言わないのは、姉ちゃんの実の母親を自殺に追いやったのがとうさんだから？　姉ちゃんは、かあさんよりもとうさんの方が憎いってこと？」

と正也はすかさず訊いてきた。鋭い指摘だった。

「夫が愛人に産ませた子をわざわざ養女にして、何食わぬ顔で育ててきたおかあさんも最低よ。でも、やっぱり一番許せないのは、その愛人が子供を産んだことも、自殺したことも知らないでのうのうと生きているおとうさんの方だわ」

美帆は言った。

「姉ちゃんもなんだかんだ言っても女だってことか」

そのとき正也はそう言ったあと、自分の口からは絶対に秘密は洩らさないと固く誓ったのだった。もちろん、彼は父が事実を知ることによって、両親の関係が決定的に損なわれるのを危惧したのだと思う。

美帆が自らの出自について知りたいと思ったのは、イギリスに行ってからだった。二人目の彼氏からのプロポーズを断り、会社も辞めて美帆は渡英した。最初の一ヵ月はロンドンで友人の家に厄介になったが、その後ブライトンに移り、部屋を借りて一人暮らしを始めた。英語学校に通い、リフレクソロジーや禅の修行に出掛けたりした。イギリスという国が性に合えば、そのまま一、二年滞在してみようかとも考えていた。

だが、実際に住んでみると侘しさが募った。言葉の壁もあったが、何より辛かったのは食事だった。食材も豊かではなかったし、まずもって毎日パン食というのが美帆には耐えられなかった。留学している日本人の中には彼らと付き合っイギリスの男たちもあまり好きになれなかった。

215

ている女性も結構いたが、美帆からすると、日本女性に近づいてくるイギリス人たちはどこか気

味の悪い人が多かった。

ありふれた話だが、海外で生活すると、否応なく自分が日本人であることを意識させられる。

孤独とさみしさの中で、自分が一体何者なのかを突き詰めないわけにはいかなくなってくる。

美帆もそういう気持ちを引きずったまま、半年足らずで日本に帰った。

ちょうど三十歳になっていた。

ふたたび上京してからは、母校での臨床心理の講義にも飽き足らず、次々に持ち込まれる仕事

をこなしているうちにフードライターとしてフリーでやっていこうという気持ちの方が強くなっ

ていった。

ここが人生の一つの節目だと感じた。美帆は意を決して本当の両親についてプロの調査員に調

べてもらうことにした。戸籍以外に手掛かりらしきものもなさそうだったが、友人の弁護士から

紹介されて永妻克子に会ってみれば、「戸籍からたぐれば大抵のことは分かります」とのことだ

った。

一ヵ月後に受け取った永妻の報告書は詳細をきわめていた。

古川美和は小柳俊彦の患者の一人だった。俊彦は東京の勤務医だった時代、看護婦として同じ

病棟で働いていた稲垣早苗と交際しながら、一方で患者の美和とも関係を持っていた。

俊彦は結局、早苗を選び、美和を捨てた。そのとき美和はすでに妊娠していた。

彼女は、昭和四十四年十二月二十四日、板橋区の産院で女の子を出産した。美帆という名前は

美和が付けた。

216

古川家は父親が早くに亡くなり、美帆の母親、つまり美帆の祖母にあたる古川美鈴が小さな食堂を営んで生計を立てていた。出産後は、美帆もその店を手伝いながら美帆を育てた。二年後の昭和四十六年七月、同じ板橋でスナックを経営していた美和の弟の隆志が、相場で大穴を開けてしまった。連帯保証人だった美鈴は息子の借金のカタになけなしの店舗兼住宅を手放さねばならない羽目に陥った。

八月、隆志も含む家族四人で区内のアパートに引っ越し、美鈴も隆志も働きに出ることになった。美和は子育ての負担の上に店を失ったショックが重なってアパートに引き籠もりの状態となった。九月、美鈴が勤め先の清掃会社で、くも膜下出血のために倒れてそのまま息を引き取った。

この母親の急逝で美和の精神状態は一気に悪化した。

翌四十七年二月十四日、美和は二歳になった美帆を連れてアパートを抜け出した。その日、隆志はすでに出勤していた。午後三時過ぎ、美和はあちこちさまよったあげく横浜市内の団地の一棟に入り、最上階九階の踊り場から身を投げた。享年二十四。

その場にいた美帆は保護され、叔父の隆志に引き渡されたが、一ヵ月後、板橋区の児童養護施設に預けられることになった。隆志が結婚詐欺で警察に逮捕されたからだった。

五月、小柳早苗がその児童養護施設を訪ねてきた。弁護士を通じて隆志の了承も得たうえで彼女は美帆を引き取った。

小柳の一家が片瀬に引きあげたのはそれから二ヵ月後のことだった。

「だけど、とうさんは知らなかったのかな」

三杯目のビールをオーダーしたあと、すこし赤みの引いた顔の正也が言った。

「何を」

美帆は問い返した。

「姉ちゃんが自分の本当の娘だったってこと」

「知らなかったんじゃない。知っていれば、私に何か言うはずだもの」

「そうかなあ。黙っていただけじゃないのかな」

「まさか」

「分からないよ。案外あの人はそういう人だったんじゃない」

正也に言われて、美帆は父が亡くなる前の晩に口にした言葉をまた思い出した。「どうしても自分の娘としか思えなかった」という一言は、美帆へのほのめかしだったのか。

「やっぱり、おとうさんは知らなかったと思う」

美帆は言った。仮に知ったとしても、父の言葉の通り、死の直前だったに違いないと美帆は思った。

正也とは二ヵ月に一回はこうして会うようにしていた。といっても正也が渡米中は、美帆が一度ニューヨークに行って会ったきりだった。そのときは、彼が黒人の女の子を連れてきて、びっくりさせられた。

帰国後の正也は多忙をきわめ、ゆっくり夕食を共にする時間は取れないようだった。毎回こうして夜中に会って二人で飲んでいた。もちろん、正也はこれから病院に戻らねばならない。

「姉ちゃん、本気で子供を産む気？」

218

正也が訊いてきた。

「当たり前でしょう。もう二十四週目に入ってるのよ」

「そうかあ」

フィッシュ・アンド・チップスをつまみながらぼやけた声を出す。

「かあさんも薄々勘づいているみたいだよ」

「嘘でしょ」

「ほんとほんと。姉ちゃんが正月に帰ったとき、そう思ったみたい。この前、僕に確かめてきたから、それはないでしょって一応否定しておいたけどね」

妊娠の事実を正也に打ち明けたのは二月に入ってからだった。その瞬間に、

「もしかして優司兄ちゃんの子?」

と言われて、美帆はどうして正也がそんなことを口にするのか不思議だった。首を振ると、明らかに落胆の表情になっていた。

「もうすこししたら、かあさんにも言うわ」

「そうしてよ」

正也が頭を下げてきた。

「姉ちゃんが産んでくれたら、甥っ子でも姪っ子でも、僕が何でも面倒見てあげるよ。かあさんだって大喜びだと思うよ」

「そうかしら」

「そりゃそうでしょう。血がつながっていないといっても、かあさんの産んだ僕とはつながって

219

るわけだし、あの人、もともと子供好きだからね」

「かあさんが子供好き?」

「そうだよ。でなきゃ、姉ちゃんのことだって引き取るわけないじゃない」

正也が、いまさら何を言ってるんだという顔で美帆を見た。

十二時ちょうどでお開きにした。お茶の水の医科歯科大病院に戻るためにタクシーを拾った正也を表参道で見送って、美帆は自宅へと向かった。

一昨年の夏から同潤会青山アパートの跡地に建設が始まった表参道ヒルズは、次第に全容を明らかにし始めていた。来年一月には完成の予定だ。目下、都内の至るところで大規模な再開発が行なわれていた。この表参道ヒルズもその一つだが、一体全体、こんな高級マンションを建てて誰が住むというのだろう。一足先に誕生した六本木ヒルズにしても、入居した人間の多くがIT長者か芸能人という有様だった。幾ら立派な器に仕上げてみても、盛りつける料理が洗練されたものでなければ意味がない、と美帆は思う。この国はここ十数年、間違ったことしかしていないのではないだろうか。

まあ、あの黒川丈二のような男が代議士を目指すような国だ。それも仕方のない話なのかもしれない。丈二からは昨年の十二月以降、何の連絡も来ない。まさかあんな形で別れた女が自分の子供を身ごもっているなどとは露ほども思っていないだろう。

結局、自分も古川美和と同じように父親のいない子供を産もうとしている。

丈二の言い草ではないが、血は争えないという気がしないでもなかった。

ただし、自分はどんなことがあっても我が子を残して自殺なんてしない。一度、産むと決意し

たからには何があっても子供と二人で生き抜いてみせる。たかが男に捨てられたくらいでくよく
よなんて絶対にしない。美帆はそう思う。

正月に会ったときの優司の言葉を借用するならば、丈二が美帆を捨てたのではない。美帆が丈
二をクビにしたのだった。

今日の昼間、永妻克子から連絡があった。

富士本美由紀の現住所が分かったという。

かすみからは、大阪の人だということしか聞いていなかったが、永妻なら住所を割り出してく
れるだろうと思っていた。それにしても相変わらず反応が素早い。調査を頼んだのは先週の金曜
日、四月一日のことだった。

富士本美由紀にどうしても会ってみたい、というわけではない。

たまたまこの週末に大阪での仕事が入っていた。先月の終わりに急に知り合いの編集者から持
ち込まれた仕事だが、義理のある相手なので断りきれなかった。関西を中心に活躍している女性
タレントが芸能生活二十五周年を記念して、料理本を出版することになり、是非手伝ってやって
ほしいというのだった。タレントはここ数年、大阪で昼間の料理番組の司会を務めており、これ
は関東でもTBS系列で放映されていた。

その仕事の打ち合わせのために、八日金曜日から急遽大阪に行くことになった。金曜はプロダ
クションの面々と会い、タレント本人とは月曜に会う予定だった。土日がぽっかり空くという迷
惑な日程だったが、それならば、富士本美由紀に会いに行ってみようかと美帆はふと考えたのだ。

かすみが美由紀と会ったのは一度きりだった。中州で腹を刺された優司は手術によって一命を

取り留めたものの、二ヵ月近く入院した。そのとき、美由紀が見舞いに来た。たまたま優司の病室でかすみは彼女と遭遇したのだった。美由紀は「大阪の富士本です」と名乗ったあと「主人が若い頃、優司君と同じ船に乗っていたんです」とつけ加えたそうだ。年齢は優司より二つ三つ上の感じだった。

「でも、優ちゃんの様子を見ていて、この人が優ちゃんの好きな人だってすぐにピンときました。どんなに親しくなっても、優ちゃんの心の中には絶対入れてくれない部屋があるって思ってましたけど、ああ、この人だけがその部屋に入れるんだなって直感したんです」

と、この前かすみは言っていた。

富士本美由紀は三日ほど優司の世話をして帰ったようだった。

「美由紀さんが帰ってしばらくして、優ちゃんがやくざから足を洗うって言い出したんです。それ聞いたとき、美由紀さんが勧めたんだなって分かりました。私にはとても勝てない相手だって身にしみて思いましたね」

かすみはそうも言っていた。

永妻の調べによると、富士本美由紀は高校生の息子と二人暮らしだった。かすみの話と相違して、優司と一緒にマグロ船に乗っていたという彼女の夫は随分前に亡くなっているようだった。

この情報を今日手に入れて、美帆は俄然美由紀に会ってみたくなった。

表参道を外れて住宅地の路地を歩く。道のそこここに桜が咲いていた。今年は月末の開花のあと花冷えになったこともあり、いまがちょうど見ごろだった。

仲間優司が密かに思いを寄せてきた相手は自分だと美帆はずっと感じてきた。

222

片瀬川で正也を救ってくれたとき、優司が病院で呟いた言葉が何よりの証拠のはずだった。これまでの優司の言動を逐一振り返ってみても、美帆のその確信を揺るがすような材料は何一つ見当たらなかった。

しかし、かすみによれば、優司が思いつづけてきたのは富士本美由紀という女性だという。このかすみの直感が間違っているとも思えなかった。優司が足を洗って始めた店の屋号に「富士本」と入れていることでも、彼の美由紀への特別な感情は十二分に察することができた。

一体、優司の気持ちはどこにあるのか。それが美帆には不可解で仕方がなかった。

むろん、自分が美由紀に嫉妬しているわけではないと思う。だが、疑問を疑問として放置しておくには、これは大きすぎる問題のようにも思えた。

仲間優司とのつながりは、ある意味では黒川丈二とのそれ以上に底深いもののように美帆には感じられた。とくに昨年再会してからは、そのことを強く意識するようになっていた。丈二との関係にしても、もし優司と出会っていなければ、あんな別れ方はしなかったような気がしている。

こうなれば、当の美由紀と直接会ってみる以外に真実に近づく方法はない、と美帆は思う。大阪行きの仕事が突然舞い込んできたのも、美由紀との対面を促す何かの計らいなのかもしれなかった。

美由紀の自宅の電話番号は調べがついていた。

先ずは明日、美由紀に電話してみよう。

路傍の満開の桜を見上げながら美帆はそう考えていた。

四月九日

携帯を鳴らすまでもなく、どの客が美由紀かはすぐに分かった。

約束通り、店内の「真ん中の一番いい席」に彼女は座っていた。

土曜日の難波界隈は人、人、人だった。東京でいえば新宿、渋谷と似たようなものだが、それにしても大阪の方が混雑の密度は高いような気がした。

地下鉄御堂筋線の心斎橋駅で降りて、心斎橋の商店街を冷やかし、戎橋を渡り、三十分ほどかけてこの千日前のお好み焼き屋にたどり着いた。道々、人込みを東京と引き比べて、要するにガヤガヤの音量が違うのだと気づいた。大阪の人たちの方が歩きながらよく喋っていた。

店も満員だった。あんないい席に座っているということはよほど前から来ていたのだろうか、と思ったが、美由紀の顔や姿を見て、この人ならそんなことをしなくても上手い具合にいくに違いないと思った。彼女は電話での印象そのままに、周囲に明るい光を放っている人だった。

美由紀も美帆にすぐに気づいた。ぱっと手を上げて合図してくる。

向かいの椅子を引くと、「ごめんなさい。こんなごみごみした場所に呼び出しちゃって」と彼女も椅子から腰を持ち上げた。顔をしかめてひどく申し訳なさそうにしていた。

「いま何ヵ月?」

美帆が腰掛けると、訊いてきた。

「七ヵ月目に入ったところです」

「そう。だったらお腹、割と大きいほうね」

「ええ。何だかすこし太り気味で」

電話でもそうだったが、美由紀はきれいな標準語を喋る。周囲のテーブルからは盛大な大阪弁が響いてきていた。

「はじめまして。富士本美由紀です」

急に彼女がぺこりと頭を下げる。美帆も慌てて「はじめまして。小柳美帆です」とお辞儀を返した。

このままだと相手のペースに乗せられそうな気がして、美帆は自分から喋ることにした。ここは大阪なのだ、と思う。

「だいぶお待たせしてしまいましたか」

約束の一時半ちょうどに店の扉を開けたのだが、とりあえず言った。

「ぜんぜん。私もさっき来たところ」

美由紀はいつの間にか広げたメニューに視線を注いだまま言った。三十秒ほどで顔を上げて、

「ねえ、美帆さん何がいい?」

とメニューを逆さにして向けてくる。

「そうですねえ」

と言うと、

225

「モダン焼きがおいしいよ」

その箇所を人差し指で示してきた。

「じゃあ、私、シーフードモダンにします」

「了解」

美由紀はメニューを閉じて、店員に合図した。

「シーフードモダンと豚モダン、それに……」

注文しながら、

「美帆さん、生ビール飲む?」

と訊いてくる。美帆が首を振ると、

「じゃあ、ウーロン茶二つ」

と言った。

店員が去って、

「すみません」

と美帆は謝った。

「いいのよ。昨日も遅くまで会社の仲間と飲み会だったんだから」

と美由紀は言い、

「妊婦があんまり気を遣っちゃ駄目だよ」

と笑った。

水曜日の夜に美由紀の自宅に電話した。美帆が名乗ると、彼女は、

226

「ああ、あなたが小柳美帆さん……」

と最初から懐かしそうな声を出した。どんなふうに話を切り出そうかと悩んでいただけに、そ
の気安い反応に美帆はやや拍子抜けしてしまった。

「どうして私のことご存知なんですか」

逆に美帆の方から訊いていた。

「小柳さんのことは優司君にむかしよく聞かされていたから」

美由紀はさらに意外なことを言った。

週末大阪に行く予定なので、土曜日か日曜日にお目にかかれないでしょうかと訊ねると、美由
紀は理由も聞かずに「いいわよ。だったら一緒にお好み焼きでも食べましょうか」と持ちかけて
きたのだった。

ウーロン茶のジョッキが届いた。

「すみませんでした。突然電話して、しかもお目にかかりたいなんてずうずうしいこと言って」

やはり最初にこの訪問の目的をきちんと説明すべきだと美帆は思っていた。

美由紀はウーロン茶を半分くらい一気飲みすると、

「いいのよ。あなたとはいつかこうして会うことになるだろうって思ってたから」

すました顔で言って、

「優司君について知りたいことがあって訪ねてきたんでしょ」

と何でもないことのようにつけ加えた。

すべてを見透かされているふうで、美帆は、つい美由紀の顔をまじまじと見た。

明るいブラウンに染めた髪は短く、横長の瞳が特徴的だった。細身の身体にグリーンのシャツ、下はジーンズという普段着のような恰好だったが、それが彼女を若々しくしていた。美帆より三つ上だと言っていたから今年で三十八歳のはずだが、そうは見えない。まして高校生の息子がいるとはとても思えなかった。

お好み焼きを食べながら一時間くらい話をした。

席を立つ際に時間を確認すると、二時四十分になっていた。

店を出て千日前の雑踏に踏み出す。

「今日も明日も大阪泊まり？」

先を歩く美由紀が振り返って言った。美帆はずっと聞き役に回っていたので、自分のことはほとんど話せなかった。

「はい」

「ホテル？」

「梅田のヒルトンです」

「だったら今夜はうちに泊まりに来ない？　息子も合宿だし、のんびりできるよ」

元太という名の息子は、昨日から学習塾の合宿で六甲に出かけ、明日の夜帰ってくるらしかった。

「うちの息子は小さい頃から勉強漬けなの。私立にやって高い学費払ってるんだから、とにかくいい大学に入ってもらわないとね」

さきほど美由紀は笑いながら言っていた。

228

「そうしなさいよ。ホテルは乾燥するから身体によくないし、このまま行っちゃおうよ」

美由紀が美帆の手を取ってきた。

「じゃあ、そうします」

美帆はその言葉に甘えることに決めた。

近鉄難波駅から奈良線に乗って鶴橋で大阪線に乗り換えた。長瀬という駅には二十分足らずで着いた。

美由紀の家は長瀬駅から歩いて十分ほどのところにあった。住宅街の中に建つ小さな一戸建てだった。

美由紀が勤める会社は環状線の京橋駅の近くだという。神戸牛や近江牛、松坂牛の卸元の会社で、彼女は大阪に出てきてすぐに勤め始め、もう勤続十七年になるとのことだった。

「とにかくおいしいお肉をお腹いっぱい食べさせて、元太を大きな強い子に育てなきゃと思ってね。親戚の紹介だったんだけど飛びついたのよ」

電車の中でも美由紀は明るい声で喋った。

美由紀が大阪に出てきたのは、夫の富士本健太を失ってすぐの平成元年四月。美帆がちょうど大学二年になったばかりの頃だった。当時美由紀は二十二歳。元太は一歳をすこし過ぎた幼児だった。

美帆は一階のリビングに通された。一階はキッチンとリビング、それに玄関を入ってすぐに四畳半の和室があった。そこが仏間になっていて、立派な仏壇が置かれていた。美帆は出されたお

茶に口をつける前に、先ずその部屋でお線香をあげさせてもらった。

二十五歳で亡くなったという富士本健太の笑顔の写真が仏壇に飾られていた。短髪の浅黒い顔は精悍で、なるほどどことなく優司に似ているような気がした。

高校を中退し、マグロ船に乗せられた仲間優司を二年近くの航海のあいだに一人前の漁師に育て上げてくれたのはこの富士本健太だった。ホオジロザメに右足を食いつかれ、その直後、横波にさらわれて海に投げ出された優司を必死になって助けてくれたのも、この健太だった。

室戸に帰投した優司は、船長、漁労長に伴われて高知に住む美由紀のもとを訪ねた。健太は「弟のような男を見つけた」と書いてきていた。

美由紀と元太と対面した彼は、健太の遺品を差し出しながら、土下座して号泣したという。

航海中に送られてくる手紙やビデオで美由紀は優司のことはよく知っていた。

身を震わせて泣くその若者の姿を見て、夫が本当に死んでしまったことを彼女は初めて実感したのだった。

焼香してリビングに戻ると、二階に行っていた美由紀がスウェットの上下を持って降りてきた。

「さあさあ、早くこれに着替えて」

ダークブルーのパンツスーツ姿の美帆に言う。

「私は元太の部屋で寝るから、美帆さんは私の部屋のベッドを使って。二階にもトイレはあるから」

と美由紀は言った。

夕食は焼肉だった。冷蔵庫の中を見せてもらうと、神戸牛の切り落としや内臓がぎっしり詰ま

っていた。リビングの座卓にホットプレートを置いて、美由紀はどんどん肉や野菜を焼いていった。神戸牛は脂と肉汁が渾然一体となってとろけるように柔らかい。溶かしバターとおろしニンニクをまぜた市販のタレで食べるだけだったが、絶品だった。美由紀は自分はビールだったが、美帆の前にはウーロン茶のグラスを置いてくれた。

「こんな美味しいお肉が手に入るなら勤め甲斐がありますね」

と美帆は言った。

「そうね。明日元太が帰ってきたら、また焼肉よ。あの子なんて平気で一キロ食べちゃうものね。あの年頃の男の子の胃袋って一体どうなってるんだろ」

美由紀はビールをぐいと飲んで言った。その飲みっぷりからしてかなりいける口のようだった。

「でも、元太君、勉強頑張ってるんですね」

「毎日毎日、塾塾塾。かわいそうだけど、そうも言ってられないしね。私なんてもっともっと勉強したかったのに貧乏だったから高校しか行けなかったし、それも普通科じゃなくて商業科にしか通わせて貰えなかった。それに比べればあの子は幸せよ。勉強だけは学生のときにやっとかないと取り返しがつかないでしょ。遊びなんていつから始めてもすぐ一人前になれるもの。優司君だって、たまにここに来れば、とにかく勉強していい大学に行けってしつこいくらいに元太に言ってるわよ。その代わり、一流大学に入れたらボーナスとして百万円くれるんだって。元太はすっかり本気にしてるのよ」

「仲間君もきっと本気にしてると思いますよ」

美帆が言うと、「おそらくね」と言って美由紀は苦笑した。

「仲間君が足を洗ったのは、美由紀さんが勧めたからだって聞きましたけど」

美帆は、誰から聞いたかをぼやかして言った。

「そんなことないわよ」

美由紀は即座に否定した。

「そうなんですか」

「私はね、優司君が刺されて大怪我したとき、病院に行って『元太に何て説明すればいいのか教えて』って言っただけ。あの事件は大阪のニュースでも流されて、小学生だった元太が偶然テレビ観ちゃったのよ。優司おじちゃんはやくざなのって半べそで訊かれて、私はきっと同姓同名の別人よって答えるしかなかった。その話を病室で優司君にしたの」

美由紀はそう言うと、手にしていたグラスをテーブルの上に戻した。

「実はね、優司君がやくざになったのは、私のせいもあると思ってるの。漁師なんて死んでしまったら何の補償もないし、主人の場合は南アでの捜索にお金がかかって、結局航海中の給料もほとんどそっちに回されてしまったの。私は幼い元太を抱えて、この先どうしていいか分からなかった。そして優司君が、お金は何とかしますって言って博多に引きあげて、一ヵ月もするとすごい大金を送ってきてくれたの。とても受け取れないって電話したら、叔父さんの借金が思ったほどじゃなくて、自分の給料がそれだけ残ったからどうしても貰ってくれの一点張りだった。でも、あのときはもうやくざの道に足を踏み入れていたんだと思う。彼がやくざになったと知ったのは、迂闊な話だけど、私たちが大阪に引っ越してずいぶん経ってからだったのよ」

「そうだったんですか」

232

美帆は呟く。

「優司君、それからもずっとうちに仕送りしてきてたの。私はそういうのの好きじゃないし、それに彼がやくざだって分かってからは本当にイヤだった。優司君は、そのお金だけはきれいな金だからって必死に言い張ってたけど、幾らきれいな金って言われても、そのぶん別のところで汚いお金を稼いでいるわけじゃない。でもね、私は彼が足を洗うまで黙って受け取ってきたの。もしこれを受け取らなかったら、優司君はもう二度と堅気の世界に戻って来れなくなるって分かってたから」

と美由紀が言った。

仲間優司にとって生涯の悔いとなった事件はケープタウンで起きた。

彼らがマグロ漁を行なっていた一九八八年当時の南アフリカは、人種隔離政策を柱とする白人独裁が終焉を迎えつつある混乱の時代だった。テロリストや黒人たちによる相次ぐテロや暴動で治安は悪化の一途をたどり、数々の外国船が入港するケープタウンはニューヨークと並ぶ犯罪都市と化していた。

入港して五日目の晩だった。

タクシードライバーだと名乗る男が血相を変えて船にやって来た。

この船の乗組員のナカマユウジという青年が酔って酒場で大暴れをしてしまい、いま警察に捕まって留置されている。保釈金を持ってすぐに来てほしいとの伝言をナカマから預かって来た、と彼は流暢な日本語で語った。

その場にちょうど居合わせた健太は、「だから、あれほど飲むなと言ったのに」と一つ舌打ち

をくれると、漁労長と相談し、余っていた入港金を摑んで男と一緒に警察署へと向かった。

酔っ払った優司が何も知らずに船に戻ったのはそれから二時間後のことだった。

そして、タクシードライバーと共に警察署へ出かけていった富士本健太はもう二度と船には戻らなかった。

酒を覚えたての優司は、飲み方を知らなかった。前の晩もケープのディスコで泥酔してしまい、店の外に出たところをチンピラたちに襲われ、あやうく財布と船員手帳を奪われそうになったばかりだった。そのときは健太たちがたまたま通りすがり、乱闘の末にギャング連中を追い払った。彼らは銃こそ出さなかったが、ナイフは振り回していた。腕におぼえのある優司はとにかく喧嘩っ早かった。モンテビデオの酒場では二メートルもあるウルグアイの大男を得意の一本背負いでぶん投げて気絶させたこともあった。

強盗騒ぎの翌日だっただけに、健太も他の乗組員もニセのタクシードライバーの持ち込んだ作り話を簡単に信じ込んでしまったのだった。

健太の捜索は一週間以上にわたってつづけられたが行方は摑めなかった。現地の警察は最初から健太がすでに殺されていると見ていた。南ア駐在の日本大使館関係者に後事を託して、優司たちの船がケープタウンを出港したのは入港から二週間後のことだった。

ビールのロング缶を二本空けて、さすがに美由紀の頰も赤く染まっていた。

いつの間にか外は暗くなっていた。春だといってもまだ日が落ちるのは早い。美由紀は立ち上がってリビングのカーテンを閉めた。住宅街なので外から聞こえる物音もなかった。席に戻って、しばらく彼女は黙っていた。

234

「予定日はいつ?」

不意に訊いてきた。

「七月の二十三日です」

「そう……」

美由紀は呟く。

「こうやって元太がいなくて、一人きりのときがたまにあるの。せいせいするんだけどね、ふっとあたりが静かになって自分の心臓の音が聞こえてきそうなときってあるじゃない。そういう瞬間、まるで一生分みたいにさみしくなるのよ。死にたくなるわけじゃないけど生きたくなくなっていうか、ああ、私のこの人生って何なんだろうって思うの。もう元太のことも、他の全部もそっちのけにして早く消えてしまいたいような、そんな気分になるの。子供ってね、親に勇気も与えてくれるし、力も与えてくれるし、すごい愛情も与えてくれるの。母親にとっては生き甲斐そのものと言ってもいいわね。でもね、やっぱり夫とは違うのよ。私みたいに夫を早く失うと分かるんだけど、どんなものより深くて太いつながりっていうのは、知り合うまで赤の他人同士だった夫との関係なのよね。大袈裟に言えばさ、何百万人何千万人の中からたった一人と一人として出会うわけでしょう。その選択っていうか偶然っていうか運命っていうか、そういうのって凄いと思う。子供は、そういう凄いことを成し遂げた人たちへの神様からのご褒美みたいなものね。だって、夫と違って、子供って自分が選んだわけじゃないしね」

この美由紀の言葉に、美帆は古川美和のことを考えた。彼女もまた俊彦に捨てられて、早く消えてしまいたかったのだろうか。

235

「じゃあ、子供が親を選ぶんでしょうか」

かつて優司が言っていた言葉も同時に美帆は思い出していた。

「どうだろ。案外、神様と相談して子供の方が親を選んで生まれてくるのかもしれないよね」

美由紀が言った。

「美由紀さんは再婚しようとか思わなかったんですか」

美帆は訊いた。

「誰と？　優司君と？」

彼女ははっきりと聞き返してくる。

「たとえば、ですけど」

美帆も誤魔化さなかった。

「どうだろ」

美由紀は瞳を凝らすような表情になった。

「もし一緒になれば彼もやくざやめてくれるだろうしって迷ったことはあったわ。ただ、優司君と一緒になるってことは、彼を元太の父親にすることだと思ったのね。そしたら、元太の父親になってもらいたいって望んでいる自分が何だかすごいずるい人みたいな気がしたんだよね。それで踏み切れなかった。彼の方はきっと私がそういう気持ちになるのを待ってたのかもしれないけどね」

美由紀は言って、美帆の目をしっかりと見た。

「でも、いま考えたらそうやって私は逃げただけかもしれないと思うの。私は本当は自分と子供

236

のことだけ考えればよかったんだよね。子供の父親なんて女が好きに選べばいいのよ。たとえその男の実の子じゃなくたって、この男が父親にするにはいいなと思えば、その人を父親にしてもいいのよ。だって子供を産むのも育てるのも私たち女なんだから」

お腹の子供のことも、その父親のことも何も話してはいないのに、美由紀は美帆の心中を見通すようなことを言った。

「昼間、お好み焼き屋でも話したけど、あなたのおかげで自分はいまこうして生きているんだって、よく優司君は言ってた。彼が心から感謝しているのはうちの主人とあなたの二人だと思うわ。優司君って生まれてすぐからずっと施設で育ってるでしょう。だから幸せになる方がよく分からないのよ。健太にもあなたにも感謝ばっかりして、そのあとどうすればいいんだか見当がつかないのね。彼、あなたのおとうさんにもあなたのことを頭を下げて頼まれたって言ってたわ。それなのに自分が極道なんかになって、何もしてやれなくなったって」

突然、父のことが出てきて、美帆はひどく驚いた。俊彦はいつそんなことをしたのだろうか。

「優司君って、不幸な人だよ」

美由紀が言った。

237

六月二十一日

美帆は五月の末に片瀬に戻ってきた。

母の早苗がどうしても片瀬で出産して欲しいと言い張ってきかなかった。

富士本美由紀と大阪で会って帰京した直後だった。妊娠を報告したのは、けていたらしく、さして驚いたふうではなかった。正也から聞いていた通りで、早苗は予想をつかった娘の妊娠にはそれほどの興味関心はないのだろう、と美帆は勘違いしてしまった。本多園長との交際もあり、自分の腹を痛め

だが、それから二日後、突然早苗が東京に出てきたのだった。

早苗からすれば、かかった魚の大きさを見て、最初からむやみに竿を振り立てるような愚を犯さなかっただけの話だった。

以来、とにかく片瀬に帰ってきてくれの一点張りだった。

美帆は仕事の都合なども持ち出して東京を離れるわけにはいかないと頑張ったが、結局は、

「だけど、それじゃあおとうさんの一周忌に出られないじゃない」

という一言で折れざるを得なかった。

たしかに俊彦の命日である七月二十日は、出産予定日の三日前だった。おまけにそのひと月後には初盆も控えていた。

238

早苗の喜びようは見ていて滑稽なくらいだった。弟の正也も「火がついたみたいだ」と呆れていたが、

「やっぱり、かあさんはとうさんのことを本当に愛していたのかもしれないな」

とも言っていた。

六月に入った途端に雨ばかりとなった。

隣接する福岡市同様、玄界灘に面した片瀬は日本海側気候だった。東京のようにからりと晴れる日は少なく、まして梅雨時ともなれば一日中、灰色の雲が空を覆っている。美帆は長い東京暮らしのあいだに、気の滅入るような故郷の天気のことをすっかり忘れていた。

半月も雨つづきの日々を過ごすと、うんざりしてきた。

お腹もどんどん大きくなり、眠っていても腰骨がきしんでたびたび目が覚めた。だいいち、自分の身体が自分の想像を超えてここまで変貌してしまうのが信じられなかった。世界中の女性がこの経験をしているのかと思うと、ちょっと唖然としてしまう。

一ヵ月も経たないうちから、美帆は片瀬に帰ってきたことを後悔しはじめていた。

その日は、十日ぶりの晴天だった。それも、めずらしいほどに空は青く高かった。美帆は早くから起き出して洗濯を済ませ、念入りな朝食を作った。窓を開けて風を入れながら箸をとると、それだけでご飯が美味しかった。食事の後、思いついて優司に電話した。

昨夕のローカルニュースで藤木町のあじさい祭が紹介されていた。あじさい寺として有名な瑞巌寺の境内に今年も一万株のあじさいが美しい花を咲かせていた。

美帆はあじさいが大好きだった。

239

晴れた空を仰いでいるうちに、瑞巌寺のあじさいをどうしても見に行きたくなった。

昼過ぎに迎えに来た優司は、

「そげん大きなお腹で、藤木みたいに遠かとこに行って大丈夫と？」

と心配顔だった。

「当たり前でしょ。仲間君は黙って私を連れて行ってくれればいいの」

優司と会うとどういうわけかわがままになった。時折、早苗に注意されたりするくらいだった。彼の店にもよく顔を出したし、買い物や気晴らしで外出したいときは運転手代わりに使っていた。

かすみやリリコと四人で会うこともたまにある。かすみはどうやら千葉に戻る決心がついたようだった。店はリリコに譲るつもりで、いまは彼女に手取り足取りママ修業をさせていた。

研一は相変わらず行方知れずだった。何度か立ち回り先を突き止められて警察が踏み込んだようだが、間一髪で逃走していた。噂では、自分を警察に売った優司に対して相当の恨みを抱いているらしかった。優司にも直接警察から身辺に気をつけるようにとの連絡が入ったらしい。リリコの話では、研一たちの悪事を暴いたのはやはり優司だったようだ。彼は、知人を介して建材会社の社長と連絡を取り、有無を言わせず被害届を警察に出させたという。

「研ちゃん、優司さんのことを父親とも兄とも慕ってたから、すっごいショックだったと思う」

リリコは自分のされたことは棚に上げて、研一に同情的だった。彼女自身、まだ研一に対して未練があるのだろうと美帆は見ていた。

240

午後一時ちょうどに出発した。

藤木町は熊本と境を接する南の町だった。茶所で有名な八女地方東部の中核都市で、お茶をは
じめとして、葡萄、桃、いちごなど果物の産地としても知られていた。片瀬からだと九州自動車
道を使っても片道二時間はかかった。

女岳のふもとに広大な敷地を有する瑞巌寺に着いたのは三時過ぎだった。優司は追い越し車線
に移ることさえほとんどしなかった。美帆の方が「もっと飛ばせばいいじゃない」とはっぱをか
けたくらいだった。

大きな駐車場の入口付近に車をとめ、あじさい庭園のある境内へと坂道をのぼった。気温は上
昇し、おそらく三十度を超えているのではないか。少し歩いただけで額に汗が滲んできた。急な
坂では優司が手を引いてくれる。優司に触れると、美帆はそれだけで気持ちが落ち着いた。

今年の正月、久留米のラブホテルで、泣き疲れてぐだぐだになった美帆を優司は帰り際に長い
時間抱き締めてくれた。上半身裸の優司に抱かれて、美帆はその胸に顔を埋めた。慶応病院で背
中の刺青に手を当てたときと同じ感触が全身に広がった。冷たくてすべすべした優司の肌は、泣
いて火照った美帆の頰に心地よかった。

そのうち不思議な感じに見舞われた。何か柔らかなものが自分と優司の身体を包み込んでくる
ようだった。美帆は目を閉じて、その感覚をさらに見極めようとした。

太く長い生き物が巻きついていた。きつくでもなくゆるくでもなく、しかししっかりと二人の
身体を縛り上げていた。

背中の一匹龍が優司の身体から抜け出したのだ、と美帆は思った。龍は鱗と鱗が擦れるシャラ

シャラという音を立てながら、美帆と優司を一つのものにしようとしていた。

小さな石橋を渡ると、山門の手前からあじさい園は始まっていた。

手毬型の大きな本あじさいは長雨で濃い紫色に染まっていた。美帆の好きな瑠璃色のひめあじさい、白やローズ色の豪華な西洋あじさいも群れをなして咲き競っていた。そんなあじさいの花壇が山門を越えて大きな本堂のそば近くまで延々とつづいていた。

火曜日の、しかも午後遅くとあって参詣人はほとんどいなかった。まるで目の前に広がるあじさいを全部独り占めにしているような気分だった。

「お参りが先やろうも」

と優司がたしなめるような口調で言った。

「この花にいまお参りしてたの」

と言うと、彼は苦笑していた。

新緑の女岳を背景に建つ大屋根の本堂は荘厳な雰囲気をたたえていた。美帆は合掌し、長いこと祈りを捧げた。隣にいた優司はさっと拝むとすぐに行ってしまった。

階段の下で待っていた優司に、

「仏様や神様にはちゃんと掌を合わせないと駄目じゃない」

と美帆は言った。さっきは参拝が先だと急かしたくせにと思っていた。

「俺は神様に顔向けできんことばしすぎとるけん怖かと」

優司がいつものぶっきらぼうな口調で言う。

242

並んであじさい園の方へ歩き始めると、優司は正面を向いたまま、

「腎臓一個なくしたくらいじゃ、とてもおっつかんよなあ」

と言った。

美帆は、何気なく洩らした彼のその一言が妙に耳に残った。

あじさい園を見て回ったあと、門前の豆腐料理の店で遅い昼食をとった。

店を出たときには、すっかり人気もなくなり、空にはいつの間にか厚い雲が垂れ込めていた。

あたりはしんとした静けさに包まれていた。時刻は四時半になるところだった。

駐車場を目指して参道を下っていると、突然、雨粒が落ちてきた。

駆け足ともいかず、次第に勢いを増していく雨に打たれながら車までたどり着いた。

「まるでペンギンやな」

がにまたでちょこちょこ走る美帆を見て優司が笑った。

車のシートに座り込んだとたん、雨脚は一気に強くなった。

優司がエンジンを掛けようとキイを差し込むと、稲光がひらめき、ものすごい雷鳴が轟いた。

直後、バケツの水でもぶちまけたような豪雨へと変わった。稲妻が走り、雷鳴が立てつづけに天に響き渡る。

「こりゃ、しばらく雨宿りやな」

優司が呟いた。

車は駐車場の入口付近にとめてあるから、瑞巌寺の幾つかの建物や背後の山々が見渡せるはずなのだが、いまは水煙のせいで何一つ見えなかった。

243

そのうち雷はおさまく雨は一向に弱まる気配を見せなかった。

優司がエアコンをつける。冷風が胸元や足元に吹きつけてきて、汗ばんだ肌に気持ちがよかった。

優司は運転席のシートを倒し、身体を斜めにした。美帆も彼に倣って助手席のシートを倒した。

しばらく二人とも無言で雨に煙る景色を眺めていた。

「先週、久しぶりに大阪に行ってきた」

不意に優司が言った。

「四月に美由紀さんと会ったんやな。大阪で初めて聞かされた」

美帆は別に美由紀に口止めしたわけではなかった。だが、優司の様子からして彼女は何も言っていないのだろうとは思っていた。

「父が、私のことを頼むって仲間君に頭を下げたってほんと?」

かねて疑問だったことを訊ねた。

「頼むっていうか、先生がヘンなことば言うたのは本当や」

「いつ」

「一度、桜花園に訪ねて来てくれたて言うたろ。あんとき」

「仲間君のためならお金でも何でも出すって言った日」

「そうや」

「ヘンなことって何」

隣の優司を見ると、苦虫を嚙み潰したような顔になっていた。

244

「何かしらんけど、いつか小柳ば嫁さんにしてやってくれみたいなことやった」

「何、それ」

「俺もよう分からん」

「ふーん」

美帆はどうしてだか自分の顔が真っ赤になっているのが分かった。胸の鼓動も早くなっていた。一度大きく息を吸った。手を口許へ持っていき、一つ咳払いをした。

「私のおかげで生きていられるってどういうこと?」

美帆はついにあのときのことを優司に向かって口にした。

「私、仲間君のこと助けてあげられなかったのに」

急に優司のシートが持ち上がった。慌てて美帆も元に戻した。

「そうやない」

怒ったような声で優司が言った。

視線は真っ直ぐにフロントガラスの先に向けていた。外の雨もだんだん小降りになってきた。

雨音も鎮まり車の中は静かだった。

「俺は、あんとき雅光兄さんの手ば自分から離したと」

美帆は思わず優司の横顔を凝視した。

「正也ば先生に渡して、雅光兄さんの腕ば摑んでだんだん身体が持ち上がっていった。ちょうど土手のへりから目のあたりまで出て、ハラハラしながら見とるお兄さんやお姉さん、子供たち、大人たち、大勢の人が見えた。そんとき、何か、俺はもうそっちの世界には戻りたくないなあっ

て思った。もう十分や、短い人生やったけど、俺にはもう腹いっぱいやって思ったと。早く静か
な世界に帰って楽になりたかなって、ふっとそういう気がした。だけん、俺は自分から雅光兄さ
んの手ば切った」

そこで優司は言葉を止め、しばらく無言だった。

「川に落ちて、流されながら手も足も動かさんかった。水に沈む直前やった。何でやろう。どうして見えたんか俺にもう分からん。
やけど沈む寸前、俺にはお前が見えた」

優司はまた言葉を止めた。正面を向いたまま、唇を嚙み締めていた。

「お前が土手から服のまま飛び込んだのを見て、俺は仰天した。一生であげん驚いたことはなか。
お前、あの日、泳いどらんかったやろ。白いワンピース着て白い傘さして河原にずっと座っとっ
ただけやったろ」

美帆は黙って優司を見つづけていた。彼の大きな瞳からわずかに涙が滲んでいるのが分かった。

「俺は動転した。こげな俺のために命は投げ出す馬鹿がおるとは思うとらんかった。俺は必死で
手足ば動かした。俺のために飛び込んだお前ばどうしても助けないかんと思った。お前だけはど
んなことがあっても死なせられんと思うた。俺は、あんときお前のために生きないかんて心底思
った。だけん、目を覚ましたときお前の姿ば見て、俺は声も出んかった。一生であれほど嬉しか
ったことはなかった。お前が生きとったこと。そして生きたお前とまた会えたこと。もうあげん
嬉しかことは二度とないと俺は思うとる」

美帆は、川に落ちていくときの優司の笑みを思い出す。咄嗟になぜあんなことをしたのか分か

246

らない。ただ、あの笑みを浮かべた少年をこのまま死なせてはいけないと思った。気づいたとき

には土手から飛んでいた。追いかけて雅光兄さんが決死の思いで飛び込み、何とか岸に連れ戻し

てくれなければ美帆は確実に溺れ死んでいただろう。

「だけど、仲間君は正也のために命を投げ出してくれた。私が仲間君のために飛び込むのは当た

り前だよ」

美帆は言った。

「そうやない」

優司はまた怒ったような声を出した。

「俺は誰よりも泳ぎが得意やった。正也が流されたのを見たときやって、俺なら追いつけるて自

信があった。やけどお前は違うやないか。体育の授業んときやって、お前は水泳はいつも休んど

ったろうが。あんときお前は俺のために死のうとした。今度は俺がお前のために死ぬのは当然の

話やろうが」

彼はそう言うと、まるで睨みつけるような目で美帆を見た。

三十分足らずで雨は嘘のように上がった。雲間からみずみずしい陽光が降り注いでいた。

「あれ」

美帆がフロントガラス越しに空の方を指差した。日が照りはじめてサングラスをかけた優司が

その方角に顔を向ける。「おう」という声が出た。

瑞巌寺のうしろの山間に美しい虹がかかっていた。

ひかりって、きれいなものをどんどんきれいにしてくれるよね――リリコの言葉をなぜか思い

出した。美しい雨上がりの茜空を、ああやってひかりが七色の虹で飾ってくれているのだろう。

美帆は助手席のドアを開けて、外に出た。

優司もすぐに降りてきた。

晴れているのに霧のような雨が降っていた。

優司がトランクから傘を出し、隣に来てさしかけてくれた。

「きれいかなあ」

サングラスを外して優司が言った。

こうして優司と二人で虹を見ている。いつかこんな日が来ることを自分はむかしから知っていたような気がする。ふと美帆はそう思った。

不意にお腹の赤ん坊が激しく動いた。

その瞬間、背後で車が急発進するときの悲鳴のような音が聴こえた。

美帆と優司が同時に振り返った。

大きなランドクルーザーが二人をめがけて突進してきた。運転席の男の姿がはっきりと見えた。

坊主頭の巨体の男。何か叫び声を上げていた。

二人にぶつかる直前、ヘッドライトが点灯した。

優司が眩しそうに顔を背けた。それが、美帆が見た最後の光景だった。

平成十九年十二月一日

「よいしょ、よいしょ」と言いながら龍司は一生懸命に階段をのぼる。

美帆の右手にしっかりと摑まっている。龍司の小さな爪が掌に食い込んでちょっと痛い。日に力が強くなる。いまでは公園を一緒にかけっこできるほど足も速くなった。日に日に力が強くなる。

「龍ちゃん、あとすこしよ、頑張って」

美帆は声を掛ける。

「うん」

顔を真っ赤にした龍司が頷いた。

ホームの階段をのぼりきると、跨線橋の上で美帆は龍司を抱き上げた。下りの階段は危ないということもあるが、つい我が子の柔らかな身体に触れたくなってしまう。

龍司は今月で二歳と五ヵ月になった。

当時の美帆は二歳と二ヵ月。女の子だからきっといまの龍司くらいにちゃんと歩けただろう。自分も母の手につながれてあのホームの階段を上がったのだろうか。

二月の風は、今日よりもさらに冷たかったはずだ。きっと母親のあたたかな手を必死に握り締めていたと思う。

まさかその同じ手が、ほどなく団地の九階の踊り場から自分を投げ捨てるなんて、露ほども思っていなかったに違いない。

想像すると身体が震えてくる。余計に龍司を強く抱き締めてしまう。

跨線橋を渡り、駅の改札を抜けて外に出た。

板橋に住んでいた母は、なぜこんな横浜のはずれまでやって来たのか。

ずっと自律神経失調症に悩んでいたという。そのために通っていた病院で父と出会った。父に捨てられ、美帆を産み、仕事と住まいをいっぺんに失い、頼りにしていた実母にまで先立たれてしまった。生きる気力を失った彼女の気持ちは分からなくはない。

だが、二歳の娘を連れて見ず知らずのこんな場所にたどり着き、しかも、自分が飛び降りる直前に我が子を先に投げ落とすなど、およそまともな人間の所業とは思えない。

母は怖かったのだ。

死にたくはあっても、死ぬのが怖かった。だから、最初に美帆を投げた。娘を殺すことで自らの退路を断とうとした。

その人間としての臆病さ、卑しさが美帆にはどうしても許せなかった。

母は芝生に仰向けに倒れた娘を見下ろして、死んだと思ったのだろうか。

おそらく、そんな確認をする間もなく身を投げたのだろう。

まさか、美帆が生きて、落下してくる自分を見ているなどとは思いもよらずに。

あの右の腿の内側にあった大きな赤い痣は生まれついてのものではなかった。

母親に投げ捨てられた美帆は、植え込みに落ち、大きく跳ねて芝の上に投げ出された。そのときどこかに打ちつけてできたのが、あの赤い痣だった。

施設に預けられたあともしばらくのあいだ腿に包帯を巻いていた。

高校二年の夏の日、美帆はその記憶を取り戻した。

250

早苗はそれを知っていたのだろうか。

だから、どうしてもあの痣を取り除きたかったのか。

駅前には大きな建物はなく、まっすぐの並木道が伸びていた。

銀杏だった。ビルに邪魔されることなく思う存分に舞っている木枯らしにハラハラと黄色い葉を散らしていた。

いまでも物寂しい風景だった。

三十五年前はもっと侘しかっただろう。　駅からつづくこの真っ直ぐな道の両脇は畑や田圃だったのかもしれない。

母は何を思ってこの道を歩いたのか。

こうして龍司を連れて同じ道を歩いてみても、美帆には想像もつかなかった。

強い風が吹くたびに、龍司が「さむい、さむい」と声を上げる。美帆は立ち止まり、首に巻いたマフラーを口許まで引き上げてやる。

龍司はだんだん父親に似てきた。寒がりなんて似なくていいのに、と思う。いや、あんな男に何一つ似る必要はないのに。

黒川丈二は二年前の郵政解散総選挙で、公認を外された現職を降して衆議院議員に当選した。

九月十一日、初当選を喜ぶ彼と夫人の姿を、生後二ヵ月になる龍司を抱いてテレビで観た。何の感慨も湧いてはこなかった。

龍司は七月二十日、父の一周忌の日に誕生した。六月の事故の影響もなく、三千二百グラムの元気な赤ちゃんだった。かすみやリリコの話によれば、龍司の産声を市民病院の分娩室前の廊下

251

で聞きつけた母は、人目もかまわず涙を流したという。

人通りの少ない道を十分ほど歩くと、大きな団地が見えてきた。

いままで何度も訪れようとして、一度も足を運ぶことのできなかった場所にようやく来ることができた。

美帆は龍司を抱き上げ、ためらうことなく団地の入口を通り過ぎた。

敷地に入ると草ぼうぼうの空き地が目立っていた。広い空き地を囲むように新しい団地が建っていた。昼時だったが、人の姿は余り見かけない。向かって左は建築途中の建物で、建築作業員たちがどこかのんびりとした様子で働いていた。

美帆は右の道を選んだ。

建物はこうして建て替わっているだろうと予想していた。だが、目指す十号棟はきっとまだあ
る。美帆には確信があった。

龍司は腕の中で眠ってしまったようだ。耳元にかすかな寝息が聞こえてくる。

さいわい風はやんでいた。風がなければ晴れ渡った空の下、ひんやりとした空気が肌に心地よかった。

ずいぶん重くなった。こうやって抱きつづけていると両腕が痺れてくる。

きっと自分は、抱かれることも眠ることもなく、母に手を引かれて従順にこの道を歩いたのだろう。

十号棟はすぐに見つかった。思ったより古びていなかった。外装や設備は幾度かあらためられたに違いない。白く塗られた

252

九階建ての建物は巨大だった。

近づいても、思い出すものは何もなかった。棟にも周辺のたたずまいにも見覚えはなかった。

だが、永妻克子の報告書によれば、母はここの九階の踊り場から身を投げて死んだ。

周囲を一巡りしてみた。外階段は建物の両端についていた。母がどちらの階段をのぼったかの見当はついた。正面玄関に向かって左端の外階段の方はポンプ室なのか電気室なのか背の低い建物が附設されていた。顔を上に向けてみた。最上階の踊り場から落ちれば、まず間違いなくあの建物の屋根に激突してしまう。

母は右の階段を選んだのだ。右には小さな公園があった。灌木のようなものはなかったが、公園との仕切りのところに幅二メートルほどの芝が植えられていた。

また上を向いてみる。あそこから身を投げれば、ちょうど芝のあたりに落下するだろう。

美帆は龍司を抱いて、芝地まで行った。下腹に負担がかからないよう慎重にしゃがんだ。

芝に手を触れる。眠っている龍司がむずかってすぐに手を戻した。この芝の上に寝そべってみたかった。仰向けに寝て自分が落とされた場所を見上げれば、忘れていた記憶の一部が甦ってくるかもしれない。

美帆は立ち上がった。また風が出てきている。あまり長居するわけにもいかない。

正面玄関から十号棟の中に入った。入ってすぐ左手にエレベーターがあった。母がエレベーターを使ったのか、それとも階段で九階まで上がったのか分からなかった。ただ、彼女も二歳の子供を連れていたのだ。恐らくエレベーターに乗って最上階のボタンを押したものと思われた。

旧式のエレベーターはゆっくりと上昇していった。九階に到着し、右の外階段を目指して開放

253

廊下を歩いた。三十メートルくらい進んだ突き当り、九〇一号室の先に階段があった。七段降り

ると そこが踊り場だった。

コンクリートの塀は美帆の胸の高さほどだった。美帆は抱いていた龍司を下ろした。龍司がい

やいやするようにしがみついてくる。

「龍ちゃん、ちょっと起きてちょうだい」

美帆はやや強い調子で言った。

「龍ちゃん、起きて」

両手で龍司の身体を引き剥がす。むずかりながらも龍司が目を開けた。とたんに不思議そうな

顔つきになって周囲を見た。

「高いところだから、ちゃんとママの手に摑まってね」

美帆は左手で龍司の右手をしっかりと握った。

母親の足元に寄り添い、龍司はぎゅっと握り返してくる。

美帆は目をつぶった。まだ身を乗り出して下を見ることはできなかった。

二歳の私。

ここで私は母に持ち上げられた。母が一体何をするつもりかなんて分からなかった。私を抱い

た母は半身を塀にくっつけるようにして、私を塀の外へと押し出すようにした。母の腕だけに支

えられ、私は中空に浮かんだ。そのときになって自分が落とされることに気づいた。私は下を見

た。恐ろしさに胸がつぶれそうになった。私の両脇を摑んでいた母の腕がゆっくりと伸びてい

く。

254

母の顔が底知れぬ苦痛に歪んでいた。　私は叫んだ。

「おかあさん、やめて！」

美帆は目を開けた。

何かが違う。何かが全然違っている。そんな気がした。

身を乗り出して下を覗いた。想像以上に高かった。公園の中の砂場、ブランコ、ベンチが掌に

すっぽりおさまる大きさに見えた。顔を上げた。古い団地はもうほとんど残っていない。この十

号棟とその隣にある二つの棟だけだった。団地の入口で建設中の建物はすでに半分ほどできあが

っていた。

顔を上に向けた。

十二月の澄んだ空が広がっていた。

透明な光が瞳の奥へと射し込んでくる。息を吸うと目の中の光は七色に変化する。

研一のランドクルーザーが突進してきたとき、美帆はお腹を守るように背を丸めた。腰のあた

りに激しい衝撃を感じた。気づいたときにはまるで鞠のように宙を飛んでいた。不思議と心は平

静だった。何かが自分とお腹の子供を包み込んでくれているのが分かった。それは、優司に強く

抱き締められたときの感覚とよく似ていた。きらきらと輝く一匹の龍が長い胴体をくねらせなが

ら、美帆の身体に巻きついていた。

目覚めたときは、病院のベッドに寝ていた。不安そうな顔の母がいた。

「赤ちゃんは？」

美帆は言った。

「大丈夫よ」

母が答えた。

二歳の私。

母と一緒に歩いていた。長い長い道。私の右手は母の左手としっかり結び合わされていた。母は歩きながら時折、私の方を見た。何か言っている。何だろう。次第に私はくたびれてきた。おかあさんはどこに行くのだろう。私はあとどれくらい歩けばいいのだろう。私は途中で足を止めたくなる。母に抱き上げてほしい。だけど、それは無理だった。どうして？　だって母は右手に大きな紙袋を提げているのだから。

踊り場に来ると、母はようやく私を抱き上げた。何度も何度も頬ずりしてくれた。何か言っている。言いながら母は泣いていた。

母と一緒に私は塀の上へと向かっていく。紙袋から出した脚立のようなものに足を掛け、母は一歩一歩上がっていく。そのたびに私の身体に冷たい風が吹きつける。私は寒くて母の胸にしがみつく。母が強く強く抱き締めてくれる。

母は塀の上に立った。すっくと真っ直ぐに立った。

私は母に抱かれて空を見ている。

真っ青な空。少し寒いけれど、もう平気だった。

母の腕に力が籠もった。母の身体が宙に浮いた。そして私の身体も。

256

私は震える声で訴えた。

「おかあさん、こわいよー」

スプーンのときとおんなじだ、と美帆は思った。全身をばたつかせながら金切り声を上げて美帆の目の前に落ちてくるスプーン。あれは美帆が勝手に作り出した心象でしかなかった。

私は母が落ちるところなど見てはいなかった。私は母に落とされたのではない。母は私を抱いてここから一緒に飛び降りたのだ。

私はどうして助かったのだろう。私の身に何が起きたのだろう。私は何も憶えていない。

ただ、母が最後の最後まで私をしっかりと包み込んでくれていたことだけは、何となく分かる。私は久しぶりにありありと思い出していた。

五年生の春に剥ぎ取られた右腿の内側のあの痣のことを。早苗が蛇のようで気味が悪いといつも言っていたあの痣の形状を。

「おかあさん」

美帆は空を見つめたまま呟く。瞳からみるみる涙が溢れ出してきた。

「おかあさん、ごめんね」

だんだん視界がぼやけてきた。

「おかあさん、一人ぼっちで死なせてごめんね。ずっと恨んできてごめんね」

美帆は顔を空に向け、立ち尽くして泣いた。声を立てず静かに、ずいぶん長い時間泣いた。

左手に強い力を感じて、我に返った。急いで涙を拭った。

龍司が不安そうな表情で見上げていた。

「ごめんね、龍ちゃん。さあ、帰ろう」

龍司が無言で頷いた。

団地を出ると、通りかかったタクシーを拾った。シートに座ると龍司を膝に載せて抱き締めた。

すこし身体が冷えているようだったが、「寒い？」と訊くと首を横に振った。

お腹にわずかな違和感があった。

冷えたのは自分の方かもしれないと美帆は思った。もうすぐ六ヵ月になる。安定期だから問題はないと思うが。

タクシーは五分ほどで駅に着いた。

降りると、美帆の手を振り切って改札口へと一目散に駆け出していった。

「龍ちゃん、走らないで」

美帆の注意など耳に入っていないようだった。龍司が駆け寄っていくと、男はしゃがんで大きく手を広げた。

改札のそばに男が立っていた。

龍司を抱き取って彼はゆっくり立ち上がった。

サングラスをかけた浅黒い顔が美帆を見ていた。

258

な口調に、あたしなんかちょっと恐怖を感じている。

〈取材協力〉

村上祥子

工藤玲子

〈参考文献〉

村上祥子・文、中山庸子・絵 『電子レンジに夢中』 (講談社)

村上祥子 『村上祥子の英語で教える日本料理』 (ランダムハウス講談社)

有元葉子 『だれも教えなかった料理のコツ』 (筑摩書房)

斎藤健次 『まぐろ土佐船』 (小学館文庫)

夏原 武 『現代ヤクザのシノギ方』 (宝島社文庫)

未生之前舊公案

中国茶叶历史资料续辑 茶书

心に龍をちりばめて

発行／2007年10月30日

著者／白石一文

発行者／佐藤隆信

発行所／株式会社新潮社

〒162-8711　東京都新宿区矢来町71

編集部　03-3266-5411

読者係　03-3266-5111

http://www.shinchosha.co.jp

印刷所／二光印刷株式会社

製本所／加藤製本株式会社

© Kazufumi Shiraishi 2007, Printed in Japan

乱丁・落丁本は、ご面倒ですが小社読者係宛お送り下さい。

送料小社負担にてお取替えいたします。

価格はカバーに表示してあります。

ISBN978-4-10-305651-5　C0093

青年のための読書クラブ　桜庭一樹

フィッシュストーリー　伊坂幸太郎

サクリファイス　近藤史恵

空色ヒッチハイカー　橋本紡

僕僕先生　仁木英之

きつねのはなし　森見登美彦

名門お嬢様学校、聖マリアナ学園。異端者だけが集う〈読書クラブ〉には、語り継がれる秘密があった。——史上最強にアヴァンギャルドな〝桜の園〟の100年間。

売れないロックバンドが最後のレコーディングで叫んだ声が、時空を越えて奇蹟を起こす。表題作他、変幻自在の筆致で編んだ、伊坂ワールドの饗宴。

レース中に起きた悲劇は、単なる事故のはずだった——。二転三転する「真相」と共に駆け抜ける物語の結末とは？　サイクルロードレースを舞台に描く青春ミステリ。

あれほど憧れた背中を追いかけて、僕は兄貴のキャデラック車で街を出た——謎の美女・杏子ちゃんと個性あふれるヒッチハイカーたちを相棒に、ただ走り続けた18歳の夏の物語。

退屈してる暇はない！　辛辣な美少女仙人・僕僕と、弱気なニート青年・王弁が、五色の雲と駿馬を走らせ、天地陰陽をひとっ飛び！〈日本ファンタジーノベル大賞受賞〉

細長く薄気味悪い座敷に棲む狐面の男。闇と夜の狭間のような仄暗い空間で囁かれた奇妙な取引——。京の骨董店を舞台にして、妖しくも美しい幻燈に彩られた奇譚集。